Early Pregnancy Ultrasound

A Practical Guide

Early Pregnancy Ultrasound

A Practical Guide

Edited by
Emma Kirk
Royal Free Hospital, London

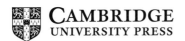
CAMBRIDGE
UNIVERSITY PRESS

CAMBRIDGE
UNIVERSITY PRESS

University Printing House, Cambridge CB2 8BS, United Kingdom

One Liberty Plaza, 20th Floor, New York, NY 10006, USA

477 Williamstown Road, Port Melbourne, VIC 3207, Australia

4843/24, 2nd Floor, Ansari Road, Daryaganj, Delhi – 110002, India

79 Anson Road, #06-04/06, Singapore 079906

Cambridge University Press is part of the University of Cambridge.

It furthers the University's mission by disseminating knowledge in the pursuit of education, learning, and research at the highest international levels of excellence.

www.cambridge.org
Information on this title: www.cambridge.org/9781316503867
DOI: 10.1017/9781316481776

First published 2017

Printed in the United Kingdom by Clays, St Ives plc

A catalogue record for this publication is available from the British Library.

Library of Congress Cataloging-in-Publication Data
Names: Kirk, Emma, editor.
Title: Early pregnancy ultrasound: a practical guide / edited by Emma Kirk.
Description: Cambridge, United Kingdom; New York, NY: Cambridge University Press, 2017. | Includes bibliographical references and index.
Identifiers: LCCN 2017034626 | ISBN 9781316503867 (paperback)
Subjects: | MESH: Ultrasonography, Prenatal | Pregnancy Trimester, First | Pregnancy Complications – diagnostic imaging | Early Diagnosis
Classification: LCC RG107.5.U4 | NLM WQ 209 | DDC 618.207/543–dc23
LC record available at https://lccn.loc.gov/2017034626

ISBN 978-1-316-50386-7 Paperback

....

Contents

Contributors

Shabnam Bodiwala, BSc MBBS, Queen Charlotte's & Chelsea Hospital, Imperial College London, Hammersmith Campus, London, UK

Cecilia Bottomley, MD MRCOG, Department of Obstetrics & Gynaecology, Chelsea & Westminster Hospital, London, UK

Tom Bourne PhD FRCOG, Queen Charlotte's & Chelsea Hospital, Imperial College London, Hammersmith Campus, London, UK

Wouter Froyman MD, Department of Obstetrics & Gynaecology, University Hospitals Leuven, Netherlands

Venetia Goodhart BSc MBBS, Department of Obstetrics & Gynaecology, University College London Hospital, London, UK

Anna Graham MBBS MA, King's College Hospital NHS Foundation Trust, London, UK

Tom Holland MD MRCOG, Department of Obstetrics & Gynecology, St Thomas's Hospital, London, UK

Jemma Johns MD MRCOG, Department of Obstetrics & Gynecology, Imperial College School of Medicine, London, UK

Davor Jurkovic MD PhD FRCOG, Department of Obstetrics & Gynaecology, University College London Hospital, London, UK

Emma Kirk BSc MD MRCOG, Department of Obstetrics & Gynaecology, Royal Free Hospital, London, UK

Dimitrios Mavrelos MD MRCOG, Department of Obstetrics & Gynaecology, University College London Hospital, London, UK

Nicola Mitchell-Jones MRCOG, Department of Obstetrics & Gynaecology, Chelsea & Westminster Hospital, London, UK

Matthew Prior MRCOG DFSRH, Department of Obstetrics & Gynaecology, University of Nottingham, UK

Nick Raine-Fenning MRCOG, Department of Obstetrics & Gynaecology, University of Nottingham Queen's Medical Centre, Nottingham, UK

Jackie A. Ross BSc FRCOG, Early Pregnancy & Gynaecology Assessment Unit, King's College Hospital NHS Foundation Trust, London, UK

Dirk Timmerman MD PhD, Department of Obstetrics & Gynecology, University Hospital Leuven, Leuven, Belgium

Aslı S. Üçyiğit BSc MRCS MRCOG, Early Pregnancy & Gynaecology Assessment Unit, King's College Hospital NHS Foundation Trust, London, UK

Preface

The use of ultrasound has revolutionised the diagnosis and management of most early pregnancy complications. It is now a key multi-disciplinary tool in the provision of early pregnancy care, with nurses, midwives, sonographers and doctors often conducting the ultrasound examinations. This book is aimed as a practical guide in this important area, not just for all those undertaking such examinations but all those with a general interest in early pregnancy. There are chapters on what to expect to see with a normal intra-uterine pregnancy as well as chapters on abnormal pregnancies and adnexal pathology. It includes sample ultrasound images, with explanatory annotated diagrams as well as expert practical advice on conducting ultrasound examinations and managing certain clinical situations. It is anticipated that the guide will be useful to both UK and international healthcare professionals. At the end of each chapter there is a list of key learning points and suggested further reading for readers who require additional information.

Introduction to Early Pregnancy Ultrasound

Emma Kirk

Ultrasound is the most commonly used medical imaging method in pregnancy. In the United Kingdom, all women are routinely offered ultrasound examinations at around 12 weeks and 20 weeks of gestation. However, the use of ultrasound prior to 12 weeks has become central to the management of women with suspected early pregnancy problems. In particular, earlier ultrasound examinations are indicated in women after assisted conception and those in whom an ectopic pregnancy or miscarriage is suspected.

The aims of an early pregnancy ultrasound scan (USS) are to confirm the presence of an intrauterine pregnancy, establish viability, determine number of embryos, determine gestational age and reassure a woman and her partner of the absence of complications.

Setting

In the United Kingdom, the majority of early pregnancy ultrasound examinations are carried out in Early Pregnancy Units. These are specialist units for the provision of care for women with suspected early pregnancy complications. It is a recommendation of the Royal College of Obstetricians and Gynaecologists that all maternity units should have such a unit. Table 1.1 summarises some of the standards that should be expected in an Early Pregnancy Unit.

Safety

In recent years, there has been much interest in the safety of early ultrasound examinations. The evidence so far suggests that ultrasound used for clinical reasons with standard presets during embryonic development (conception to ten weeks' gestation) is safe and the benefits outweigh any theoretical risks. It is, however, essential that whoever is carrying out the ultrasound examination is aware of the safety indices and scanning modes. A fundamental approach to the safe use of diagnostic ultrasound is to use the lowest output power and the shortest scan time consistent with acquiring the required diagnostic information. This is referred to as the ALARA ('as low as reasonably achievable') principle.

Safety Indices

Ultrasound examination of the developing embryo or fetus exposes it to both mechanical and thermal stress. The potential effects of these forms of stress are represented by the mechanical index (MI) and thermal index (TI) respectively. These two indices are summarised in Table 1.2. They are displayed on the ultrasound screen during the examination, as shown in Figure 1.1.

Scanning Modes

Evidence suggests that the most commonly used B-Mode ultrasound is safe in early pregnancy when using standard obstetric presets on modern machines. Colour Doppler and pulsed wave Doppler involve greater average intensity and power outputs as shown by higher TIS (TI soft tissue) levels compared to B-Mode imaging. There is therefore a greater risk to the developing fetus of overheating. If Doppler ultrasound is used in early pregnancy, the operator should aim to keep the TIS < 1.0 and limit the scan exposure time. Currently it is not recommended that Doppler be routinely used in early pregnancy ultrasound assessments. The M-Mode is a low-energy alternative to pulsed wave Doppler, which can be used to insonate the embryonic heart if required in early pregnancy.

There is no current evidence that three-dimensional (3D) ultrasound leads to higher ultrasound exposure than two-dimensional (2D) examinations. In fact, scanning and exposure times may actually be reduced, as the data set can be analysed offline. The routine use of 3D examinations, however, is also not routinely recommended.

Table 1.1 Standards for provision of care in early pregnancy units

		Essential	**Desirable**
Accessibility		• Minimum five-day opening. • Access to transvaginal and transabdominal ultrasound. • Acceptance of direct referrals from general practitioners (GPs), accident and emergency responders and other health care professionals seeing women in early pregnancy. • Acceptance of self-referrals from women with a previous history of ectopic pregnancy or recurrent miscarriage.	• Is Open seven days a week. • Accepts self-referral from all women.
Environment		• Units should have a designated reception and waiting area. • Appropriately furnished room for breaking bad news and counseling. • System for capturing all patient information and creating written reports.	• Unit separate from the main maternity unit.
Process		• Clear protocols for carrying out a pregnancy test and performing an ultrasound examination in any woman of reproductive age presenting with any type of abdominal pain, irregular vaginal bleeding or amenorrhoea. • Direct laboratory access to same-day serum human chorionic gonadotropin (hCG) and blood group results. • Clear guidelines and algorithms for the management of pregnancies of unknown location and of uncertain viability. • A full range of management options (expectant, medical and surgical) for women diagnosed with miscarriage or ectopic pregnancy.	• Serum hCG results available within two hours. • Access to serum progesterone levels.
Communication		• Clear patient information leaflets. • A written report of the outcome of a woman's ultrasound examination, with a copy sent to their GP or referring health professional.	• Direct access to bereavement counselling.

Source: Adapted from Moody, ed., *RCOG Standards for Gynaecology*, 2008.

Table 1.2 Ultrasound safety indices

		Explanation	**Recommended levels ***
Mechanical index	**MI**	MI is an on-screen indicator of the relative potential for ultrasound to induce an adverse bioeffect by a nonthermal or mechanical mechanism. This includes cavitation (which refers to the development of gas bubbles in an acoustic field at high negative pressures) and streaming (the expansion and contraction, or collapse, of gas bubbles during the oscillatory cycle).	An MI of < 1.0 indicates that effects arising from acoustic cavitation are very unlikely. Ideally aim for levels < 0.7 in early pregnancy scanning.
Thermal index	**TI**	TI provides an indication of the relative potential for a rise in tissue temperature. It is intended to give a rough guide to the likely maximum temperature rise that might be produced after long exposure. There are three types: **TIS** – thermal index for soft tissue. The index used during scanning < ten weeks of gestation. **TIB** – thermal index for bone. **TIC** – thermal index for cranial bone.	The higher the TI, the shorter the ultrasound exposure should be. TIS < 0.7 – no restriction on scan time. TIS 0.7–1.0 – restrict scan time to < 60 minutes. TIS 1.0–1.5 – restrict scan time to < 30 minutes. TIS > 3.0 – scanning not recommended.

* Recommended by the British Medical Ultrasound Society.

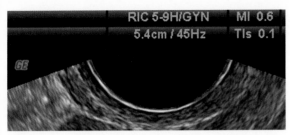

Figure 1.1 Image showing on-screen display of mechanical index (MI) and thermal index (TI).

Scanning Route

There are a number of advantages of the transvaginal route over the transabdominal route in early pregnancy, as indicated in Table 1.3. There is plenty of evidence in the literature suggesting that in the early first trimester a transvaginal scan (TVS) can reliably identify normal and abnormal pregnancies and various developmental markers at an earlier stage than a transabdominal scan (TAS). A TVS has been shown to be acceptable to women attending Early Pregnancy Units and in fact some women do actually prefer it to a TAS. The reasons for this include the discomfort and time needed to fill the bladder to adequately examine the pelvis abdominally. TVS is also superior in obese patients and those with a retroverted uterus.

Occasionally it may be necessary to perform a transrectal ultrasound scan. This may be used as an alternative to a TVS if either a TVS is not possible and insufficient information is obtained by a TAS.

Ultrasound Technique

Whether performing a TVS or TAS, it is essential that the examination is performed in a systematic fashion and the image is optimised to enable the examiner to get the most information from the procedure.

Image Orientation

There is a general agreement that when in transverse section, the patient's right side should be seen on the left side of the ultrasound screen. With a TAS, in the longitudinal view the cranial structures should be seen on the left side of the screen and the caudal structures on the right side. Superficial structures should be seen on the top half of the screen and deeper structures on the bottom half, as indicated in Table 1.4.

With TVS, there is no agreement on image orientation. Some scan with the transducer head in the upper part of the screen and some with it at the bottom.

Similarly, when examining in the longitudinal plane, some will have the bladder on the left and some will have it on the right, as indicated in Table 1.4. The most important thing is that the examiner is aware of his or her own orientation when performing the ultrasound examination.

Image Optimisation

Whilst most modern ultrasound machines are now programmed with suggested presets for the examination type intended in order to obtain the best images, there are still some things that usually need to be changed during every examination.

1. Depth

Usually the examination is started using high depth or a low magnification. Increasing the depth allows deeper structures to be viewed. Reducing the depth allows more superficial structures to be viewed.

2. Magnification

For superficial structures it is usually easiest to magnify the image by reducing the depth of the image. For deeper structures or to get an even bigger image, the zoom function can be used. This zoom function just takes a portion of the screen and magnifies it. It can be used whilst scanning or whilst the image is frozen.

3. Focus

The focus can be adjusted to manipulate the pulse of the ultrasound to be at its narrowest at a particular depth. This means that the image quality is maximised at this level. It allows the best lateral resolution (ability to see two things as two things) to be achieved.

4. Gain

The overall brightness of the image can be adjusted by altering the gain. This is usually one of the most important changes to make to optimise the image, as if the image is too light or too dark, it is difficult to see subtle changes in texture.

The ultrasound waves change and get smaller as they pass through tissues (attenuation). In order to make structures look the same even if they are located in different depths, the time gain compensation (TGC) can be adjusted. Usually there is lower gain superficially and higher gain deeper in the image where the image quality is weaker.

Table 1.3 Advantages and Disadvantages of Transvaginal Sonography and Transabdominal Sonography

	Advantages	Disadvantages
Transvaginal (TVS)	• Higher frequencies • Superior resolution of images *Less ultrasound penetration is needed as probe is closer to pelvic structures, therefore higher frequencies can be used to obtain higher resolution of images.* • Requires an empty bladder, so often more comfortable. • The probe can be used to exert localised pressure on the pelvic organs to test for pain. • The pelvic organs can be moved with the probe to see if they slide easily. If the organs do not slide easily, this suggests that adhesions may be present. The TVS can actually be combined with a bimanual examination. The examiner can place his or her hand on the patients abdomen while operating the vaginal probe with the other. • The probe can be moved in and out of the vagina to adjust the depth of the organs on the screen. • Allows better imaging in obese patients.	• Depth of penetration is limited due to high-frequency of the ultrasound • Lack of probe mobility. Due to the confines of the introitus and vagina, the probe cannot be moved in all dimensions
Transabdominal (TAS)	• May allow better visualisation of a pregnancy in a large fibroid uterus.	• Decreased resolution. This is due to: 1. The lower frequency of abdominal probes compared to vaginal probes 2. The scan being performed through the abdominal wall which contains fat, muscle and tendons which distorts the ultrasound image 3. The relative greater distance bowel which may contain air and block visualisation of deeper structures. • Often requires a full bladder. • Poor views in obese patients.

5. Frequency

The highest ultrasound frequency possible should be chosen. However, the higher the frequency, the lower the depth of penetration. Therefore, if the object of interest is situated far away from the transducer, the frequency may need to be reduced to get the best image. A disadvantage of the lower frequency, however, is a reduction in the image resolution.

Transvaginal Scan (TVS)

A TVS should be performed when the patient has an empty bladder. The procedure should be explained to the woman and consent taken. The probe should be thoroughly cleaned by a gloved operator, ideally in front of the patient, before the procedure. The probe should be covered with a protective sheath. There should be a layer of ultrasound gel between the transducer head and the probe cover, with all air expelled. Extra lubricating gel should then be put on the covered probe. The operator should introduce the probe slowly into the vagina whilst watching the screen. It is sometimes helpful to ask the woman to take a deep breath at this point. The scan should then be performed in a systematic manner. A suggested method of doing this is shown in Table 1.5. After the examination is completed, the probe should be removed from the vagina, the probe cover removed and the probe cleaned.

If a transrectal scan is performed, the same examination technique should be used as for a TVS.

Table 1.4 Image orientation

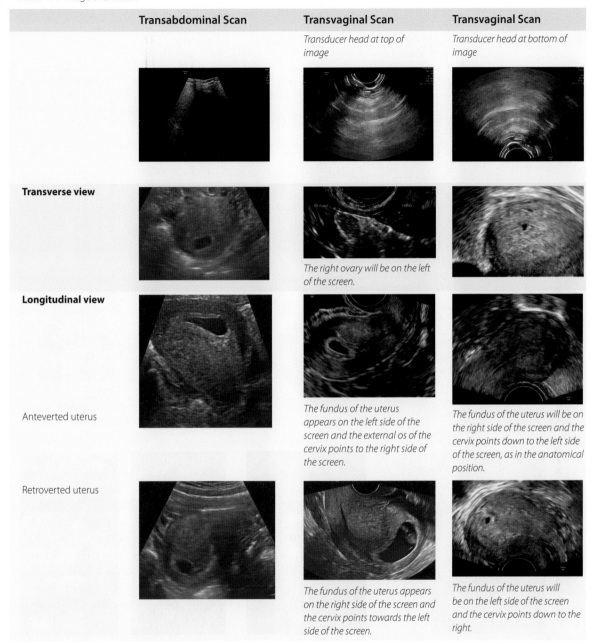

	Transabdominal Scan	Transvaginal Scan	Transvaginal Scan
		Transducer head at top of image	*Transducer head at bottom of image*
Transverse view			
		The right ovary will be on the left of the screen.	
Longitudinal view			
Anteverted uterus		*The fundus of the uterus appears on the left side of the screen and the external os of the cervix points to the right side of the screen.*	*The fundus of the uterus will be on the right side of the screen and the cervix points down to the left side of the screen, as in the anatomical position.*
Retroverted uterus		*The fundus of the uterus appears on the right side of the screen and the cervix points towards the left side of the screen.*	*The fundus of the uterus will be on the left side of the screen and the cervix points down to the right.*

Transabdominal Scan (TAS)

A TAS should be performed when the patient has a full bladder. A full bladder displaces the bowel and allows the ultrasound beam to travel through the urine until it reaches the uterus and ovaries. Again, it should be performed in the same systematic way suggested for TVS (see Table 1.5).

Documentation and Storage of Images

It is important to carefully document all findings in a systematic fashion when providing a report of the ultrasound examination. Suggested information to include in a report is given in Table 1.6. It is also important to store copies of the USS images taken. When writing the report and storing images, it is

Table 1.5 Systematic approach to the TVS

		Ultrasound image	Schematic drawing	Details
1.	Longitudinal View of the Uterus			• It is important to obtain a longitudinal view of the uterus, ideally visualising the whole of the endometrial cavity down to the cervix. • The uterus should be scanned from one side to the other in the longitudinal plane. • An image should be saved, showing, if present, the intrauterine gestational sac within the endometrial cavity, which should be seen continuous with the cervical canal (thus confirming an intrauterine pregnancy). • If no intrauterine pregnancy is visualised, the endometrial thickness should be measured where it appears to be at its thickest. • The endometrium should be measured from the endometrial-myometrial border on one side to that on the other.
2.	Transverse View of the Uterus			• After examination in the longitudinal plane, the probe should be rotated 90° so that the uterus can be examined in the transverse plane. • The uterus should then be scanned from the fundus down to the cervix. • Even if a gestational sac is immediately visible, it is important to pan through the uterus in the longitudinal and transverse planes to check for the presence of an additional sac, fibroids or uterine anomalies. • State if the sac appears low in the cavity.
3.	Visualisation of the Gestational Sac			• The gestational sac should be visualised and measured in the longitudinal and transverse planes. • The height and length of the sac should be measured in the longitudinal plane and the width of the sac in the transverse plane. • It should be stated if the sac appears low in the cavity.
4.	Assessment of Embryonic Structures			• The sac should be examined in both planes for the presence or absence of a yolk sac, embryo/fetus and amniotic sac. • Measurements should be taken if present.

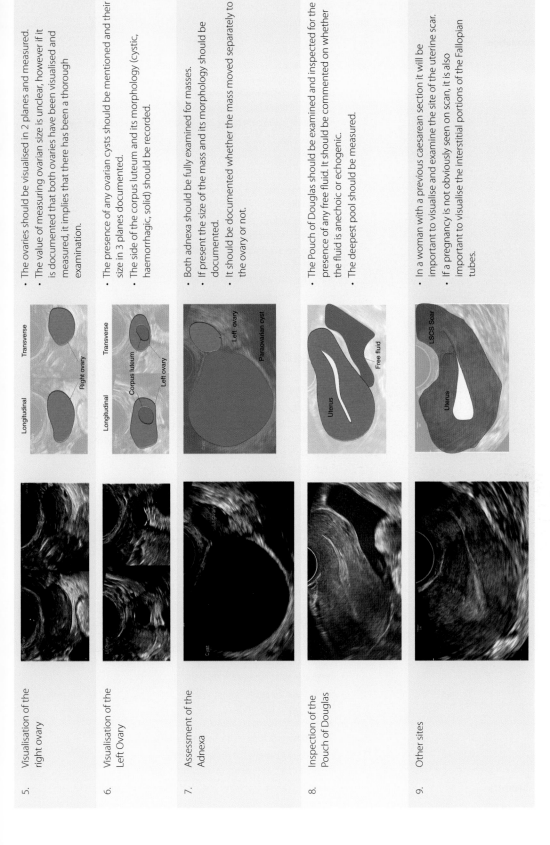

5. Visualisation of the right ovary

- The ovaries should be visualised in 2 planes and measured.
- The value of measuring ovarian size is unclear, however if it is documented that both ovaries have been visualised and measured, it implies that there has been a thorough examination.

Longitudinal   Transverse

Right ovary

6. Visualisation of the Left Ovary

- The presence of any ovarian cysts should be mentioned and their size in 3 planes documented.
- The side of the corpus luteum and its morphology (cystic, haemorrhagic, solid) should be recorded.

Longitudinal   Transverse

Corpus luteum

Left ovary

Left ovary

7. Assessment of the Adnexa

- Both adnexa should be fully examined for masses.
- If present the size of the mass and its morphology should be documented.
- It should be documented whether the mass moved separately to the ovary or not.

Left ovary

Paraovarian cyst

8. Inspection of the Pouch of Douglas

- The Pouch of Douglas should be examined and inspected for the presence of any free fluid. It should be commented on whether the fluid is anechoic or echogenic.
- The deepest pool should be measured.

Uterus

Free fluid

9. Other sites

- In a woman with a previous caesarean section it will be important to visualise and examine the site of the uterine scar.
- If a pregnancy is not obviously seen on scan, it is also important to visualise the interstitial portions of the Fallopian tubes.

LSCS Scar

Uterus

Table 1.6 Suggested information to be included in the structured ultrasound report

General information

	Maternal age	
	Previous obstetric history	• Parity – include live births and stillbirths • Number of miscarriages • Number of terminations of pregnancy • Number of ectopic pregnancies – include mode of management
	Conception	• Spontaneous • Assisted

Pregnancy

	Gestational age	• According to last menstrual period (LMP) or USS measurements as appropriate
	Gestational sac	• Present or absent • Number of gestational sacs • Intrauterine or extrauterine (and site – tubal, interstitial, Caesarean section scar, cervical etc.) • Size in three orthogonal dimensions
	Yolk sac	• Present or absent • Size
	Amniotic sac	• Present or absent • Size • Present or absent • number
	Embryo/fetus	• Measurement of crown rump length (CRL)
	Fetal cardiac pulsations	• Present or absent (may include heart rate)

	Other	• Presence of retained products of conception in the uterine cavity
		• Documentation if any tissue appears cystic and suggestive of a possible molar pregnancy
		• Presence or absence of a:
		  ○ Subchorionic haematoma
		  ○ Chorionic bump
		  ○ Caesarean section scar niche
		• Presence of fluid in the Pouch of Douglas, measurement of the deepest pool, and a description of whether it appears anechoic or echogenic

Maternal structures

	Uterus	• Anteverted • Retroverted • Axial • Presence of a uterine anomaly • Fibroids – including location and size • Intrauterine contraceptive device (IUCD) if present with exact location and relationship to pregnancy • Cervical length if clinically indicated
	Ovaries	• Size in three dimensions • Side of corpus luteum • Morphology of corpus luteum • Size and morphology of any ovarian cysts if present
	Other	• Presence of a paraovarian/fimbrial cyst • Presence of a hydrosalpinx or other tubal pathology

Serum biochemistry

	• Serum hCG and progesterone levels if clinically indicated and known

Table 1.6 (continued)

Diagnosis	
	• Single/multiple viable intrauterine pregnancy
	• Intrauterine pregnancy of uncertain viability
	• Missed miscarriage
	• Incomplete miscarriage
	• Complete miscarriage (only if the patient had a previously visualised pregnancy on USS)
	• Pregnancy of unknown location
	• Ectopic pregnancy
	• Suspected molar pregnancy
Follow-up/recommendation	
	• Further follow-up scan if indicated and suggested time interval
	• Recommendations for serial hCG or progesterone estimations if indicated
	• Advice to book for antenatal care if indicated
	• Referral to discuss management of ectopic pregnancy or miscarriage

important to document all findings and to label all images taken and stored.

Specialist computer programs are available that allow the storage of USS images and offer the ability to generate a structured report as soon as the examination is complete. As all reports and images are saved under a patient's particular identification number, all previous scan images and reports can be reviewed easily. This is extremely useful when a patient is returning for a follow-up scan after a previous inconclusive scan. Normal values for USS measurements such as gestational sac size and crown rump length (CRL) are contained within the programs, allowing them to assist with pregnancy dating. Another advantage of such a program is that they can enable a clinic to run efficiently by becoming paperless. However, the most important thing is that they allow a patient to leave the clinic with a written report in her hand.

Auditable Standards

It is good practice for all those performing ultrasound examinations in early pregnancy to attend regular departmental meetings to review guidelines and protocols and discuss difficult cases. Regular audits should also be performed on the rates of pregnancy of unknown locations and number of ectopic pregnancies diagnosed on ultrasound prior to treatment.

Learning Points

- The aims of an early pregnancy ultrasound scan are to confirm pregnancy location, establish viability, determine number of embryos, and determine gestational age.
- Ideally all women with suspected complications should be seen in a dedicated Early Pregnancy Assessment Unit.
- Ultrasound used with standard presets for clinical reasons during embryonic development (conception to ten weeks' gestation) is safe and the benefits outweigh any theoretical risks.
- A transvaginal scan has a number of advantages over a transabdominal scan in early pregnancy.
- It is essential to provide a structured written report of the ultrasound scan examination findings.

Further Reading

1. Moody J, ed. (2008). *RCOG Standards for Gynaecology.* RCOG Press.

2. Joy J, Cooke I, Love M (2006). Is ultrasound safe? *The Obstetrician & Gynaecologist* 8: 222–227.

3. RCOG ultrasound from conception to 10+0 weeks of gestation. Scientific Impact Paper No. 49. March 2015.

4. World Federation for Ultrasound in Medicine and Biology. Safety statements. www.wfumb.org/about/statements.aspx. Accessed 20 October 2014.

5.   British Medical Ultrasound Society. Statement on the safe use, and potential hazards of diagnostic ultrasound. https://www.bmus.org/static/uploads/resources/STATEMENT_ON_THE_SAFE_USE_AND_POTENTIAL_HAZARDS_OF_DIAGNOSTIC_ULTRASOUND.pdf

6.   Kaur A. (2011). Transvaginal ultrasonography in first trimester of pregnancy and its comparision with transbdominal ultrasonography. *J Pharm Bioallied Sci* 3: 329–338.

7.   Dutta R L, Economides D L. (2003). Patient acceptance of transvaginal sonography in the early pregnancy unit setting. *Ultrasound Obstet Gynecol* 22: 503–507.

Chapter 2

The Normal Early Intrauterine Pregnancy 4–11 Weeks

Aslı' S. Üçyiğit and Jackie A. Ross

The use of transvaginal ultrasound (TVS) has facilitated the earlier detection and assessment of the first-trimester intrauterine pregnancy, such that evidence of a normally developing pregnancy may be seen as early as four weeks and three days of gestation. An appreciation of the normal landmarks and characteristic features of a normal early pregnancy is essential for enabling the accurate diagnoses of early pregnancy complications and for the communication of the ultrasound findings to patients.

It is widely accepted that measurement of the crown rump length (CRL) in the first trimester is the most accurate parameter for the ascertainment of embryonic age, and that the transvaginal scanning route will usually detect pregnancies at an earlier gestation than the transabdominal route. Symptomatic women are at risk of early pregnancy complications, so care must be taken to first identify the normal pelvic anatomy before focusing on the pregnancy; otherwise, the risk is that accurate measurements of the embryo are made without appreciating that the pregnancy is abnormally located.

Landmarks for Diagnosis

A normally developing early intrauterine pregnancy will display specific ultrasound features that can be used as the landmarks for diagnosis. These are summarised in Table 2.1.

Early Pregnancy Ultrasound Measurements

The gestational (chorionic) sac should be measured in three planes, from the inner edges of trophoblast. The maximum and mean diameters should be recorded and the volume can be calculated using the formula for ellipsoid (V = A x B X C x 0.523).

The yolk sac should be measured by taking three perpendicular diameters from the centre of the yolk sac wall. The amniotic sac is comparatively thinner, and therefore three perpendicular diametres should be measured from the centre of the membrane, and the mean diametre calculated.

The 'crown' and 'rump' are not distinguishable in very early pregnancy and therefore the crown rump length (CRL) should be taken as the greatest measurable length of the embryo. From seven weeks onwards, the measurement should be obtained in the sagittal section of the embryo, ensuring that the yolk sac is *not* included in the length. Useful lengths to recall are listed in Table 2.2.

Embryonic cardiac activity is generally evident as soon as the embryo itself is visible. Heart rate measurements should be obtained using the M-mode feature in the first trimester, as the time-averaged acoustic intensity delivered to the embryo is lower with M-mode than with spectral Doppler. The embryonic heart rate peaks at 9^{+0} to 10^{+0} weeks at around 170–180 beats per minute (bpm) (Figure 2.1).

Diagnosis of Multiple Pregnancy

In early multiple pregnancy, the chorionicity can simply be determined by counting the number of gestational sacs (in Figure 2.2). Undercounting can occur if the endometrial cavity is not systematically examined, so care should be taken to pan through the uterus both transversely and longitudinally so as not to miss higher-order multiple pregnancies. Between 7 and 12 weeks, the chorionic and amniotic membranes are yet to fuse, thereby enabling clear visualisation of the amniotic cavity and diagnosis of amnionicity (in Figure 2.3). An image demonstrating both embryos on the screen at the same time should be obtained when possible.

The number of yolk sacs in monochorionic pregnancies is variable and should not be used for diagnosis. It is important to note that dichorionic twins are not always dizygotic (nonidentical), as up to 15 per cent

Table 2.1 Week-by-week landmarks for the diagnosis of early pregnancy on scan

Gestation	Ultrasound findings	Ultrasound image	Diagram
4^{+3} to 5^{+0}	A small gestation sac (GS) (2–5 mm) is visible within the endometrium. It is spherical, regular in outline and surrounded by an echogenic ring of trophoblast. It is eccentrically located towards the fundus and implanted just beneath the endometrial surface (midline echo).		
5^{+1} to 5^{+5}	The GS should be visible by 5^{+2}. The yolk sac becomes visible within the GS (chorionic cavity). The yolk sac should be seen when the mean GS diameter is > 12 mm.		
5^{+6} to 6^{+0}	The embryonic pole is visible as a straight line, adjacent to the YS. It measures 2–4 mm in length. Fetal heart activity is detectable. The embryo is usually visible with a mean GSD > 18 mm.		
6^{+1} to 6^{+6}	The embryo appears kidney bean-shaped. It is separated from the YS by the vitelline duct. The CRL measures 4–10 mm. Care should be taken not to include the YS when measuring the CRL. Fetal heart activity should be detectable.		
7^{+0} to 7^{+6}	The CRL measures 11–16 mm. The rhombencephalon is visible (diamond-shaped), enabling distinction of cephalad and caudal ends. The spine is visible as double echogenic parallel lines. The amniotic cavity is visible within the chorionic cavity and contains the embryo. The umbilical cord can be seen.		

Table 2.1 (continued)

Gestation	Ultrasound findings	Ultrasound image	Diagram
8^{+0} to 8^{+6}	The CRL measures 17–23 mm. The forebrain, midbrain, hindbrain, and skull are distinguishable. The limb buds and first movements are seen. The umbilical cord and vitelline duct lengthen. The chorion frondosum and chorion laevae are visible.		
9^{+0} to 10^{+0}	The CRL measures 23–32 mm. The limbs lengthen and hands, feet, and eyes are visible. The midgut hernia is present. Choroid plexae can be seen.		

Abbreviations: GS = gestational sac; YS = yolk sac; GSD = gestational sac diameter; CRL = crown rump length.

Table 2.2 Mean CRL in relation to gestational age

CRL	Gestational age
10 mm	= mean for 7^{+2} weeks
20 mm	= mean for 8^{+5} weeks
30 mm	= mean for 10^{+0} weeks
40 mm	= mean for 10^{+6} weeks

of dichorionic twins are monozygotic (identical), depending on how early cleavage occurs. The presence of a single or two ovarian corpora lutea may provide an insight into the zygosity of the pregnancy. Table 2.3 depicts the ultrasound findings expected according to gestational age in a normally developing twin pregnancy.

Variants of Normal

The following ultrasound features are less commonly seen variants of the normal intrauterine pregnancy (IUP), and if they have not been seen previously by the operator can lead to diagnostic confusion and uncertainty.

(a) Chorionic bumps (Figure 2.4)
- ○ Appear as cystic areas within chorion
- ○ Evolve to become echogenic
- ○ Usually resolve spontaneously
- ○ Cause gestational sac to appear irregular
- ○ May be associated with an increased risk of miscarriage

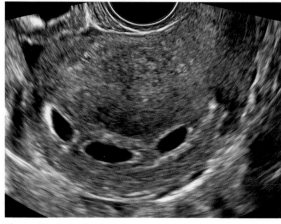

Figure 2.2 Trichorionic triplet pregnancy.

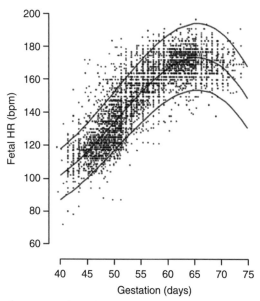

Figure 2.1 Relationship between embryonic heart rate and gestational age; median, 95th and 5th centiles [3]. (Relevant permissions obtained from copyright holder.)

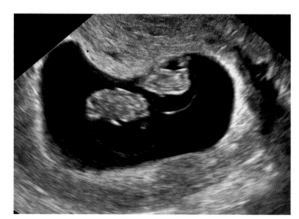

Figure 2.3 Monochorionic diamniotic pregnancy.

(b) Umbillical cord cysts (Figure 2.5)
- ○ Overall incidence in first trimester of 3–4 per cent
- ○ Incidence may be as high as 25 per cent at eight to nine weeks

Table 2.3 Schematic depicting the ultrasound diagnosis of chorionicity and amnionicity in early twin pregnancy (○ = chorionic cavity; ● = amniotic cavity; ● = embryo)

Multiple pregnancy diagnosis

Gestation	Dichorionic diamniotic	Monochorionic diamniotic	Monochorionic monoamniotic
5+0 to 5+6	◯ ◯	◯	◯
6+0 to 6+6	◉ ◉	◉◉	◉◉
7+0 to 7+6	◉ ◉	◉◉	◉◉

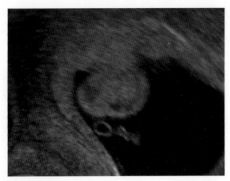

Figure 2.4 Chorionic bump producing an irregularly shaped gestation sac contour.

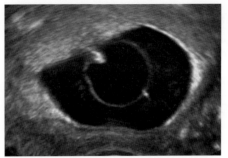

Figure 2.6 Echogenic coelomic fluid seen throughout the gestation and amniotic sacs.

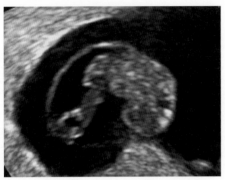

Figure 2.5 Cross section of umbilical cord (left) containing cystic structure within.

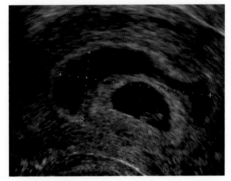

Figure 2.7 Fluid collection in endometrial cavity, surrounding an IUP.

○ Unlikely to be clinically significant unless large and multiple or if they persist into the second trimester and are associated with other structural abnormalities

(c) Echogenic coelomic fluid (Figure 2.6)

○ Fluid within the gestation and amniotic sacs appears echogenic as opposed to anechoic

○ Underlying process unknown but may be due to preceding haemorrhage

○ Not known to be associated with an increased risk of miscarriage

(d) Fluid in endometrial cavity (Figure 2.7)

○ This may be a 'subchorionic haematoma' in women who have experienced vaginal bleeding, but may be seen in women with no bleeding, probably due to secretions within the endometrial cavity

○ Can be variable in position and amount

○ Not thought to have an effect on outcome of pregnancy

Learning Points

• The landmarks for diagnosis of normal early pregnancy must be learned prior to performing first-trimester ultrasound scans, so that the ultrasound findings may be explained.

• A systematic approach to the ultrasound evaluation and measurement of an early intrauterine pregnancy will ensure a correct assessment and conclusion.

• Accurate diagnosis of multiple pregnancy may require repeated scans, depending on the gestation at initial presentation.

Further Reading

1. Verhaegen J, Gallos ID, van Mello NM, Abdel-Aziz M, Takwoingi Y, Harb H et al. (2012). Accuracy of single progesterone test to predict early pregnancy outcome in women with pain or bleeding: meta-analysis of cohort studies. *BMJ* 345: e6077

2. Jurkovic D, Gruboeck K, Campbell S (1995). Ultrasound features of normal early pregnancy

development. *Curr Opin Obstet Gynecol* Dec;7(6): 493–504.

3. Papaioannou G, Syngelaki A, Poon L, Ross A, Nicolaides K (2010). Normal ranges of embryonic length, embryonic heart rate, gestational sac diameter and yolk sac diameter at 6–10 weeks. *Fetal Diagn Ther* 28: 207–219.

4. Arleo EK, Dunning A, Troiano RN (2015). Chorionic bump in pregnant patients and associated live birth rate: a systematic review and meta-analysis. *J Ultrasound Med* Apr;34(4): 553–557.

5. Ross JA, Jurkovic D, Nicolaides K (1997). Coelocentesis: a study of short-term safety. *Prenat Diagn* Oct;17(10): 913–917.

Diagnosis of Miscarriage

Nicola Mitchell-Jones and Cecilia Bottomley

Miscarriage is the most common complication of early pregnancy. Ultrasound is now pivotal in modern-day practice for its diagnosis and management of miscarriage.

Terminology

When diagnosing miscarriage or possible miscarriage in patients following ultrasound assessment, it must be remembered that the diagnosis is highly emotive and has wide-reaching psychological consequences. The terminology used to describe miscarriage can be confusing for patients. Preferred terms are described in Table 3.1, and Figure 3.1 shows the types of miscarriage.

Aetiology

The prevalence of miscarriage is commonly quoted as one in five pregnancies, with higher rates of pregnancy loss if 'biochemical pregnancies' are included (where miscarriage occurs before a pregnancy is visible on scan). Around 70 per cent of miscarriages are attributed to chromosomal abnormalities (most

Table 3.1 Terminology used in early pregnancy assessment

Term	Definition	Notes
Miscarriage	Pregnancy loss at < 24 weeks' gestation	'Spontaneous miscarriage' is used where the pregnancy has been expelled from the uterus. 'Delayed' or 'missed' miscarriage is used where the pregnancy has ceased to develop but a spontaneous miscarriage is yet to occur.
Late miscarriage	Pregnancy loss between 12 and 24 weeks gestation	Used where fetal demise occurs in the second trimester. Pregnancy loss < 24 weeks where signs of life are noted at delivery is termed a neonatal death.
Live intrauterine pregnancy	Intrauterine pregnancy with visible embryo and heart pulsations or fetal heartbeat (FH)	May also be referred to as a 'viable' pregnancy.
Intrauterine pregnancy of uncertain viability (IPUV)	Intrauterine pregnancy where viability is yet to be determined (FH not seen on initial scan)	May represent a normal early pregnancy of 5–6 weeks' gestation or a failed pregnancy with arrested growth.
Inevitable miscarriage	A pregnancy destined to end in miscarriage; the cervix is open, but the pregnancy has yet to be expelled	An active miscarriage is in progress, products of conception are seen within the cervix on ultrasound and/or clinical examination.
Incomplete miscarriage/ retained products of conception (RPOC)	RPOC (well-defined mixed echoes) within the uterine cavity with no identifiable gestation sac	The presence of vascularity within this tissue helps confirm the diagnosis and differentiate from intrauterine blood clot (although RPOC may be avascular). If uncertainty and an intrauterine pregnancy has not previously been seen, the findings are classified as 'pregnancy of unknown location'.
Complete miscarriage	Ultrasound finding of empty uterus with no retained tissue identified, where an intrauterine pregnancy has previously been visualized	If an intrauterine pregnancy has not previously been seen, this term cannot be applied, and the findings are classified as 'pregnancy of unknown location'.

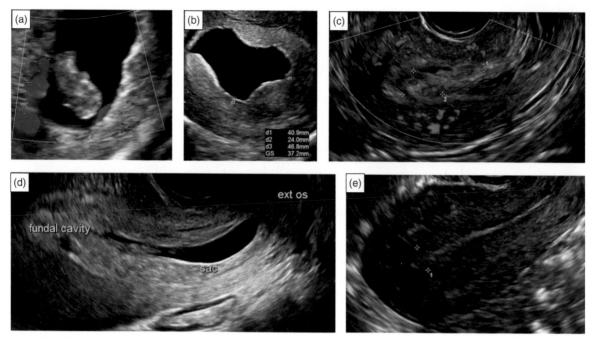

Figure 3.1 Types of miscarriage. A and B: Delayed miscarriage. Embryo with CRL of 19 mm. Fetal heart pulsations are absent, as demonstrated with colour doppler (image A). Empty gestation sac with a mean sac diametre of 37 mm (image B). **C:** Incomplete miscarriage. Heterogeneous material of mixed echoes within the uterine cavity in keeping with retained products of conception. Some vascularity is seen within this tissue helping to differentiate between this and a blood clot within the cavity. **D:** Inevitable miscarriage. Gestation sac within the cervix (cervical ectopic pregnancy must be excluded). **E:** Complete miscarriage. The endometrial cavity is empty. This term may only be applied where an intrauterine pregnancy has been confirmed previously (otherwise, use 'pregnancy of unknown location').

Bleeding Score: *please circle as appropriate*

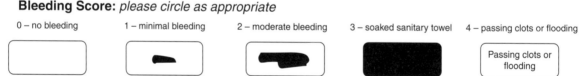

Figure 3.2 Pictorial blood loss assessment chart. Taken from Higham J, O'Brien P, Shaw R (1990). Assessment of menstrual blood loss using a pictorial chart. *BJOG* 97(8): 734–739.

commonly trisomy). The risk of miscarriage increases more significantly after the age of 35 due to a higher frequency of chromosomal abnormalities. Other aetiological factors include thrombophilias, maternal systemic disease or its treatment, uterine anomalies, and endometrial environmental factors.

Presentation

Vaginal bleeding is the most common symptom preceding a diagnosis of miscarriage. This can be objectively assessed using a pictorial blood loss assessment chart (Figure 3.2). Many women, however, have no symptoms at the time of diagnosis. Ultrasound is the primary diagnostic tool for a diagnosis of miscarriage.

More rarely, a clinical diagnosis of miscarriage may be made where the cervical os is open and products of conception have been passed or are seen within the cervix.

Ultrasound Diagnosis

The diagnosis of miscarriage may in some circumstances be made at the initial ultrasound scan (Table 3.2). These ultrasound criteria have been determined such that both the specificity and positive predictive value are 100 per cent and there is allowance for interobserver variability in measurements. A miscarriage must not be diagnosed where there is any perceived possibility that the pregnancy is ongoing,

Table 3.2 Ultrasound criteria for diagnosis of miscarriage (where these criteria are not fulfilled, a repeat scan is indicated, as in Figure 3.3. MSD: mean gestation sac diameter (mean of three orthogonal measurements)

Diagnostic criteria	Gestation by Last Menstrual Period (LMP)	Explanation
Visible embryo with CRL ≥ 7 mm without fetal heart pulsations	At any gestation	Colour Doppler may be applied to confirm the absence of heart pulsations.
Gestation sac with MSD ≥ **25 mm** without visible yolk sac (YS) or embryo	At any gestation	Previously referred to as an 'anembryonic pregnancy' or 'blighted ovum'. This pregnancy has stopped developing in the early stages before the embryo is visible (or the embryo has become nonvisible following demise) and may be described as an 'empty sac'.
Embryo with absent fetal heart pulsations, where previous scan demonstrated heart pulsations	At any gestation	Applies for any CRL (though caution if CRL is small, where a repeat scan may be considered to confirm the diagnosis).
Visible embryo with CRL ≥ **3 mm** without fetal heart pulsations OR Gestation sac with MSD ≥ **18 mm** without visible embryo	At ≥ **70** days gestation	Diagnostic for miscarriage only if dates known for certain (usually reserved for women following assisted reproduction treatment).

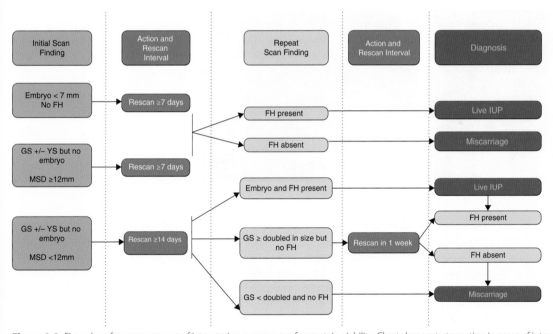

Figure 3.3 Flow chart for management of intrauterine pregnancy of uncertain viability. Chart demonstrates action in cases of intrauterine pregnancy of uncertain viability (where initial scan does not demonstrate a embryo with heart pulsations). A second scan is required at an interval determined by the initial scan findings. In some cases, a third interval scan is required.

as this could result in the termination of a potentially viable pregnancy.

If a live pregnancy (fetal heart pulsations present) or a failed pregnancy fulfilling the diagnostic criteria of miscarriage (Table 3.2) is not found on initial scan,

then an interval scan is required to assess ongoing pregnancy development. The timing of the repeat scan (7 or 14 days) is dependent on the initial findings (Figure 3.3).

If a woman has fetal cardiac activity noted on an initial scan and re-presents, then the absence of cardiac

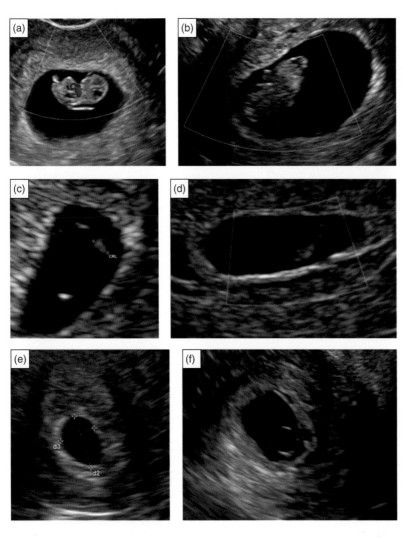

Figure 3.4 Diagnosing miscarriage. A & B: This patient was initially seen at 10 weeks' gestation by menstrual dates with a complaint of light vaginal bleeding; initial scan (A) demonstrated a live IUP of eight weeks gestation by CRL measurement. Further bleeding prompted a second scan (B), at which fetal heart pulsations were no longer present. **C & D:** This patient underwent initial scan at nine weeks gestation by menstrual dates due to moderate vaginal bleeding; on the first occasion (C), a gestation sac with a 3 mm embryo was seen, and no fetal heart pulsations were present. Repeat scan seven days later (D) demonstrates no significant change in measurements, and again no fetal heart pulsations were present. **E & F:** This patient underwent viability assessment due to a history of recurrent miscarriage. The initial scan (E) was performed at six weeks' gestation by menstrual dates; an intrauterine gestation sac with an MSD of 12 mm was seen. A repeat scan (F) was performed 14 days later; the MSD was 19 mm, and a yolk sac was visible; however, no embryo was identified.

activity on repeat assessment is diagnostic of miscarriage without the need to fulfil measurement criteria.

To minimise the risk of termination of an ongoing pregnancy, the diagnosis of miscarriage should be confirmed by two operators or on two separate occasions. Figure 3.4 shows some scan images in patients who were diagnosed with a miscarriage.

Soft Markers and Prediction of Miscarriage

Where fetal heart pulsations are not seen on initial scan (IPUV), clinicians may use ultrasound findings and clinical information to help counsel women regarding the likely pregnancy outcome. Soft markers (Table 3.3) are not diagnostic but suggestive of

an increased chance of miscarriage. Other factors associated with increased risk of miscarriage are discordance between embryo size and menstrual dates, moderate or heavy vaginal bleeding and increasing maternal age (a woman aged 40 has up to a 45 per cent chance of miscarriage).

Caution

As detailed, the diagnosis of miscarriage may often need to be deferred for up to three weeks, where repeat scan is necessary. Strict adherence to the guidelines is essential to avoid termination of a potentially viable pregnancy. However, careful counselling of women in such a situation is important to manage expectations and prepare them for possible bleeding or spontaneous miscarriage in the meantime.

Table 3.3 Soft markers of miscarriage: ultrasound findings that are not diagnostic of miscarriage but may present an increased risk of miscarriage; in all cases, a repeat scan in 7–14 days is recommended to assess ongoing viability

Soft marker	Image	Description
Empty amnion		The presence of an amniotic sac without visible embryo seen within. Referred to as the 'empty amnion sign' and usually associated with a nonviable pregnancy.
Subchorionic haematoma		Hypoechoic, crescent-shaped area separating the uterine wall and chorion. Frequently associated with vaginal bleeding. Also associated with adverse perinatal outcome.
Chorionic bumps		Irregular, hyperechogenic bulge from the choriodecidual surface into the gestation sac. Associated with first- and second-trimester miscarriage.
Large yolk sac		YS diameter of ≥ 5 mm is commonly a pathological sign.
Early embryonic growth restriction		Significant discrepancy between the expected size of the embryo (from LMP dates) and the observed sized on scan (in women with certain menstrual dates).
Bradycardic fetal heart pulsations		Fetal heart pulsations < 100 bpm are predictive of miscarriage (except in very small embryos (2–5 mm), which are expected to have a fetal heart rate of < 100 bpm).

Learning Points

- Ultrasound diagnosis of miscarriage is made using objective measurements and pathways.
- Frequently an interval scan is required.
- The diagnostic criteria are altered after 70 days (10 weeks) of gestation where gestational age of the pregnancy is certain (usually only in pregnancies conceived via in vitro fertilization.
- The diagnosis of miscarriage should be confirmed by two practitioners or on two separate occasions.
- Several ultrasound 'soft markers' are associated with an increased risk of a failing pregnancy, but these are not diagnostic of miscarriage and should be used only to inform that a repeat scan is required and for counselling.
- The likelihood of impending miscarriage diagnosis may be predicted using a combination of maternal history, the presence of symptoms, bleeding score, and ultrasound findings.

Further Reading

1. Abdallah Y, Daemen A, Kirk E, Pexsters A, Naji O, Stalder C, Gould D, Ahmed S, Guha S, Syed S, Bottomley C, Timmerman D, Bourne T (2011). Limitations of current definitions of miscarriage using mean gestational sac diameter and crown–rump length measurements: a multicentre observational study. *Ultrasound Obst Gynecol* 38: 497–502.

2. Bottomley C, Bourne T (2009). Diagnosing miscarriage. *Best Practice & Research Clinical Obstetrics and Gynaecology* 23: 463–477.

3. Doubilet P, Benson C, Bourne T, Blaivas M (2013). Diagnostic criteria for nonviable pregnancy early in the first trimester. *N Eng J Med* 369: 1443–1451.

4. National Institute for Health and Care Excellence (NICE) (2012). Ectopic pregnancy and miscarriage: diagnosis and initial management in early pregnancy of ectopic pregnancy and miscarriage. NICE Clinical Guideline 154.

5. Jeve Y, Rhana R, Bhide A, Thangaratinam (2011). Accuracy of first-trimester ultrasound in the diagnosis of early embryonic demise: a systematic review. *Ultrasound Obstet Gynecol* 38: 489–496.

6. Newbatt E, Beckles Z, Ullman R, Lumsden MA, on behalf of the Guideline Development Group (2012). Ectopic pregnancy and miscarriage: summary of NICE guidance. *BMJ* 345: e8136.

7. Preisler J, Kopeika J, Ismail L, Vathanan V, Farren J, Abdallah, Y, Battacharjee P, Van Holsbeke C, Bottomley C, Gould D, Johnson S, Stalder C, Van Calster B, Hamilton J, Timmerman D, Bourne T (2015). Defining safe criteria to diagnose miscarriage: prospective observational multicentre study. *BMJ* 351: h4579.

Gestational Trophoblastic Disease

Anna Graham and Jemma Johns

Gestational trophoblastic disease (GTD) is the collective term for a number of conditions, including hydatidiform mole (HM) (complete and partial), invasive mole, choriocarcinoma, and placental site trophoblastic tumour (PSTT) (Table 4.1). GTD is characterised by abnormal proliferation of the trophoblast layer of the placenta; if there is any evidence of persistent elevation of beta human chorionic gonadotrophin (hCG), the condition is referred to as gestational trophoblastic neoplasia (GTN).

Epidemiology

The United Kingdom has a national register for HM pregnancies, and all cases are managed from two centres: the Sheffield Trophoblastic Disease Centre and the Charing Cross Hospital Trophoblastic Disease Service. This ensures that central histopathological review occurs and hCG surveillance is consistent. The reported incidence in the United Kingdom for CHM is 1 per 1,000 pregnancies and 3 per 1,000 for PHM (Table 4.2). Most other countries have less rigorous reporting systems, but rates have historically been reported as higher in Asian countries, with GTD occurring in 2 per 1,000 pregnancies.

Maternal age is a risk factor for a HM, with women over 35 years having an elevated relative risk of 1.9 for a CHM compared to under 35 year olds; this rises to 7.5 times higher in the over 40 group. This is consistent with the reduced quality of a woman's ova as she ages and the subsequent predisposition to abnormal fertilisation. Additionally, a previous molar pregnancy (partial or complete) carries a risk of recurrent molar pregnancy of 1–2 per cent. This increases to 15–20 per cent after two HMs, and the risk is not decreased by a change in partner.

Genetics

In a normal pregnancy, a spermatozoon with 23 chromosomes fertilises an oocyte with 23 chromosomes to produce a diploid zygote (46XX or 46XY). This then undergoes mitosis and develops into a normal fetus and placenta. HMs are genetically abnormal pregnancies and are categorised by their genetic and histopathological features into CHMs and PHMs. These genetics are summarised in Figure 4.1.

Rarely, a CHM and twin pregnancy coexist (approximately 1/20,000–100,000 pregnancies). They occur when two oocytes are fertilised: one abnormally (from an empty oocyte), as shown in Figure 4.1, producing a CHM; and one normally, producing a normal pregnancy.

Histopathology

HMs arise from abnormal trophoblast hyperplasia (Figure 4.2). The trophoblast is the outer layer of cells of the blastocyst. In a normal pregnancy, the trophoblast will develop into the placenta. The trophoblast has two layers: the inner cellular layer is the cytotrophoblast, and the outer layer is the syncitiotrophoblast. In HMs, both of these layers develop with abnormal proliferation and vesicular swelling of placental villi. CHMs show diffuse trophoblastic hyperplasia and swelling of the villi, whereas PHMs tend to have focal areas of abnormal change. A histopathological diagnosis is required in all cases of HM, as other methods are unreliable.

Human Chorionic Gonadotrophin and Hydatidiform Moles

hCG is produced by the syntotrophoblast of the placenta. In GTD, there is abnormal trophoblastic hyperplasia, and therefore significantly more hCG is produced than in a normal pregnancy. Approximately 50 per cent of CHMs will have preevacuation levels of hCG > 100,000 mIU/mL, in comparison to less than 10 per cent of PHMs.

Table 4.1 Comparison of the main features of GTD

GTD	Overview
Complete Hydatidiform Mole (CHM)	Genetically abnormal pregnancy – 46XX/XY No fetus Vaginal bleeding in 1st or 2nd trimester; medical complications common 15% progress to GTN
Partial Hydatidiform Mole (PHM)	Genetically abnormal pregnancy – 69XXX/XXY/XYY Abnormal fetus Missed miscarriage, vaginal bleeding, medical complications rare 0.5% progress to GTN
Invasive mole	Benign tumor Derived from myometrial invasion of HM 15% metastasise to lungs or vagina Persistently elevated hCG following HM
Choriocarcinoma	Malignant disease Occurs following any pregnancy: 25% post miscarriage or ectopic, 25% post normal pregnancy, 50% post HM Metastasise to lungs, brain, liver, pelvis, vagina, kidney, intestines, and spleen
Placental Site Trophoblastic Tunour (PSTT)	Malignant disease Very rare – arises from the placental implantation site Occurs following nonmolar pregnancies more commonly than HM Lymphatic metastasis

Table 4.2 Epidemiology of GTD

	Gestational trophoblastic disease			
	Incidence in U.K. per 1,000 pregnancies	Risk factors for GTD	Risk of developing to GTN (%)	Risk of repeat HM (%)
CHM	1	• Increased maternal age • Previous HM • Asian	15	1–2
PHM	3	• Increased maternal age • Previous HM • Asian	0.5	1–2

Clinical Presentation

HMs were historically diagnosed in the mid trimester; however, with the introduction of nuchal scanning at 11–14 weeks' gestation and widespread access to early pregnancy units with scanning facilities, this is now rarely the case. The average gestational age at evacuation in the United Kingdom is now less than 10 weeks, and the classic symptoms described in textbooks – including hypertension, hyperthyroidism, the passing of grapelike products and abdominal distention secondary to bilateral multiple ovarian theca lutein cysts – are now rare. The most common presenting symptom in both CHMs and PHMs is vaginal bleeding in early pregnancy, which in most cases leads to an early pregnancy ultrasound scan and diagnosis of a nonviable pregnancy; see Table 4.3.

Clinical Presentation – CHMs

Eighty to ninety per cent of CHMs present with vaginal bleeding between 6 and 16 weeks' gestation. The other classic signs and symptoms are less common, such as uterine enlargement greater than expected for gestational dates, which occurs in 25 per cent of cases; hyperemesis, which appears in 10 per cent; and pregnancy-related hypertension in the first or second trimester, which occurs in around 1 per cent (Table 4.3). There remain rarer presentations, such as hyperthyroidism, early onset preeclampsia,

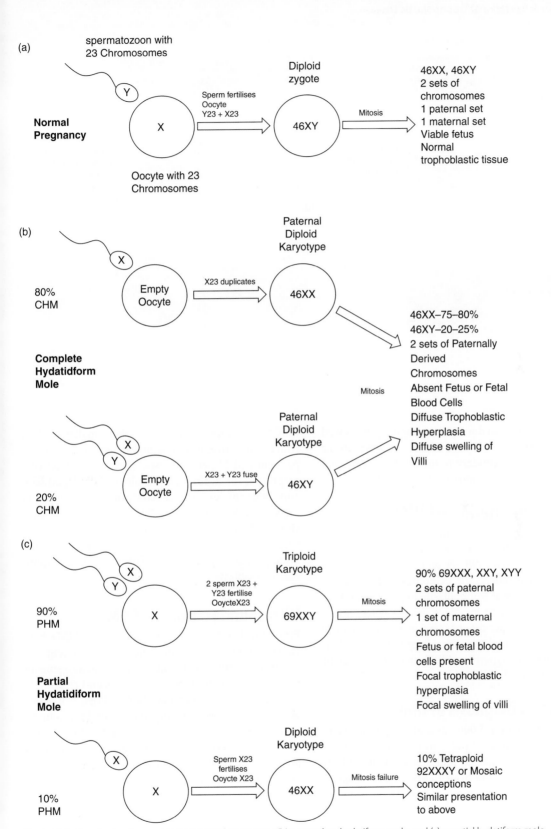

Figure 4.1 Genetic development in (a) a normal pregnancy; (b) a complete hydatiform mole; and (c) a partial hydatiform mole.

(a)

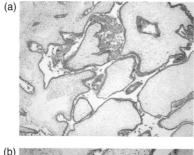

(b)

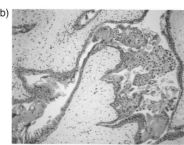

Complete hydatidiform mole shows enlarged and bulbous villi with branching and budding, cistern formation and, focally, circumferential trophoblastic hyperplasia.

(c)

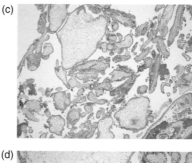

(d)

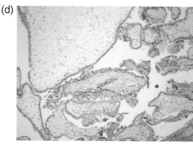

Partial hydatidiform mole shows mixed dilated, oedematous and sclerosed irregular villi with occasional trophoblast hyperplasia.

Figure 4.2 Gestational trophoblastic disease: (a) complete hydatidiform mole; (b) partial hydatidiform mole. Images courtesy of Dr Abdel-Ghani Selim, MBBCh, MSc, PhD, FRCPath Consultant Histopathologist and Cytopathologist, King's College Hospital, National Health Service Foundation Trust.

abdominal distention due to theca lutein cysts, as well as acute respiratory failure or neurological symptoms such as seizures (secondary to metastatic disease), all of which warrant exclusion of HM.

Clinical Presentation – PHMs

PHMs tend to present later than CHMs but also present with vaginal bleeding (75 per cent) or incomplete or missed miscarriage (90 per cent). Other symptoms are rarer, which reflects the pathology of PHM compared to CHM; focal trophoblastic hyperplasia rather than diffuse produces excessive uterine enlargement in only around 10 per cent of cases; hCG is raised only marginally compared to normal pregnancies, leading to hyperemesis, hyperthyroidism, and theca lutein cysts very rarely (Table 4.3).

Ultrasound Diagnosis of HMs

A U.K. study of over 1,000 cases at a regional referral centre found that 79 per cent of complete moles and 29 per cent of partial moles were suspected on ultrasound examination prior to histological diagnosis. The overall rate of detection was 44 per cent. In addition to this, 10 per cent of cases that were thought to be molar on USS were diagnosed as nonmolar hydropic abortions on histological review. These findings are supported by two other smaller studies, which found overall ultrasound detection rates of 56 per cent and 44 per cent respectively. As with all USS diagnoses, the accuracy of results is user dependent, and operator experience contributes to detection rates. Therefore, although USS assists in the diagnosis of HMs, the products obtained from all medical or surgical miscarriages of all failed pregnancies should undergo histological assessment to exclude trophoblastic neoplasia.

Ultrasound Features – CHMs

From the late first trimester onwards, CHMs have classic ultrasound scan findings, including an enlarged uterine cavity filled with a heterogeneous mass containing multiple cystic areas and referred to as a 'snowstorm' appearance (Table 4.4a); a lack of evidence of fetal development; and bilateral theca lutein cysts in 15 per cent of cases (Table 4.4). The differential diagnosis on USS is of retained placental tissue that has undergone hydropic degeneration (Table 4.5). The history from the patient may help to distinguish between the two; the CHM will have had minimal bleeding, whereas the hydropic retained products of conception (RPOC) are likely to describe an incomplete miscarriage with heavier bleeding.

Table 4.3 A comparison of clinical presentation and USS findings of CHM and PHM

	1st trimester, 2nd trimester	USS findings and hCG levels	USS diagnosis
CHM	80–90% vaginal bleeding 6–16 weeks 40% asymptomatic 25% uterine enlargement 10% hyperemesis 5% anaemia 1–2% preeclampsia Rare passing of 'grapelike' products Rare hyperthyroidism	• Heterogenous Mass – 'snowstorm' • Multiple cystic spaces • No fetus • 15% theca lutein cysts • 50% hCG > 100,000 mIU/ml	79%
PHM	75% vaginal bleeding Missed/incomplete miscarriage 10% uterine enlargement 2.5% preeclampsia	• Echogenic placental tissue • Multiple cystic areas • Fetus present • Rarely theca lutein cysts • Increase in transverse diametre of GS • 10% hCG > 100,000 mIU/ml	29%

Table 4.4 (a) CHM at 12 weeks; and (b) theca lutein cysts

	History and clinical presentation	USS	USS features
CHM	33 yo P2 + 1 (termination) 12 + 2/40 Brown PV discharge Attended for nuchal scan Dx: CHM or hydropic RPOC		• Diffuse heterogeneous mass • Uterus enlarged to 18 weeks' size • Multiple cysts within the mass • No fetus
CHM	32 yo P1 Bilateral multifollicular cysts in 13/40 CHM hCG: 905193 Dx: Theca lutein cysts or hyperstimulated ovaries		• Enlarged ovaries bilaterally • Multiple follicles

USS features are less apparent earlier than this, and although the scan may be suspicious of a HM, the differential diagnosis is often an early intrauterine pregnancy (IUP) or a pregnancy of unknown location (PUL) (Table 4.6). A CHM twin pregnancy will be more difficult to diagnose. There will be a heterogenous mass with cystic areas; however, there will also be a fetus with or without fetal heart pulsations (Tables 4.7 and 4.8). The RCOG recommends that prenatal invasive testing for fetal karyotype should be considered where it is unclear whether the pregnancy is a complete mole with a coexisting normal twin or a partial mole.

Ultrasound Features – PHMs

PHMs have less distinctive features on USS in either the first and second trimester compared to CHMs; however, USS remains helpful in facilitating their diagnosis. There is likely to be a gestational sac, but there may also be a thickened trophoblastic layer containing multiple avascular cystic spaces (Table 4.8). PHMs often present as an incomplete or missed miscarriage, and the findings on USS may be just this, with no evidence of HM on the scan (Table 4.8). The differential diagnosis is a CHM and coexistent twin (Table 4.7).

Table 4.5 Hydropic retained products of conception

	History and clinical presentation	USS	USS features
Hydropic RPOC	39 yo P1 7 + 2/40 Pelvic pain No PV bleeding Dx: CHM or hydropic RPOC		• Diffuse heterogeneous mass • Multiple cysts within the mass • No fetus

Table 4.6 (a) Pregnancy of unknown location (PUL); (b) rescanned a week later with a molar pregnancy suspected

	History and clinical presentation	USS	USS features
CHM	23 yo P1 + 1 (termination) 6 + 4/40 PVB 2/7 Classified as a PUL hCG and progesterone requested Dx: PUL		• Heterogeneous mass • Small cystic area within the mass • No fetus
CHM	Pt above rescanned at 7 + 4/40 hCG: 49061 Dx: CHM or hydropic RPOC		• Diffuse heterogeneous mass • Few cysts within the mass • No fetus

Table 4.7 CHM and coexistent twin pregnancy

	History and clinical presentation	USS	USS features
CHM + Twin	32 yo P2 + 3 miscarriages 12 + 1/40 Asymptomatic Attended nuchal scan Dx: CHM + twin or PHM		• Diffuse heterogenous mass • Multiple cysts within the mass • Live fetus with fetal heart pulsations

Table 4.8 (a) PHM at 13 weeks; (b) PHM at 16 weeks with no evidence of HM on USS

	History and clinical presentation	USS	USS features
PHM	27 yo P0 13 + 3/40 Asymptomatic Attended nuchal scan Dx: Early embryonic demise or PHM		• GS present • Embryo present (not visible in this image) • No FH • Thickened placental tissue • Cystic areas within placenta
PHM	35 yo P2 + 1 (miscarriage) 16 + 2 Asymptomatic Routine scan Dx: Early embryonic demise		• Thickened placental tissue • Nonviable fetus present • No evidence on USS of HM

Management of HMs

It is essential that when a nonviable pregnancy is diagnosed and molar pregnancy is suspected (clinically, with USS and hCG) that surgical management is recommended and the products of conception are sent for histological analysis (Figure 4.3). This is to ensure that the correct diagnosis is established and the patient can be monitored for subsequent progression to GTN. It is widely accepted that surgical management should be performed via suction aspiration rather than sharp curette to reduce the risk of perforation. Ultrasound examination throughout this procedure also aids in reducing the risk of perforation and ensuring that the uterine cavity is completely evacuated.

The overall preevacuation rate of HM diagnosis on USS is under 50 per cent, and given that the great majority of PHM are not even suspected, it is essential that products from all miscarriages are sent for histological diagnosis to exclude molar pregnancy. This does not exclude expectant or medical management of miscarriage but does imply the need for collection of products by the patient to be sent for histology. In reality, this rarely occurs.

It could also be argued that all specimens removed at a termination of pregnancy (TOP) should also be analysed for HM, but given the large numbers being performed in the United Kingdom, around 200,000 per year, this would be unfeasible. The RCOG does not recommend screening for GTD; however, it does advise that an intrauterine pregnancy should be visualised on USS prior to a TOP. This is likely to identify or raise suspicions of a CHM, which would then warrant a referral. The rate of progression to GTN following a TOP has been estimated to be 1/20,000, but due to late diagnosis, this leads to poor prognosis. It is recommended that women undergoing a TOP are counselled to be assessed for ongoing pregnancy symptoms and to perform a urine pregnancy test at three to four weeks postprocedure if in any doubt.

The CHM twin pregnancy poses a management dilemma, because if the CHM is treated surgically this will inevitably end the healthy pregnancy; however, if the pregnancy is allowed to continue then the woman is at risk of both the previously discussed complications as well as malignant disease. The RCOG Green-Top Guideline quotes live birth rates of around 25 per cent, but Sebire et al. showed healthy birth rates to be around 40 per cent in a case series of 77 pregnancies. This study also showed that there was no increase in the risk of developing GTN despite continuing with the pregnancy until term. Women should be counselled about the risks, including the increased risk of early fetal loss (40 per cent), premature delivery (36 per cent), and preeclampsia (4–20 per cent); however, ultimately the clinician should support the woman's choice as this is likely to vary significantly due to her personal history, age, fertility potential, and other children.

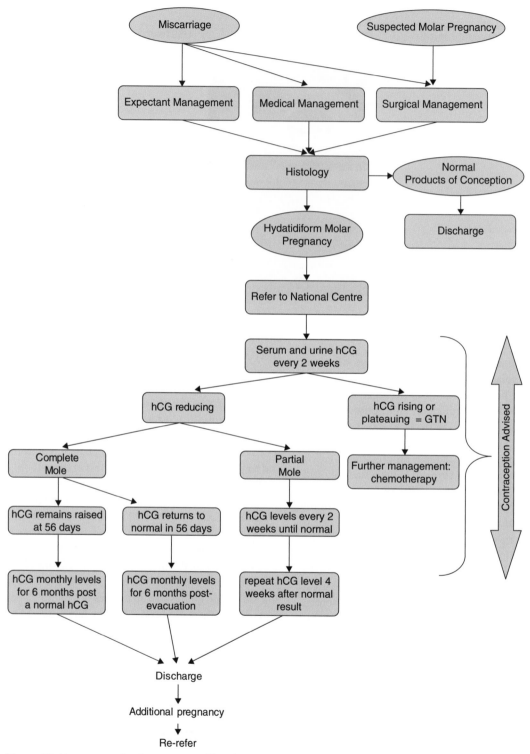

Figure 4.3 Management of molar pregnancies (Flow chart developed from Royal College of Obstetricians and Gynaecologists (February 2010). The management of gestational trophoblastic disease. *Green-Top Guideline* 38).

Monitoring Post-HM Evacuation

All patients with identified HM should be referred to one of the U.K. centres for histopathological review and placed on the national registry for hCG follow-up. An overview of hCG follow-up is given in Figure 4.3. During the hCG follow-up period, women are advised to use reliable contraception. Traditionally barrier methods were recommended, but now in the United Kingdom the national centres advise that oral contraceptives after molar evacuation, before hCG returns to normal, can be used safely. Studies have shown no increase in development of invasive mole or choriocarcinoma in women taking oestrogen and or progestogens during this time. Following a diagnosis of GTD, even when the hCG has normalised, if the patient becomes pregnant again, she is once again at risk of developing GTN. Therefore, hCG levels should be checked after every pregnancy to ensure no reactivation of previous HM.

Gestational Trophoblastic Neoplasia

Molar pregnancies are followed up so closely due to the risk of development to GTN, which can be fatal if left untreated. The rate of development from a complete molar pregnancy is around 15 per cent and from a partial hydatidiform mole 0.5 per cent. The diagnosis of GTN is made on the basis of an elevated hCG plateau or rising hCG titres over a period of several weeks. GTN is scored and staged using the International Federation of Gynaecology and Obstetrics (FIGO) (2000) scoring system for GTN. Approximately 95 per cent of patients will have low-risk, low-resistant disease and will be treated with monotherapy chemotherapy (methotrexate); if this fails, a second line chemotherapy can be used (actinomycin D or EMA/CO [etoposide, methotrexate, actinomycin D, cyclophosphamide, vincristine]). This group has an overall survival rate of nearly 100 per cent.

High-risk disease occurs in only 5 per cent of cases and usually presents with many metastases months or years after the causative pregnancy. They are at a high risk of developing resistant disease and therefore require treatment with multi-agent chemotherapy. Even in this high-risk group there is a cure rate of around 84 per cent.

Learning Points

- Molar pregnancies have an incidence of 1 in 1,000 pregnancies for complete hydatidiform moles and 3 in 1,000 for partial hydatidiform moles.
- The risk of progression to gestational trophoblastic neoplasia is 15 per cent for complete hydatidiform moles and 0.5 per cent for partial hydatidiform moles.
- Hydatidiform moles rarely present with the classical symptoms described in textbooks and are far more likely to present with vaginal bleeding or missed or incomplete miscarriage in the first trimester.
- The majority of complete hydatidiform moles will be suspected on ultrasound prior to histological diagnosis. Ultrasound has a lower sensitivity for the diagnosis of partial molar pregnancies, and they are often diagnosed as missed miscarriages.
- Suspected molar pregnancies should be managed surgically with suction aspiration, and all miscarriage products should be sent for histological diagnosis to exclude molar pregnancy.
- Upon diagnosis, all HMs should be referred to the national centre for central histopathological review and hCG follow-up.
- In the United Kingdom, if gestational trophoblastic neoplasia develops, 95 per cent will be low risk and have close to 100 per cent cure rates, and 5 per cent will be high risk and have 84 per cent cure rates.

Further Reading

1. Royal College of Obstetricians and Gynaecologists (February 2010). The management of gestational trophoblastic disease. *Green-Top Guideline* 38.

2. Seckl MJ, Sebire NJ, Berkowitz RS (2010).Gestational trophoblastic disease. *Lancet* 376: 717–729.

3. Ngan H, Kohorn E, Cole L, Kurman R, Kim S, Lurain J, Seckl M, Sasaki S, Soper J (2012). Figo Cancer Report. Trophoblastic disease. *International Journal of Gynecology and Obstetrics*: S130–S136.

4. Lurain J (2010). Gestational trophoblastic disease I: epidemiology, pathology, clinical presentation and diagnosis of gestational trophoblastic disease, and management of hydatidiform mole. *AJOG*. Dec: 531–539.

5. Parazzini F, LaVecchia C, Pampallona S (1986). Parental age and risk of complete and partial hydatidiform mole. *Br J Obstet Gynecol* 93: 582–585.

6. Sebire NJ, Foskett M, Fisher RA, et al. (2002). Risk of partial and complete molar pregnancy in relation to maternal age. *Br J Obstet Gynecol* 109: 99–102.

7. Sebire NJ, Fisher RA, Foskett M, Rees H, Seckl MJ, Newlands ES (2003). Risk of recurrent hydatidiform mole and subsequent pregnancy outcome following complete or partial hydatidiform molar pregnancy. *BJOG* 110: 22–26.

8. Sebire NJ, Jauniaux E (2012). Gestational trophoblastic disease: the role of ultrasound imaging. *Ultrasound Clin* 7: 33–45.

9. Fowler D, Lindsay I, Seckl M, Sebire N (2006). Routine pre-evacuation ultrasound diagnosis of hydatidiform mole: experience of more than 1000 cases from a regional referral centre. *Ultrasound Obstet Gynecol* 27(1): 56–60.

10. Johns J, Greenwold S, Buckley S, Jauniaux E (2005). A prospective study of ultrasound screening for molar pregnancies in missed miscarriages. *Ultrasound Obstet Gynecol* 25: 493–497.

11. Kirk E, Papageorghiou AT, Condous G, Bottomley C, Bourne T (2007). The accuracy of first trimester ultrasound in the diagnosis of hydatidiform mole. *Ultrasound Obstet Gyecol* 29: 70–75.

12. Royal College of Obstetricians and Gynaecologists (2011). *The Care of Women Requesting Induced Abortion. Evidence-based Clinical Guidance No 7.* London: RCOG.

13. Sebire NJ, Foskett M, Paradinas FJ, et al. (2002). Outcome of twin pregnancies with complete hydatidiform mole and healthy co-twin. *Lancet* 359: 2165–2166.

Pregnancy of Unknown Location

Shabnam Bodiwala and Tom Bourne

The term pregnancy of unknown location (PUL) describes the clinical scenario that arises when a woman has a positive urinary pregnancy test, but a pregnancy cannot be visualised on a transvaginal ultrasound scan (TVS).

Clinical Outcomes

It is important to emphasise that the term PUL is not a diagnosis and that all women need follow-up to determine a final clinical outcome. The final outcome in women classified as having a PUL is either *intrauterine pregnancy, failed PUL, ectopic pregnancy, or persistent PUL*:

- **Intrauterine pregnancy (IUP):** This includes women with a very early IUP, where an embryo or yolk sac is not visible on an initial scan and so was classified as a PUL. Between 30–40 per cent of women with a PUL are usually subsequently diagnosed with an IUP.
- **Failed PUL (FPUL):** This includes all women initially classified as a PUL with a probable complete miscarriage where an IUP had not been previously visualised using ultrasound *or* a failing pregnancy undergoing spontaneous resolution (this may be intrauterine or ectopic). In the region of 50–70 per cent of women with a PUL will be a failing PUL.
- **Ectopic pregnancy (EP):** This category includes all women initially classified as a PUL where the ectopic pregnancy was not visualised on the initial TVS. Evidence suggests that 6–20 per cent of women classified as having a PUL will subsequently be diagnosed with an ectopic pregnancy.
- **Persistent PUL (PPUL):** This is a PUL that is followed with serial serum hCG levels, but a pregnancy is not visualised on TVS and does not resolve spontaneously. Often, the hCG change over three consecutive tests (each 48 hours apart)

is < 15 per cent each time. This is likely to be an ectopic pregnancy that is never visualised on TVS.

The PUL rate can vary significantly depending on the unit in question and has been reported to be anywhere between 5 and 42 per cent. This rate is largely dependent upon the quality of ultrasound scanning within a unit. The more ectopic and intrauterine pregnancies that are definitively visualised on TVS, the lower the PUL rate. A designated early pregnancy unit equipped with specialists adequately trained in TVS should aim for a rate of < 15 per cent, as suggested by the International Society of Ultrasound in Obstetrics and Gynaecology.

The current management of PUL is based on stratifying women as being either at 'low risk' (IUP and FPUL) or 'high risk' of complications (EP or PPUL). See Figure 5.1. Women with low-risk PUL (IUP and FPUL) generally need minimal follow-up, whilst high-risk PUL (EP and PPUL) will need repeat hCG levels measured and further ultrasound scans until the final location and outcome of the pregnancy is known.

Presentation

Women usually present for assessment in early pregnancy with vaginal bleeding and/or pelvic pain. Other reasons include previous poor outcome (ectopic pregnancy/miscarriage/molar pregnancy), maternal anxiety, and hyperemesis gravidarum. It is important to note that with the advent of earlier scans being offered and women expecting their pregnancy to be visualised at earlier gestations, PUL is to an extent an iatrogenic phenomenon. The trade-off when performing ultrasonography at earlier gestations lies between increasing the PUL rate, with the result that women undergo unnecessary blood tests and follow-up, and missing the opportunity to manage ectopic pregnancies more conservatively because they were examined too late. There is evidence to suggest that, in asymptomatic

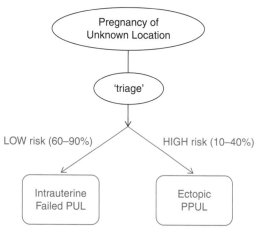

Figure 5.1 Low-versus high-risk triage of women with a PUL.

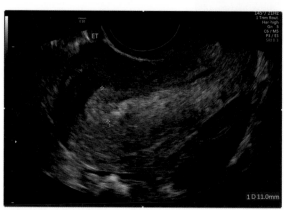

Figure 5.3 Transvaginal ultrasound image of a more thickened and heterogeneous endometrium.

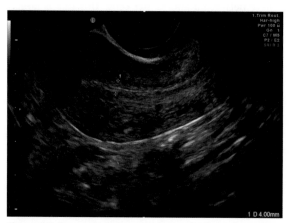

Figure 5.2 Transvaginal ultrasound image of a thin endometrium. The calipers are measuring the endometrial thickness.

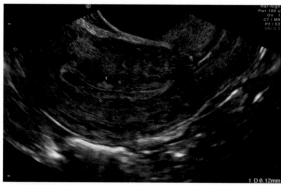

Figure 5.4 Transvaginal ultrasound image of a fluid in the endometrial cavity – often called a pseudosac. Note the presence of a previous Caesarean section scar that is also visible on this image.

women, the best time to perform a TVS whilst minimising the chances of morbidity and mortality associated with a ruptured ectopic pregnancy is at seven weeks (49 days).

Ultrasound Findings

TVS remains the gold standard investigation in early pregnancy. By definition, an intrauterine gestation sac cannot be visualised if the pregnancy has been classified as a PUL. There may be a thin endometrium similar to that seen in the nonpregnant state (Figure 5.2) or a more thickened and heterogenous appearance (Figure 5.3). However, endometrial thickness has not been found to be a useful predictor of PUL outcome when used in isolation, and it is contentious as to whether it has real clinical utility when used in logistic regression models with other variables.

The term *pseudosac* is an outdated term referring to a collection of fluid in the endometrial cavity (Figure 5.4). It tends to have a central location within the endometrial cavity (whereas an intrauterine gestation sac (IUGS) tends to be eccentrically placed). A pseudosac has also been described as having a 'pointy edge'. It does not have the usual hyperechoic decidual reaction around it, as seen with an IUGS (Figure 5.5). It may also be transient and change shape during scanning and/or when pressure is exerted. Note that an early intrauterine gestational sac may be easily confused with a pseudosac, and the presence of a hypoechoic area in the endometrial cavity is more likely to be an early intrauterine gestational sac rather than a marker of an ectopic pregnancy. In fact, in the absence of an adnexal mass, a fluid-filled structure within the uterus has a '0.02% probability of

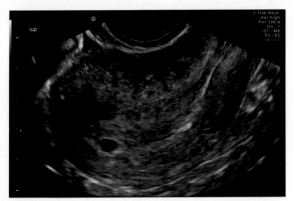

Figure 5.5 Transvaginal ultrasound image of an early intrauterine gestation sac. Note the hyperechogenic ring, and that neither a yolk sac or fetal pole is visible.

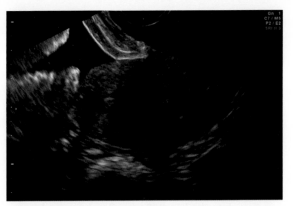

Figure 5.6 Blood in the pelvis. Note the blood that can be seen in the utero-vesical pouch, as well as the Pouch of Douglas.

ectopic pregnancy' (and 99.98 per cent probability of IUP) according to a study by Benson et al. *This must be remembered in order to avoid unnecessary intervention with methotrexate and inadvertent termination of an intrauterine pregnancy.*

Even when the pregnancy cannot be visualised, there may be other ultrasound findings that influence management. This includes the presence of blood in the pelvis, which may represent a ruptured ectopic pregnancy. There is no consensus on what is 'significant' blood on ultrasound, but it can be defined as when blood in the Pouch of Douglas (a potential space between the posterior part of the uterus and the rectum) tracks posteriorly all the way to the fundus of the uterus and/or blood is seen in the utero-vesical pouch. If blood is seen in Morison's pouch (a potential space separating the liver from the right kidney that is not filled with any fluid in normal conditions) on transabdominal ultrasound, this also indicates a worrying amount of blood loss. Blood usually has a typical 'ground glass' appearance, whilst clear fluid will have an anechoic (black) appearance. Note that the gain on the ultrasound machine must be adjusted appropriately to make this distinction. Figure 5.6 demonstrates the preceding findings.

Management

Clinical information has not been found to be diagnostically useful for predicting the final outcome of PUL, and diagnosis is largely based on serum biochemistry results. Measuring serum hCG and/or serum progesterone is the current mainstay of managing women with a PUL.

Serum Progesterone

A serum progesterone levels has been shown to be a good predictor of pregnancy viability. Some units use a serum progesterone level as a single-visit strategy. One such recognised protocol involves discharging women if their initial progesterone level is ≤ 10 nmol/l, with a urine pregnancy test in two weeks to confirm a negative result. In a study by Cordina et al., using this strategy allowed 37 per cent of PUL to be discharged with minimal follow-up. Of course, a drawback of such a study will be that some ectopic pregnancies are misclassified, and in this study five ectopic pregnancies (two needing surgical intervention) were inadvertently classified as low risk and discharged.

Serum hCG

Single measurements of serum hCG perform poorly as a predictor of PUL outcome, and management should be based on serial hCG measurements. The concept of the 'discriminatory zone' (that the PUL is less likely to be an ectopic pregnancy if the hCG is < 1,000 IU/L) is an outdated one and should not be relied upon in clinical practice. This is because the majority of ectopic pregnancies diagnosed in developed countries have serum hCG levels below 1,000 IU/L. Where single levels may be helpful is to flag cases that need senior review. If a woman is classified as a PUL with an initial hCG of over 1,000 IU/L, it is sensible to have the ultrasound findings checked, as most intrauterine pregnancies will be visualised at hCG values above this level, and so the possibility of an ectopic pregnancy that has been missed should be considered.

hCG Ratio

The hCG ratio (hCG at 48 hours/hCG at 0 hours) is a commonly used algorithm to manage PUL. If the hCG ratio is < 0.87, the final outcome is likely to be a failing PUL (low risk); if it is > 1.66, the final outcome is likely to be an ongoing IUP (low risk), and if the hCG ratio is ≥ 0.87 – ≤ 1.66, the final outcome is likely to be an ectopic pregnancy (high risk). See Figure 5.7.

Risk Prediction Models

The use of risk prediction models to help manage PUL was first described in 2004 by Condous et al., who developed the M4 model. The model was then validated on nearly 2,000 prospectively collected cases of

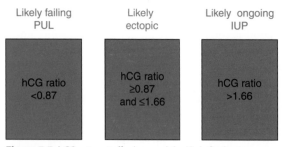

Figure 5.7 hCG ratio cutoff values and the likely final outcomes with a PUL.

PUL. The M4 model utilises the patients' initial hCG and the hCG ratio to assign risk (where high risk of an ectopic pregnancy is defined as being ≥ 5 per cent). It has been demonstrated to perform better than a single-visit strategy using serum progesterone levels and the hCG ratio.

A newer risk prediction model (the M6 model) utilises initial progesterone as well as the initial hCG and hCG ratio and has been developed on a much larger cohort of PUL. It has been found to be superior in performance to the M4 model and works as a two-step process; see Box 5.1.

It is important to state that the use of a model does not replace careful clinical assessment, and if there is any concern about the patient clinically, then management should be altered as deemed appropriate. Neither a normally rising or falling serum hCG excludes an ectopic pregnancy, and the patient must be counselled to seek medical advice if she experiences abdominal pain until an intrauterine pregnancy has been demonstrated on an ultrasound scan or the patient has a negative pregnancy test.

Persistent PUL

This is defined as a PUL that is followed with three successive 48-hour serum hCG levels that vary less than 15 per cent and where a pregnancy is never

Box 5.1: M6 Model to Predict PUL Outcome

Step 1: if the initial serum progesterone is ≤ 2 (irrespective of the initial hCG), a 48-hour blood test is not performed, as the final outcome is highly likely to be a failed PUL. The patient is advised to perform a urine pregnancy test in two weeks to confirm a negative result. If the result is positive, then the patient is asked to attend a follow-up serum hCG +/– transvaginal ultrasound.

Step 2: For all women with an initial progesterone of > 2, a 48-hour serum hCG level is performed, and the model assigns risk depending on the result. Two submodels have been created, as although step 1 can be used in women using progesterone supplementation, the initial progesterone level is likely to be artificially raised in this group of patients and would skew the results of a model that includes the serum progesterone level.

The two submodels use the following variables:

M6P model: uses the initial progesterone, initial hCG and the hCG ratio (for women *not* using progesterone supplementation).

M6NP model (NP = no progesterone): uses the initial hCG and the hCG ratio (for women using progesterone supplementation).

If the PUL is assigned as 'high risk', a repeat ultrasound scan and serum hCG level is recommended in 48 hours. If the risk prediction is 'low risk, likely failing PUL', a urine pregnancy test in two weeks is recommended, and if the prediction is 'low risk, likely intrauterine pregnancy', a repeat scan in one week is recommended. See Figure 5.8. The management of PUL can often be haphazard and prolonged; this model allows significant streamlining and rationalising of the care for women in this situation. To facilitate its use, the M6 model is available for clinical use at no charge at www.earlypregnancycare.org. It can also be downloaded as an app for smartphones (search 'early pregnancy Leuven').

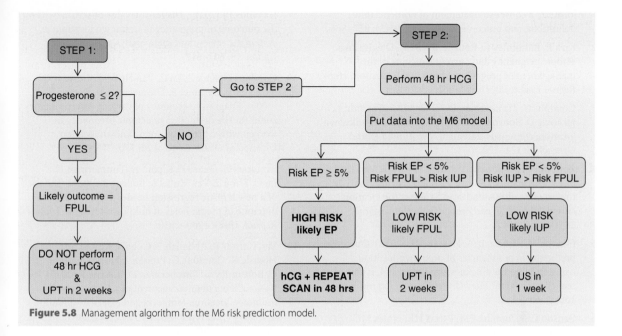

Figure 5.8 Management algorithm for the M6 risk prediction model.

visualised on TVS. This may represent a failed intra-uterine pregnancy or an ectopic pregnancy that has not been visualised. There is no data to support any one management option. This may involve expectant management, medical treatment with methotrexate or surgical management via uterine curettage/hysteroscopy.

In an international consensus document, Barnhart et al. described four possible outcomes in a patient with a persistent PUL:

- *Nonvisualised EP* (defined as a rising serum hCG level after uterine evacuation).
- *Treated persistent PUL* (defined as those who are treated medically [with methotrexate] without confirmation of the location of the gestation by TVS, laparoscopy, or uterine evacuation).
- *Resolved persistent PUL* (defined as resolution of serum hCG levels after expectant management or after uterine evacuation [without medical therapy] without evidence of chorionic villi on pathology).
- *Histological IUP* (defined as identification of chorionic villi in the contents of the uterine evacuation).

Summary and Learning Points

- The term PUL is an intermediate classification and not a final diagnosis.

- The concept of a 'discriminatory zone' may be useful in highlighting cases that require senior review but should not be used as cutoffs to rule in or out either an ectopic or an intrauterine pregnancy.
- The management of PUL can often be haphazard and lack an evidence base. There is therefore a clinical need to rationalise the management of PUL.
- Management is dictated by triaging women into either a low-risk or high-risk of complications group.
- Various management protocols exist to triage PUL, including the following:
  - Initial progesterone levels and a single-visit strategy for those with a progesterone of ≤ 10 nmol/l
  - hCG ratio (hCG at 48 hours/hCG at 0 hours)
  - Risk prediction models utilising hCG +/− progesterone levels

Further Reading

1. Barnhart K, van Mello NM, Bourne T, Kirk E, Van Calster B, Bottomley C, Chung K, Condous G, Goldstein S, Hajenius PJ, Mol BW, Molinaro T, KL O'Flynn O'Brien KL, Husicka R, Sammel M, Timmerman D (2011). Pregnancy of unknown

location: a consensus statement of nomenclature, definitions, and outcome. *Fertil Steril.* 95(3): 857–866.

2. Kirk E, Bottomley C, Bourne T (2014). Diagnosing ectopic pregnancy and current concepts in the management of pregnancy of unknown location. *Hum Reprod Update* 20(2): 250–261.

3. Condous G, Timmerman D, Goldstein S, Valentin L, Jurkovic D, Bourne T (2006). Pregnancies of unknown location: consensus statement. *Ultrasound Obstet Gynecol* 28: 121–122.

4. Bottomley C, Van Belle V, Mukri F, Kirk E, Van Huffel S, Timmerman D, Bourne T (2009). The optimal timing of an ultrasound scan to assess the location and viability of an early pregnancy. *Hum Reprod* 24(8): 1811–1817.

5. Ellaithy M, Abdelaziz A, Hassan MF (2013). Outcome prediction in pregnancies of unknown location using endometrial thickness measurement: is this of real clinical value? *Eur J Obstet Gynecol Reprod Biol.* 168(1): 68–74.

6. Benson CB, Doubilet PM, Peters HE, Frates MC (2013). Intrauterine fluid with ectopic pregnancy: a reappraisal. *Ultrasound Med* 32: 389–393.

7. Condous G, Van Calster B, Kirk E, Haider Z, Timmerman D, Van Huffel S, Bourne T (2007). Clinical information does not improve the performance of mathematical models in predicting the outcome of pregnancies of unknown location. *Fertil Steril.* 88: 572–580.

8. Cordina M, Schramm-Gajraj K, Ross JA, Lautman K, Jurkovic D (2011). Introduction of a single visit protocol in the management of selected patients with pregnancy of unknown location: a prospective study. *BJOG* 118(6): 693–697.

9. Van Mello N, Mol F, Opmeer BC, Ankum WM, Barnhart K, Coomarasamy A, Mol BW, van der Veen F,

Hajenius PJ (2012). Diagnostic value of serum hCG on the outcome of pregnancy of unknown location: a systematic review and meta-analysis. *Hum Reprod Update* 18: 603–617.

10. Condous G, Kirk E, Lu C, Van Huffel S, Gevaert O, De Moor B, De Smet F, Timmerman D, Bourne T (2005). Diagnostic accuracy of varying discriminatory zones for the prediction of ectopic pregnancy in women with a pregnancy of unknown location. *Ultrasound Obstet Gynecol* 26: 770–775.

11. Condous G, Okaro E, Khalid A, Timmerman D, Lu C, Zhou Y, Van Huffel S, Bourne T (2004). The use of a new logistic regression model for predicting the outcome of pregnancies of unknown location. *Hum Reprod.* 19(8): 1900–1910.

12. Van Calster B, Abdallah Y, Guha S, Kirk E, Van Hoorde K, Condous G, Preisler J, Hoo W, Stalder C, Bottomley C, Timmerman D, Bourne T (2013). Rationalizing the management of pregnancies of unknown location: temporal and external validation of a risk prediction model on 1962 pregnancies. *Hum Reprod.* 28(3): 609–616.

13. Guha S, Ayim F, Ludlow J, Sayasneh A, Condous G, Kirk E, Stalder C, Timmerman D, Bourne T, Van Calster B (2014). Triaging pregnancies of unknown location: the performance of protocols based on single serum progesterone or repeated serum hCG levels. *Hum Reprod.* 29(5): 938–945.

14. Van Calster B, Bobdiwala S, Guha S, Van Hoorde K, Al-Memar M, Harvey R, Farren J, Kirk E, Condous G, Sur S, Stalder C, Timmerman D, Bourne T (2016). Managing pregnancy of unknown location based on initial serum progesterone and serial serum hCG: development and validation of a two-step triage protocol. *Ultrasound Obstet Gynecol* [Epub ahead of print].

Tubal Ectopic Pregnancy

Emma Kirk

An ectopic pregnancy is any pregnancy implanted outside of the endometrial cavity. The most common site is the Fallopian tube. However, other sites include the cervix, ovary, Caesarean section scar, and abdomen (see Figure 6.1).

The incidence of ectopic pregnancy varies from 11–20 per 1,000 live births. Around 2–3 per cent of women attending early pregnancy units will be diagnosed with an ectopic pregnancy.

Risk Factors

The highest risk is associated with tubal damage following surgery or infection (especially *Chlamydia trachomatis*). Other risk factors include smoking, use of an intrauterine contraceptive device, in vitro fertilisation (IVF), and increased maternal age. However, the majority of women with an ectopic pregnancy have no identifiable risk factor.

Aetiology

The exact aetiology remains poorly defined, but with tubal ectopic pregnancies, it is likely to be a combination of impaired embryo-tubal transport and alterations in the tubal environment allowing early implantation.

Presentation

Amenorrhoea, pain, and vaginal bleeding are the classic triad of symptoms reported to occur with an ectopic pregnancy. There may also be a history of shoulder tip pain and syncope. However, now, history and physical examination alone rarely lead to a diagnosis or exclusion of an ectopic pregnancy.

It has been reported that up to one-third of women with an ectopic pregnancy have no clinical signs or symptoms, as they tend to present earlier in the course of the disease. The symptoms may also be very non-specific and difficult to differentiate from those of

other gynaecological, gastrointestinal, or urological disorders, including urinary tract infection, appendicitis, gastroenteritis, miscarriage, and ovarian cyst accident.

A diagnosis of ectopic pregnancy should be considered in all women of reproductive age who present with a history of sudden onset abdominal pain or gastrointestinal symptoms. This is especially the case if the woman is not aware she has a positive pregnancy test when she presents. Abdominal distension, tenderness, signs of peritonism, and hypovolaemic shock should raise the suspicion of a ruptured ectopic pregnancy.

Diagnosis of Ectopic Pregnancy

Ultrasound Diagnosis

Transvaginal ultrasound (TVS) is now accepted as the diagnostic tool of choice for ectopic pregnancy. The aim of TVS is to positively identify the ectopic pregnancy rather than just excluding the presence of an intrauterine pregnancy.

The majority of tubal ectopic pregnancies can be visualised on TVS prior to treatment. In the published literature, TVS has reported sensitivities of 87.0–99 per cent and specificities of 94.0–99.9 per cent for the diagnosis of tubal ectopic pregnancy. Most should be visualised on the initial TVS examination performed, but the remainder will be initially classified as a pregnancy of unknown location (PUL) and diagnosed on subsequent TVS examinations or at the time of surgery. In one study, almost 75 per cent of tubal ectopic pregnancies were visualised on the initial TVS performed and the remainder initially classified as PULs. Overall, > 90 per cent of the tubal ectopic pregnancies were visualised on TVS prior to treatment.

Sonographic criteria for the diagnosis of ectopic pregnancies have now been described (see Table 6.1).

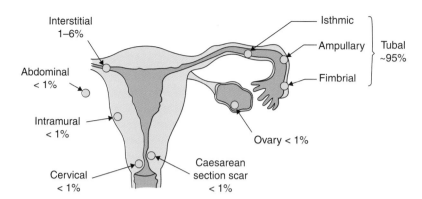

Figure 6.1 Sites for an ectopic pregnancy.

Further details of nontubal ectopic pregnancies are given in Chapter 7.

Inhomogeneous Mass

An inhomogeneous or noncystic adnexal mass that moves separate from the ovary is the most common finding in 50–60 per cent of cases of tubal ectopic pregnancy (see Figure 6.2). The mass is generally spherical and seen medial to the ovary, although it may have a more tubular appearance if bleeding creates a haematosalpinx. A consensus on nomenclature proposed that these inhomogeneous masses should be termed 'probable ectopic pregnancies' rather than 'definite ectopic pregnancies'. There is of course the risk that a false positive diagnosis of ectopic pregnancy is made, with the mass actually being, for example, a pedunculated or broad ligament fibroid or highly exophytic ovarian cyst. A more conservative approach is linked to the need for a very high level of diagnostic certainty in the event that medical management is being considered. Administration of methotrexate to a false positive diagnosis of ectopic pregnancy could potentially lead to inadvertent termination of an undetected intrauterine pregnancy (IUP) or severe abnormality in any surviving pregnancy.

Empty Gestational Sac or Gestational Sac with or without Yolk Sac or Fetal Pole

An empty gestational sac in the adnexal region will be visualised in around 20–40 per cent of cases of tubal ectopic pregnancy (see Figures 6.3, 6.4, 6.5). In another 15–20 per cent, this sac will contain either a yolk sac or fetal pole. There are reported cases of molar ectopic pregnancies and multiple gestation

ectopic pregnancies (see Figure 6.6). The term 'viable ectopic pregnancy' is applied when fetal heart pulsations is visualised.

There are also a number of nonspecific findings that may be indicative but not diagnostic of an ectopic pregnancy; see Table 6.2.

Endometrium

There is no specific endometrial appearance or thickness that supports a diagnosis of tubal ectopic pregnancy. Table 6.3 illustrates the variation in the appearance of the endometrial cavity in women diagnosed with a tubal ectopic pregnancy. In up to 20 per cent of cases, a collection of fluid may be seen within the endometrial cavity. This is classically referred to as a 'pseudosac'; see Chapter 5, page 33.

In addition to an ectopic pregnancy, there may be a coexistent IUP. This is referred to as a heterotopic pregnancy. A heterotopic pregnancy should be considered in all women presenting after IVF when more than one embryo has been transferred. It should also be considered in those women with an IUP who have persistent pain and in those with a persistently raised hCG after a miscarriage or termination of pregnancy. The incidence of heterotopic pregnancy in natural conceptions was originally estimated on a theoretical basis to be 1 in 30,000 pregnancies but in real life is likely to be more like 1 in 7,500.

Free Pelvic Fluid

A small amount of anechoic free pelvic fluid can be found in both intrauterine and extrauterine pregnancies and is often of no significance. The presence of echogenic fluid has been reported in up to about one-half of all tubal ectopic pregnancies and often signifies haemoperitoneum. Although this may be due to tubal

Table 6.1 Sonographic criteria for the diagnosis of ectopic pregnancies

Type of ectopic pregnancy	USS image	Diagram	Sonographic criteria	Additional information
Tubal				
Inhomogeneous mass			1. Empty uterine cavity 2. An inhomogeneous adnexal mass seen separate to the ovary	The most common finding in 50–60% of cases.
Empty gestational sac			1. Empty uterine cavity 2. An empty extrauterine gestation sac seen separate from the ovary	Present in around 20–40% of cases of tubal ectopic pregnancy.
Sac with yolk sac/fetal pole			1. Empty uterine cavity 2. A yolk sac or fetal pole ± cardiac activity in an extrauterine sac.	Seen in 15–20% of cases. The term 'viable ectopic' is often applied when fetal heart pulsations are visualised.
Interstitial			1. Empty uterine cavity 2. Products of conception/gestation sac located in the interstitial (intramyometrial) portion of the tube surrounded by a continuous rim of myometrium 3. Interstitial line sign (thin echogenic line extending from central uterine cavity echo to periphery of interstitial sac)	Use of 3D ultrasound to obtain a coronal view of the uterus can be useful. The added information given with this view means that a connection may be seen between the endometrial cavity and interstitial portion of the Fallopian tube.

(continued)

Table 6.1 (continued)

Type of ectopic pregnancy	USS image	Diagram	Sonographic criteria	Additional information
Cornual			1. A single interstitial portion of Fallopian tube in the main uterine body 2. Products of conception/gestation sac mobile and separate from the uterus surrounded by myometrium 3. No communication between the gestation sac and the unicornuate uterus cavity 4. Vascular pedicle joining the gestational sac to the unicornuate uterus.	Interstitial pregnancies are often referred to as cornual pregnancies. However, a true cornual pregnancy occurs when implantation occurs in the noncommunicating horn associated with a unicornuate uterus.
Cervical			1. Empty uterine cavity 2. Barrel-shaped cervix 3. Products of conception/gestation sac below the level of the internal cervical os 4. Negative sliding organ sign	The exact aetiology is unknown. One theory is that there is rapid transport of the fertilised ovum to the cervical canal before it is capable of nidation. Recognised predisposing factors include trauma to the cervical canal caused by previous surgical instrumentation, anatomical anomalies, IVF, and use of an intrauterine contraceptive device.
Caesarean section scar			1. Empty uterine cavity 2. Products of conception/gestation sac located anteriorly at the level of the internal os covering the presumed site of the previous lower segment Caesarean section scar 3. Negative sliding organ sign 4. Evidence of peritrophoblastic flow on colour Doppler examination	Results from implantation of a pregnancy within a lower uterine segment Caesarean section scar. They have been reported to occur in 1 in 1800–2200 pregnancies of all pregnancies and to comprise 6% of ectopic pregnancies in women with a previous Caesarean section. The obvious risk factor is a previous history of Caesarean section, but why implantation in the scar occurs in some women is poorly understood. Myomectomy, uterine curettage, manual removal of placenta, IVF, and adenomyosis have been identified as other possible risk factors.

Ovarian

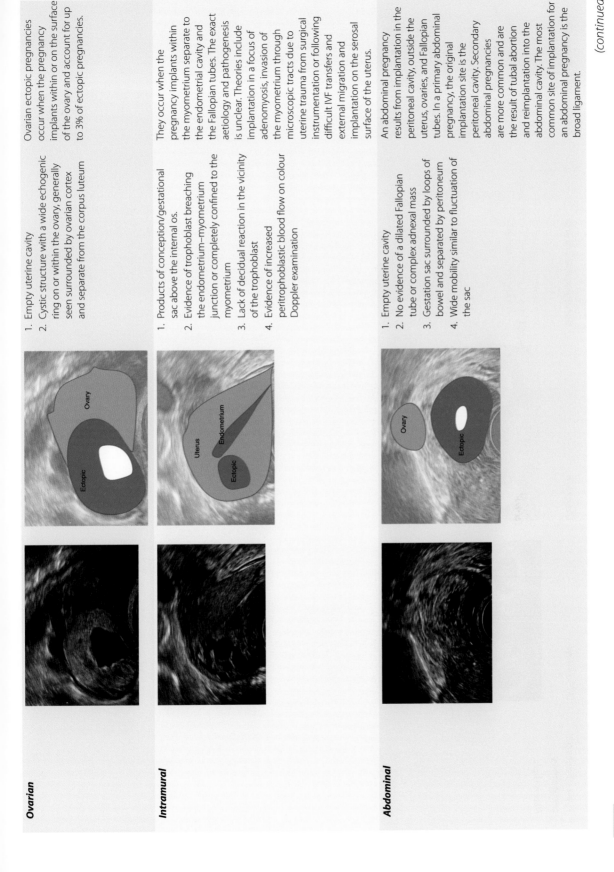

1. Empty uterine cavity
2. Cystic structure with a wide echogenic ring on or within the ovary, generally seen surrounded by ovarian cortex and separate from the corpus luteum

Ovarian ectopic pregnancies occur when the pregnancy implants within or on the surface of the ovary and account for up to 3% of ectopic pregnancies.

Intramural

1. Products of conception/gestational sac above the internal os.
2. Evidence of trophoblast breaching the endometrium–myometrium junction or completely confined to the myometrium
3. Lack of decidual reaction in the vicinity of the trophoblast
4. Evidence of increased peritrophoblastic blood flow on colour Doppler examination

They occur when the pregnancy implants within the myometrium separate to the endometrial cavity and the Fallopian tubes. The exact aetiology and pathogenesis is unclear. Theories include implantation in a focus of adenomyosis, invasion of the myometrium through microscopic tracts due to uterine trauma from surgical instrumentation or following difficult IVF transfers and external migration and implantation on the serosal surface of the uterus.

Abdominal

1. Empty uterine cavity
2. No evidence of a dilated Fallopian tube or complex adnexal mass
3. Gestation sac surrounded by loops of bowel and separated by peritoneum
4. Wide mobility similar to fluctuation of the sac

An abdominal pregnancy results from implantation in the peritoneal cavity, outside the uterus, ovaries, and Fallopian tubes. In a primary abdominal pregnancy, the original implantation site is the peritoneal cavity. Secondary abdominal pregnancies are more common and are the result of tubal abortion and reimplantation into the abdominal cavity. The most common site of implantation for an abdominal pregnancy is the broad ligament.

(continued)

Table 6.1 (continued)

Type of ectopic pregnancy	USS image	Diagram	Sonographic criteria	Additional information
Heterotopic	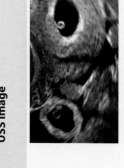		1. Intrauterine pregnancy and 2. Any of the previously mentioned ectopic pregnancies	A heterotopic pregnancy occurs when any of the previously mentioned forms of ectopic pregnancy is found simultaneously with an intrauterine pregnancy. The incidence of heterotopic pregnancy in natural conceptions was originally estimated on a theoretical basis to be 1 in 30,000 pregnancies but in real life is likely to be more like 1 in 7,500. The incidence is thought to be 1 to 3 in 100 pregnancies if conception is due to assisted reproductive techniques The risk increases in proportion to the number of embryos transferred with IVF.

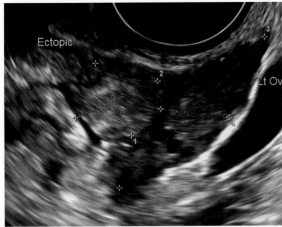

Figure 6.2 Image of a tubal ectopic pregnancy showing an inhomogeneous mass.

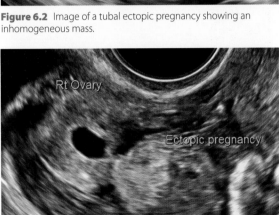

Figure 6.3 Image of a tubal ectopic pregnancy showing an empty gestational sac in the adnexa.

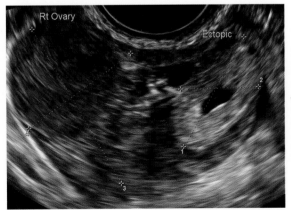

Figure 6.4 Image of a tubal ectopic pregnancy sharing an embryo generated sac.

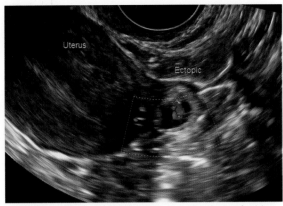

Figure 6.5 Image of a tubal ectopic Doppler sharing fetal heart pulsations

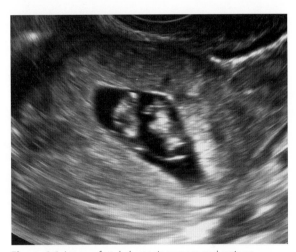

Figure 6.6 Image of a tubal ectopic pregnancy showing a gestational sac with two fetal poles (monochorionic diamniotic twin ectopic).

rupture, it may be more commonly due to leakage of blood from the fimbrial end of the tube. The amount of fluid is thought to be significant if it reaches above the fundus of the uterus or is visualised in Morison's Pouch. This is the space between the kidney and the liver in the right-upper quadrant of the abdomen. This simple examination performed using an abdominal probe forms part of the Focussed Assessment by Sonography for Trauma (FAST) scan used in emergency departments.

Biochemical Investigations

No biochemical investigations by themselves should be used to make a diagnosis of tubal ectopic pregnancy.

Table 6.2 Nonspecific findings that may be indicative of an ectopic pregnancy

USS finding	USS images	Description	Additional information
Echogenic free fluid		• Echogenic fluid may signify haemoperitoneum secondary to tubal rupture or tubal miscarriage. • The amount is thought to be significant if it reaches above the level of the fundus of the uterus or if it is present in Morison's Pouch.	Other nonectopic causes of haemoperitoneum include a ruptured haemorrhagic ovarian cyst.
Fluid within the endometrial cavity		• This is a collection of fluid within the endometrial cavity. • It is usually possible to distinguish if from an early intrauterine gestational sac, which is seen as an eccentrically placed hyperechoic ring within the endometrial cavity.	This is often referred to as a 'pseudosac'. It has been reported to be present in up to 20% of cases of ectopic pregnancy. The presence of a collection of fluid within the endometrial cavity alone, however, should not be used solely to diagnose an ectopic pregnancy.

Table 6.3 Endometrial appearances in women with a tubal ectopic pregnancy (all images taken from real cases where a tubal ectopic pregnancy was also visualised on the same TVS examination)

Appearance	Description
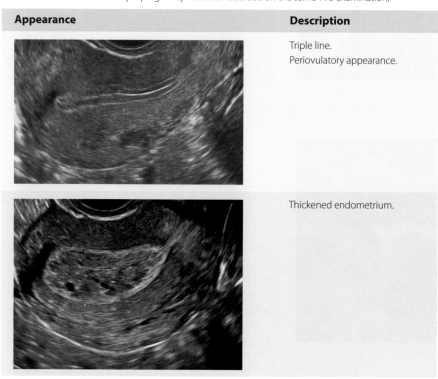	Triple line. Periovulatory appearance. Thickened endometrium.

Table 6.3 (continued)

Appearance	Description
	Thin endometrium.
	Disrupted endometrium.
	Collection of fluid in the endometrial cavity.
	Coexistent intrauterine pregnancy.
	Intrauterine contraceptive device (IUCD) in place within the endometrial cavity.

Table 6.4 Factors helping decide on most appropriate management of a tubal ectopic pregnancy

	Expectant management	Medical management	Surgical management
Patient	• Haemodynamically stable • Pain-free • Willingness to attend for follow-up	• Haemodynamically stable • Pain-free • Willingness to attend for follow-up • No contraindication to methotrexate	• Haemodynamicallly unstable • Pain
Ultrasound Findings	• No fetal cardiac activity	• No fetal cardiac activity • Certainty that there is no intrauterine pregnancy	• Haemoperitoneum • Fetal cardiac activity • Large ectopic mass (> 3.5 cm)
Serum Biochemistry	• hCG ideally < 1,500 IU/L • Decreasing hCG levels	• hCG ideally < 1,500 IU/L but up to 5,000 IU/L • Rising hCG levels	• hCG > 5,000 IU/L • Rising hCG levels

However, as discussed in Chapter 5, serum hCG and progesterone levels can be used to help predict ectopic pregnancy in women classified with a pregnancy of unknown location (PUL).

A serum hCG level is useful in planning the management of an ultrasound visualised tubal ectopic pregnancy. An hCG level of > 3,000–5,000 IU/L is usually an indication for surgical management. At lower levels of hCG, expectant or medical management may be appropriate. However, the hCG level alone cannot be used to plan the most suitable treatment; the ultrasound appearance of the ectopic pregnancy should also be taken into consideration (see Table 6.4).

Surgical Diagnosis

Laparoscopy with histological confirmation was previously regarded as the gold standard for diagnosis of tubal ectopic pregnancy. Most surgical procedures now for tubal ectopic pregnancies are carried out as a therapeutic procedure after the ectopic pregnancy has been diagnosed on TVS. Diagnostic surgery is generally reserved for women presenting with signs of an acute abdomen and hypovolaemic shock. A surgical diagnosis may also be made in women with a PUL who become symptomatic.

Laparoscopy has been quoted has having a ~ 5 per cent false negative and ~ 5 per cent false positive rate. Given this, the high positive predictive values for TVS and the now widespread use of conservative management strategies for tubal ectopic pregnancies, laparoscopy is now no longer considered the gold standard.

Learning Points

- The majority of ectopic pregnancies should be visualised on TVS prior to treatment.

- Diagnosis should be based on positive visualisation of an ectopic pregnancy rather than the inability to visualise an intrauterine pregnancy.
- Specific sonographic criteria now exist for all types of ectopic pregnancies.

Further Reading

1. Elson CJ, Salim R, Potdar N, Chetty M, Ross JA, Kirk EJ on behalf of the Royal College of Obstetricians and Gynaecologists (2016). Diagnosis and management of ectopic pregnancy. *BJOG* 123: e15–e55.

2. Bouyer J, Coste J, Shojaei T, Pouly JL, Fernandez H, Gerbaud L, Job-Spira N (2003). Risk factors for ectopic pregnancy: a comprehensive analysis based on a large case-control, population-based study in France. *Am J Epidemiol.* 157: 185–194.

3. NICE (December 2012). Ectopic pregnancy and miscarriage: diagnosis and initial management in early pregnancy of ectopic pregnancy and miscarriage. NICE Clinical Guideline 154.

4. Kirk E, Bottomley C, Bourne T (2014). Diagnosing ectopic pregnancy and current concepts in the management of pregnancy of unknown location. *Hum Reprod Update* 20(2): 250–261.

5. Confidential Enquiry into Maternal Deaths in the United Kingdom (CMACE) (2011). *The Eighth Report of the Confidential Enquiries into Maternal Deaths in the United Kingdom.* CMACE 118.

6. Benson CB, Doubilet PM, Peters HE, Frates MC (2013). Intrauterine fluid with ectopic pregnancy: a reappraisal. *J Ultrasound Med.* 32: 389–393.

7. Condous G, Okaro E, Khalid A, Lu C, Van Huffel S, Timmerman D, Bourne T (2005). The accuracy of transvaginal sonography for the diagnosis of ectopic pregnancy prior to surgery. *Hum Reprod* 20: 1404–1409.

8. Kirk E, Papageorghiou AT, Condous G, Tan L, Bora S, Bourne T (2007). The diagnostic effectiveness of an initial transvaginal scan in detecting ectopic pregnancy. *Hum Reprod* 22: 2824–2828.

9. Brown DL, Doubilet PM (1994). Transvaginal sonography for diagnosing ectopic pregnancy: positivity criteria and performance characteristics. *J Ultrasound Med* 13: 259–266.

10. Kirk E, Daemen A, Papageorghiou AT, Bottomley C, Condous G, De Moor B, Timmerman D, Bourne T (2008). Why are some ectopic pregnancies characterized as pregnancies of unknown location at the initial transvaginal ultrasound examination? *Acta Obstet Gynecol Scand.* 87: 1150–1154.

11. Elson J, Tailor A, Banerjee S, Salim R, Hillaby K, Jurkovic D (2004). Expectant management of tubal ectopic pregnancy: prediction of successful outcome using decision tree analysis. *Ultrasound Obstet Gynecol* 23: 552–556.

12. Lipscomb GH, Mc Cord ML, Stovall TG, Huff G, Portera SG, Ling F (1999). Predictors of success of methotrexate treatment in women with ectopic pregnancies. *N Engl J Med* 341: 1974–1978.

13. RCOG (2016). Diagnosis and management of ectopic pregnancy. *Green-Top Guideline No. 21.*

Chapter

7

Nontubal Ectopic Pregnancy

Dimitrios Mavrelos and Davor Jurkovic

Nontubal ectopic pregnancies are relatively rare and account for less than 5 per cent of the total number of pregnancies, which are partially or completely located outside the uterine cavity (see Figure 6.1). They are often difficult to differentiate from pregnancies that are located normally within the uterine cavity. Their rarity and variable location add further to diagnostic difficulties.

Nontubal ectopic pregnancies can be divided into two broad categories: those that are partially or completely confined to the uterus, which include interstitial, cervical, Caesarean scar and intramural pregnancies; and those that are located within the peritoneal cavity, which include ovarian and abdominal pregnancies.

Intersitial, Cornual, Cervical, Caesarean Scar, and Intramural Pregnancies

Interstitial Ectopic

Interstitial pregnancy represents a subset of tubal ectopic pregnancies where implantation has occurred in the proximal part of the Fallopian tube as it travels through the myometrium. As a consequence of their location, interstitial ectopics are associated with relatively high mortality since the myometrial mantle supports more advanced development of the pregnancy before rupture occurs and rupture is associated with more rapid blood loss. Risk factors for interstitial pregnancy include ipsilateral salpingectomy, previous ectopic pregnancy, and in vitro fertilisation (IVF). The surgical management of an interstitial ectopic pregnancy is different from that of a more distal Fallopian tube ectopic and may require more advanced laparoscopic skill. It is thus critical that practitioners of early pregnancy ultrasound are aware of the diagnostic criteria for an interstitial ectopic and are able

to differentiate this from a tubal pregnancy. The term 'cornual pregnancy' should be restricted for pregnancy in a functional rudimentary cornu of a unicornuate uterus to avoid errors in communication.

Diagnosis of Interstitial Ectopic Pregnancy

The ultrasound diagnostic criteria for an interstitial ectopic pregnancy (Figure 6.2) are the following:

1. Empty uterine cavity
2. Gestational sac in the lateral aspect of the uterine fundus surrounded by myometrium
3. A thin interstitial line adjoining the gestational sac and the endometrial cavity

The main differential diagnoses of an interstitial ectopic pregnancy include an intrauterine pregnancy (IUP) implanted high and lateral in the endometrial cavity (previously known as 'angular pregnancy'), an IUP in a uterus with a congenital uterine anomaly such as a bicornuate or septate uterus or a proximal tubal ectopic pregnancy located in the isthmic part of the tube. The first step in making the diagnosis is identification of an empty uterus. The uterus should be scanned in the transverse plane in order to follow the endometrium up to the uppermost lateral aspect to the internal tubal ostia (Figure 7.1). If an interstitial pregnancy exists, following the interstitial portion of the tube in this way will lead to visualisation of a gestational sac, which will be covered by myometrium and is connected to endometrial cavity by a thin echogenic line, the 'interstitial line' (Figure 7.2). Visualisation of the 'interstitial line' connecting the pregnancy with the endometrial cavity excludes an IUP in a congenitally anomalous uterus or a pregnancy implanted high and laterally but still in the endometrial cavity. In both of these instances, the connection between pregnancy and endometrial cavity will be much wider than the 'interstitial line'. If a three-dimensional (3D) ultrasound is available, a coronal plane view of the uterus can increase diagnostic

(a) (b)

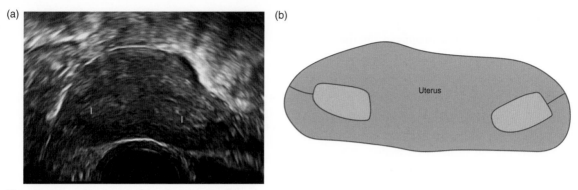

Figure 7.1 Interstitial portion of tube in transverse plane.

(a) (b)

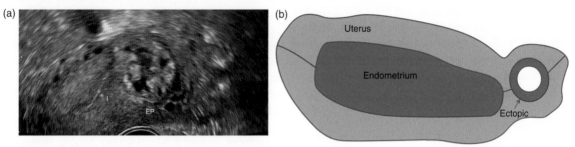

Figure 7.2 Interstitial ectopic demonstrating two-dimensional (2D) interstitial line.

(b)

(a)

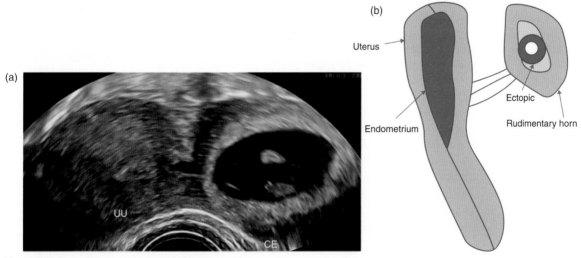

Figure 7.3 Cornual pregnancy surrounded by myometrium.

confidence (Figure 7.3). Once the diagnosis is made, it is useful, from a surgical perspective, to describe the relative proximity of the gestational sac to the endometrial cavity; the more distal the pregnancy, the likelier it is that a loop can be passed around it and excision performed. More proximal pregnancies will require more dissection to remove the pregnancy and suturing of the myometrial incision in a fashion similar to a myomectomy. As the tube is effectively occluded by the sutures, we advocate removal of the distal part of the Fallopian tube as well to prevent ipsilateral tubal ectopics in the future.

Cornual Pregnancy

A cornual pregnancy is a pregnancy in the non-communicating functional rudimentary horn of a unicornuate uterus. A unicornuate uterus with a non-communicating rudimentary horn represents around 4 per cent of anomalous uteri. A functional noncommunicating horn contains endometrium and has an attached Fallopian tube. Over half of the women with this anomaly present with severe dysmenorrhea due to retrograde menstruation from the blind ending horn. The rest, however, remain asymptomatic and may present with a pregnancy in the noncommunicating horn, a cornual pregnancy. Undiagnosed cornual pregnancies can advance well into the second trimester and present with abdominal pain on average at 21 weeks. Rupture at such advanced gestation can be catastrophic, with severe intra-abdominal bleeding. The majority of cornual pregnancies are currently diagnosed at rupture even though diagnostic criteria to make this diagnosis early in the first trimester have been formulated.

Diagnosis of Cornual Pregnancy

The uterus is scanned in the transverse plane to identify both the interstitial portions of the Fallopian tubes, as outlined in the preceding. The first clue for the diagnosis of a unicornuate uterus is the finding of a single interstitial portion of Fallopian tube. Suspicious practitioners will then examine the adnexae to identify a rudimentary horn. This is often found lateral to the unicornuate uterus but medial to the ovary and has the echotexture similar to myometrium. Once the rudimentary horn is found, it can be established whether it contains a functional cavity with endometrium and thus whether a cornual pregnancy is present. The diagnostic criteria are as follows:

1. Unicornuate uterus with a single interstitial portion of Fallopian tube
2. A gestational sac surrounded by a myometrial mantle
3. No communication between the gestational sac and the unicornuate uterus cavity
4. A vascular pedicle feeding into the noncommunicating functional rudimentary horn

The main differential diagnoses are an interstitial pregnancy and an IUP in an anomalous uterus, such as a bicornuate uterus. It is of course critical that the differentiation is made, as the first requires a different surgical approach and the second is potentially viable IUP. The differential centres on the connection between gestational sac. As outlined in the preceding, an interstitial pregnancy will have a thin, narrow, echogenic line connecting the gestational sac with the endometrial cavity, representing the proximal Fallopian tube (Figure 7.2). In contrast, a cornual pregnancy will be completely surrounded by myometrium (Figure 7.3), while an IUP in an anomalous uterus will have a wide connection between gestational sac and endometrial cavity.

Cervical Pregnancy

The cervix contains relatively little contractile tissue compared to the myometrium, so implantation here can have serious consequences when a pregnancy is terminated and the cervix is unable to stem bleeding. Early diagnosis of a cervical pregnancy allows early and effective treatment as opposed to later diagnosis, when a hysterectomy may become necessary due to intractable haemorrhage. The internal cervical os is identified by TVS as the point of insertion of the uterine arteries. To find this level when scanning, the cervical canal is visualised in the transverse plane and then scanned slowly cranially. The uterine arteries are seen as prominent vessels in the lateral aspect of the uterus entering the myometrium. Doppler examination can help to identify this vascularity clearly. Implantation of a pregnancy below this level represents a cervical pregnancy. A cervical pregnancy becomes likelier if there has been previous instrumentation of the cervix, a previous Caesarean section or the pregnancy is achieved following in vitro fertilisation and embryo transfer.

Diagnosis of Cervical Pregnancy

The diagnosis of cervical pregnancy centres on demonstrating a gestational sac or trophoblastic tissue in the cervical canal and differentiating between ongoing pregnancy and the cervical phase of a miscarriage. There are important differences that can help practitioners make the correct diagnosis; in a miscarriage, the internal cervical os is open, the gestational sac has become irregular and there is no heartbeat. In contrast, a spherical gestational sac in the cervical canal with a closed internal cervical os is strongly suggestive of a cervical pregnancy, and if a viable embryo is seen within the sac, the diagnosis is confirmed (Figure 7.4). It may be, however, that the pregnancy is too early to contain an embryo, while the internal cervical os can only be established by approximation as described previously. To improve diagnostic confidence, patience and the 'sliding organ sign' can be employed. A pregnancy that has reached the cervical stage of a miscarriage will have become detached from its original implantation point in contrast to an ongoing cervical pregnancy. Thus patient observation of the gestational sac or trophoblast under examination will reveal whether the tissue is moving within the canal, in which case a miscarriage is more likely. Moreover, gentle palpation with the probe in a miscarriage will demonstrate sliding of the sac on the cervical canal surface, the 'sliding organ sign'. In contrast, a cervical pregnancy remains implanted and thus will not slide but move in concert with surrounding cervical tissue. In an ongoing cervical pregnancy, Doppler examination can be used to demonstrate vessels crossing from the cervix into the trophoblastic tissue of the gestational sac, which will be absent in a miscarriage. In a more advanced pregnancy, the cervical canal expands and the internal cervical os remains closed, giving an hourglass appearance that is typical of a cervical ectopic pregnancy. Later in pregnancy, the uterine fundus is pushed superiorly and thus harder to identify by TVS. In these circumstances, a transabdominal scan can be performed to gain additional more information.

Caesarean Scar

A lower segment Caesarean section involves a transverse incision on the uterus posterior to the bladder usually just above the level of the internal cervical os. In some women, particularly those with a retroverted uterus, the Caesarean scan can become deficient, which is visualised on TVS as a hypoechoic discontinuity of the anterior uterine wall and cervix bulging towards the bladder (Figure 7.5). It is possible for a pregnancy to implant within the scar, which if undiagnosed or untreated may then develop later in pregnancy into a morbidly adherent placenta with

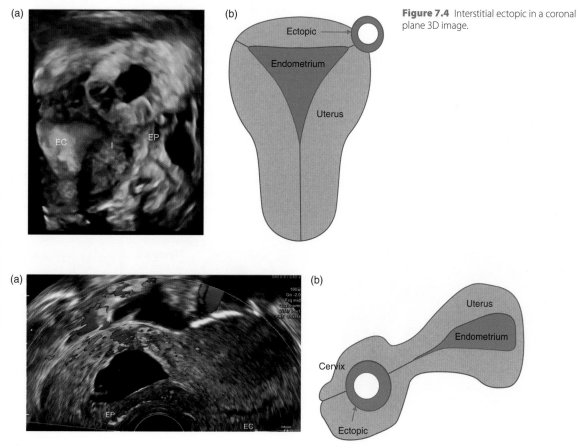

Figure 7.4 Interstitial ectopic in a coronal plane 3D image.

Figure 7.5 Cervical pregnancy with spherical gestational sac below the internal cervical os.

attendant risks to mother and baby. As expected, multiple previous Caesarean sections increase the likelihood of a deficient scar, which in turn increases the likelihood of a Caesarean scar pregnancy and abnormal implantation.

Diagnosis of Caesarean Scar Ectopic Pregnancy

The diagnosis of Caesarean scar ectopic pregnancy shares some features with cervical ectopic pregnancy previously described. Again, the main differential is the cervical phase of a miscarriage. On TVS, the aim is to demonstrate a pregnancy implanted at the level of the internal cervical os covering the Caesarean section scar. Similar to when suspecting a cervical ectopic, gentle pressure can be applied with the probe to explore whether the pregnancy slides over the surface of the Caesarean section scar or whether it moves in concert with surrounding tissues, the 'sliding organ sign'. Doppler examination can be used to identify peritrophoblastic blood vessels crossing into the pregnancy from the scar, which will be absent in a detached sac in the process of miscarrying (Figure 7.6). Jurkovic et al. suggested the following criteria for the diagnosis of Caesarean section scar ectopic:

1. Empty uterine cavity
2. Gestational sac located at the level of the internal os covering the visible or presumed site of the previous lower uterine segment Caesarean section scar
3. Evidence of functional trophoblastic/placental circulation on Doppler examination
4. Negative sliding organs sign, that is, inability to displace the gestational sac from its position with gentle pressure by the transvaginal probe

Figure 7.7 shows a USS image of a pregnancy implanted in a Caesarean section scar. Once the diagnosis is made, operators should try to establish the relationship between gestational sac and the bladder as well as herniation into the broad ligament, as this information can inform subsequent surgical management.

Intramural Pregnancy

Only a few case reports exist in the literature of intramural pregnancy. This is a pregnancy that has become enveloped by the myometrium beneath the endometrial–myometrial junction. Previous uterine surgery such as myomectomy or adenomyosis may predispose to this abnormal implantation by creating access to the myometrium and an environment that allows myometrial implantation and pregnancy growth.

Diagnosis

Recently the ultrasound diagnostic criteria for the diagnosis of intramural pregnancy have been formulated, as follows (see Figure 7.8):

1. Gestational sac/products of conception above the internal os
2. Evidence of trophoblast breaching the endometrium–myometrium junction or completely confined to the myometrium
3. Lack of decidual reaction in the vicinity of the trophoblast
4. Evidence of increased peritrophoblastic blood flow on colour Doppler examination

The differential diagnosis includes invasive gestational trophoblastic disease, which can also present with foci of trophoblastic tissue invading deep into

(a)

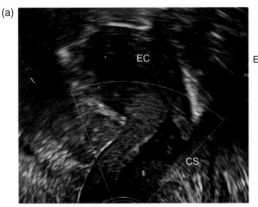

(b)

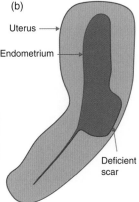

Uterus

Endometrium

Deficient scar

Figure 7.6 Deficient Caesarean scar on 2D transvaginal ultrasound.

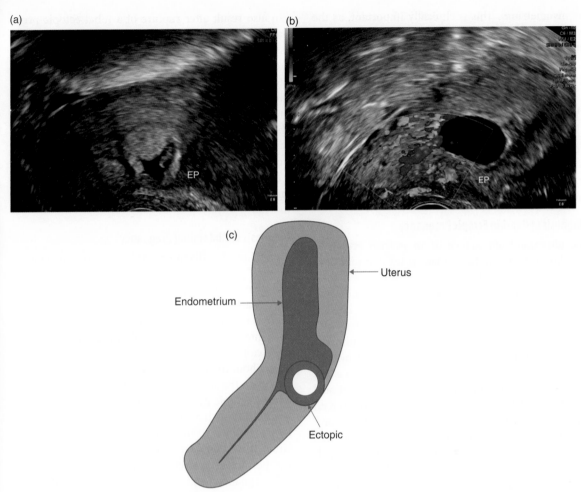

Figure 7.7 Pregnancy implanted into deficient Caesarean section scar with Doppler.

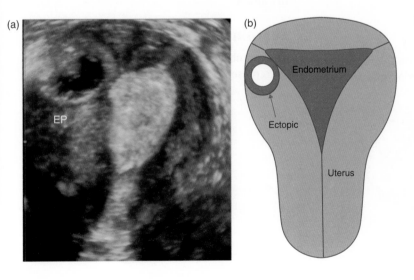

Figure 7.8 Myometrial pregnancy.

the myometrium. This is clinically important, as the trophoblastic disease requires referral to a dedicated oncology unit.

Ovarian and Abdominal Pregnancies

Ovarian Ectopic

It is possible for a pregnancy to implant on the surface of the ovary, giving rise to the rare diagnosis of ovarian ectopic. Pregnancy after assisted conception or conception with a contraceptive coil in situ make this type of ectopic pregnancy more likely.

Diagnosis of Ovarian Ectopic Pregnancy

The ultrasound appearance of an ovarian ectopic is an echogenic ring in the ovarian cortex that may have circumferential blood flow on Doppler examination (Figure 7.9). As such, it is not easy to differentiate an ovarian ectopic pregnancy from a corpus luteum, although the visualisation of two structures with appearances similar to a cystic corpus luteum within the ovary should always give rise to suspicion of an ovarian ectopic. It has been suggested that corpus luteum is less echogenic than the trophoblastic tissue of a gestational sac. If the gestational sac contains a yolk sac or even an embryo, then the diagnosis is more straightforward. The main differential diagnosis of an ovarian ectopic is a tubal ectopic pregnancy that is fixed to the ovary by pelvic adhesions. The sliding organ sign can be employed to attempt to make this differentiation; an ovarian ectopic will move in concert with the ovary on pressure with the ultrasound probe, while a tubal ectopic can be shown to slide on the ovary on pressure.

Abdominal Ectopic Pregnancy

A pregnancy can implant directly on the surfaces and organs in the abdominal cavity. Abdominal pregnancy can also result after rupture of a tubal ectopic pregnancy and subsequent reimplantation. The commonest sites for abdominal ectopic pregnancy implantation are the pouches around the uterus (Pouch of Douglas/uterovesical pouch), broad ligament, and the serosal surfaces of the uterus and tubes. More advanced pregnancies can involve the omentum and bowel. An abdominal pregnancy is the rarest form of nontubal ectopic pregnancy, and as a consequence most practitioners may not come across this diagnosis more than a few times in their career. Nevertheless, it is important to be aware of this entity, as it carries significant mortality.

Diagnosis of Abdominal Pregnancy

Achieving the diagnosis of abdominal pregnancy in early gestation is often difficult. An empty uterus will give rise to suspicion of ectopic pregnancy, and if a gestational sac is then seen in an unusual location such as the Pouch of Douglas or vesicouterine pouch, with intact Fallopian tubes and ovaries, then the diagnosis can be made (Figure 7.10). In one published case of an abdominal pregnancy diagnosed at eight weeks' gestation, the authors were able to differentiate it from a tubal ectopic by identifying that the gestational sac was in the Pouch of Douglas and surrounded by bowel loops. Doppler examination can be used to demonstrate the trophoblast induced vascularisation from the peritoneal surface. In more advanced abdominal pregnancy (> 20 weeks' gestation), the diagnosis centres on identification of an empty uterus, abnormal fetal lie, oligohydramnios, and poor placental definition.

Learning Points

- Nontubal ectopic pregnancies are rare and represent < 5 per cent of all ectopic pregnancies.

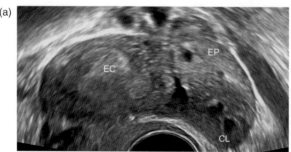 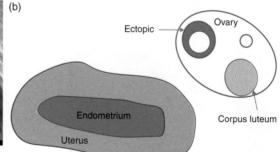

Figure 7.9 Ovarian ectopic pregnancy.

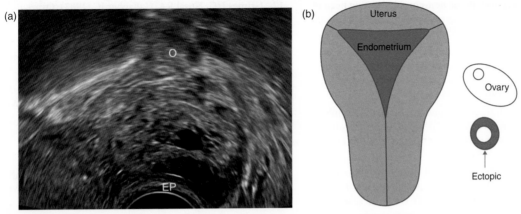

Figure 7.10 Abdominal pregnancy in the Pouch of Douglas.

Table 7.1 Summary table of ultrasonic criteria for the diagnosis of nontubal ectopic pregnancy

		Empty endometrial cavity	Myometrial mantle	Connection with endometrial cavity	Internal cervical os
Uterine					
	Interstitial	√	√	Thin	N/A
	Cornual	√	√	None	N/A
	Cervical	√	√	None	below
	Intramural	√	√	None	above
	Caesarean scar	√	√	Cervical canal	at level of
Nonuterine					
	Ovarian	√	X	X	N/A
	Abdominal	√	X	X	N/A

- The first step in achieving the diagnosis is common in all ectopic pregnancies: the identification of an empty uterus.
- Examiners must then carefully examine all potential sites of ectopic pregnancy, including the entire Fallopian tube from interstitium to fimbriae, the ovaries, the uterus, cervix and Caesarean scar as well as the Pouch of Douglas and vesicouterine pouch.
- There are now recognised sonographic criteria for all nontubal ectopic pregnancies; see Table 7.1.

Further Reading

1. Mavrelos D, Sawyer E, Helmy S, Holland TK, Ben-Nagi J, Jurkovic D (2007). Ultrasound diagnosis of ectopic pregnancy in the non-communicating horn of a unicornuate uterus (cornual pregnancy). *Ultrasound Obstet Gynecol* 30(5): 765–770.

2. Sagiv R, Debby A, Keidar R, Kerner R, Golan A (2013). Interstitial pregnancy management and subsequent pregnancy outcome. *Acta Obstet Gynecol Scand* 92(11): 1327–1330.

3. Jurkovic D, Mavrelos D (2007). Catch me if you scan: ultrasound diagnosis of ectopic pregnancy. *Ultrasound in Obstetrics & Gynecology: The Official Journal of the International Society of Ultrasound in Obstetrics and Gynecology* 30(1): 1–7.

4. Ackerman TE, Levi CS, Dashefsky SM, Holt SC, Lindsay DJ (1993). Interstitial line: sonographic finding in interstitial (cornual) ectopic pregnancy. *Radiology* 189(1): 83–87.

5. Stiller RJ, de Regt RH (1991). Prenatal diagnosis of angular pregnancy. *JCU* 19(6): 374–376.

6. Mavrelos D, Sawyer E, Helmy S, Holland TK, Ben-Nagi J, Jurkovic D (2007). Ultrasound diagnosis of

ectopic pregnancy in the non-communicating horn of a unicornuate uterus (cornual pregnancy). *Ultrasound Obstet Gynecol* 30(5): 765–770.

7. Jurkovic D, Hacket E, Campbell S (1996). Diagnosis and treatment of early cervical pregnancy: a review and a report of two cases treated conservatively. *Ultrasound Obstet Gynecol* 8(6): 373–380.

8. Timor-Tritsch IE, Monteagudo A, Santos R, Tsymbal T, Pineda G, Arslan AA (2012). The diagnosis, treatment, and follow-up of cesarean scar pregnancy. *Am J Obstet Gynecol* 207(1): 44 e41–13.

9. Timor-Tritsch IE, Monteagudo A, Cali G, Palacios-Jaraquemada JM, Maymon R, Arslan AA, Patil N, Popiolek D, Mittal KR (2014). Cesarean scar pregnancy and early placenta accreta share common histology. *Ultrasound Obstet Gynecol* 43(4): 383–395.

10. Jurkovic D, Hillaby K, Woelfer B, Lawrence A, Salim R, Elson CJ (2003). First-trimester diagnosis and management of pregnancies implanted into the lower uterine segment Cesarean section scar. *Ultrasound in Obstet Gynecol* 21(3): 220–227.

11. Memtsa M, Jamil A, Sebire N, Jauniaux E, Jurkovic D (2013). Diagnosis and management of intramural ectopic pregnancy. *Ultrasound in Obstet Gynecol* 42(3): 359–362.

12. Grimes HG, Nosal RA, Gallagher JC (1983). Ovarian pregnancy: a series of 24 cases. *Obstetrics and Gynecology* 61(2): 174–180.

13. Joseph RJ, Irvine LM (2012). Ovarian ectopic pregnancy: Aetiology, diagnosis, and challenges in surgical management. *Journal of Obstetrics & Gynaecology* 32(5): 472–474.

14. Comstock C, Huston K, Lee W (2005). The ultrasonographic appearance of ovarian ectopic pregnancies. *Obstetrics and Gynecology* 105(1): 42–45.

15. Poole A, Haas D, Magann EF (2012). Early abdominal ectopic pregnancies: a systematic review of the literature. *Gynecol Obstet Invest* 74(4): 249–260.

16. Sandro G, Dario R, Gabriela B, Graziano C, Vittorio U, Gian Carlo Di R (2004). Early ultrasonographic diagnosis and laparoscopic treatment of abdominal pregnancy. *European Journal of Obstetrics & Gynecology and Reproductive Biology* 113(1): 103–105.

17. Varma R, Mascarenhas L, James D (2003). Successful outcome of advanced abdominal pregnancy with exclusive omental insertion. *Ultrasound in Obstet Gynecol* 21(2): 192–194.

The Adnexa and Other Pathology

Wouter Froyman and Dirk Timmerman

With the introduction of routine obstetric ultrasound examination, adnexal masses are increasingly being incidentally detected during pregnancy. The incidence of adnexal pathology diagnosed in the first trimester varies from 0.2 to 6 per cent. The overall incidence of malignancy in adnexal masses identified in pregnancy ranges from 1 to 8 per cent. In general, adnexal tumours can be accurately classified using transvaginal ultrasound (TVS). Different algorithms exist to differentiate between benign and malignant tumours or to stratify the risk of malignancy, using elements such as the tumour size, morphology, and the presence of colour Doppler flow.

As the majority of cysts (up to 72 per cent) detected at the time of a first-trimester ultrasound examination spontaneously resolve and therefore are considered to be physiological in nature, expectant management is advocated. Characteristics favourable for spontaneous regression include simple morphology on ultrasound, size less than 5–6 cm in diameter and diagnosis before 16 weeks of gestation. Larger masses or those with a more complex morphology are less likely to resolve spontaneously and may represent a neoplastic process.

The risk of ovarian torsion decreases as the gestational age increases. In the literature, rates of 1–3 per cent are reported. When they are symptomatic, simple cysts diagnosed during pregnancy can be successfully and safely treated with ultrasound-guided cyst aspiration. However, in the few cases where the nature of the cyst is uncertain, the risks to the pregnancy from surgical intervention must be weighed against the risk of malignancy.

During pregnancy, the same ovarian masses can be found as in the nonpregnant population. Additionally, a number of pregnancy-associated masses may occur (see the section 'Nonneoplastic Ovarian Lesions' later in this chapter). When a patient presents with a symptomatic adnexal mass in early pregnancy, first an ectopic pregnancy (and the rarely occurring heterotopic pregnancy) must always be ruled out (see Chapters 6 and 7).

Benign Adnexal Lesions

Non-neoplastic Ovarian Lesions

As described previously, functional ovarian cysts represent the largest group of lesions detected during pregnancy.

Follicular cysts/simple cysts have their origin in anovulatory follicles (Figure 8.1). They are unilocular and thin-walled with anechoic contents. They rarely exceed 8–10 cm in diameter and typically resolve spontaneously within six weeks.

Corpus luteum cysts are formed following ovulation (Figure 8.2). They are thick-and hyperechoic-walled cysts that often show circumferential blood flow, sometimes described as the 'ring of fire'. The cyst contents typically have a spider-web-like appearance due to internal haemorrhage, but may frequently show different features including blood clots within the cyst, resembling solid components. In these cases, Doppler examination (a clot will have no blood flow) and 'pushing' the lesion with the probe (a clot will have typical jellylike movement) can be used to help in differentiating between clots and solid parts. During pregnancy, these cysts usually resolve after the first 14–16 weeks of gestation.

Luteomas are rare solid ovarian tumours that occur exclusively in pregnancy (Figure 8.3). They are generally asymptomatic and are often found incidentally. Maternal hirsutism or virilisation has been seen in approximately 30–35 per cent of reported cases of pregnancy luteoma. Approximately 75 per cent of female infants born to virilised mothers with luteomas are virilised, whereas in the absence of maternal virilisation, fetuses are not virilised. On ultrasound examination, luteomas appear as unilateral or bilateral (almost half of cases) heterogeneous solid masses,

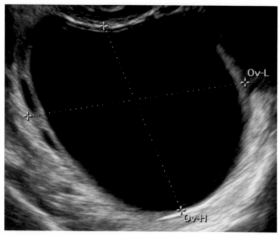

Figure 8.1 Simple cyst. Unilocular and thin-walled appearance, anechoic content.

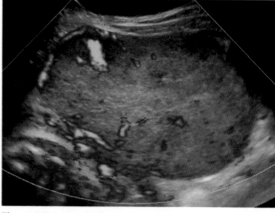

Figure 8.3 Luteoma of pregnancy. Heterogeneous solid mass, often highly vascularised.
Image is courtesy of Professor Lil Valentin.

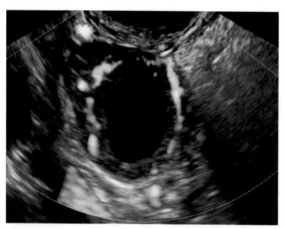

Figure 8.2 Corpus luteum gravidarum. Thick- and hyperechoic-walled cyst, circumferential blood flow ('ring of fire').

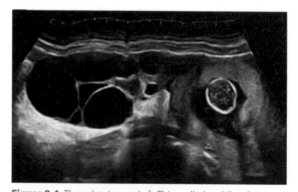

Figure 8.4 Theca-lutein cyst. Left: Thin-walled multilocular cyst with anechoic content ('spoke wheel' appearance).
Right: Intrauterine pregnancy.
Image originally published in Van Holsbeke C, Amant F, Veldman J, De Boodt A, Moerman P, Timmerman D (2009). Hyperreactio luteinalis in a spontaneously conceived singleton pregnancy. *Ultrasound Obstet Gynecol* 33: 371–373.
Reproduced with permission from John Wiley and Sons

predominantly hypoechoic compared with the surrounding normal ovarian tissue. They are often highly vascularised, mimicking ovarian neoplasms. However, they spontaneously regress when the pregnancy has ended.

Theca-lutein cysts (Figure 8.4) are seen in cases of hyperreactio luteinalis (due to very high endogenous or exogenous β-hCG stimulation, as in multiple pregnancies, gestational trophoblastic disease and fertility treatment). Depending on the size of the masses, patients are either asymptomatic or they present with pain due to intra-abdominal pressure, torsion or intracystic haemorrhage. Virilisation due to hyperandrogenism can occur in as many as 25 per cent of affected patients. These lesions usually present as

bilateral thin-walled multilocular cysts with anechoic content ('spoke wheel' appearance). Ascites may be present. Most theca-lutein cysts spontaneously regress later in pregnancy or after delivery.

Benign Ovarian Neoplasms

Mature teratomas/dermoid cysts are the most common nonfunctional ovarian masses in premenopausal women (Figure 8.5). They mostly have a unilocular cystic appearance with mixed echogenicity, due to different tissue components such as fat, bone, hair and fluid. Acoustic shadowing is typical and often prevents the cyst from being completely visualised ('tip of the

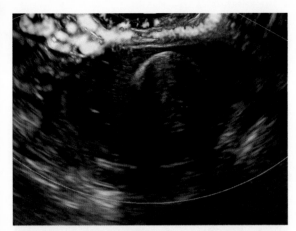

Figure 8.5 Dermoid. Unilocular cystic appearance with mixed echogenicity, hyperechoic tissues packed together into a Rokitansky nodule. Minimal vascularisation.

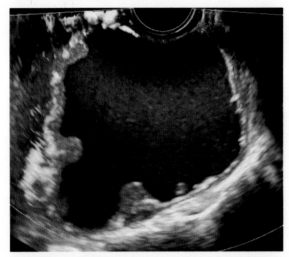

Figure 8.7 Decidualisation. Appearance of rounded vascularised papillary projections with smooth contours.

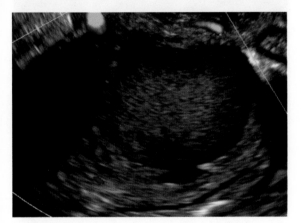

Figure 8.6 Endometrioma. Unilocular tumour, low-level echogenic content ('ground glass') and limited vascularity.

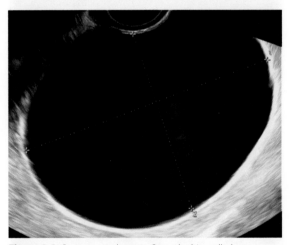

Figure 8.8 Serous cystadenoma. Smooth, thin walled, anechoic cyst.

iceberg' phenomenon). Different hyperechoic tissues often pack together into a Rokitansky nodule, and the presence of hair, is often seen as multiple stripy hyperechoic interfaces ('dermoid mesh'). In general, vascularity is minimal.

Endometriomas are typically unilocular tumours with a low-level echogenic content representing old blood ('ground glass' appearance) and limited vascularity (Figure 8.6). However, atypical features may be present. Debris within the cyst may give the impression of solid components.

Due to high progesterone levels, these lesions may undergo decidualisation during pregnancy (Figure 8.7). The appearance of vascularised papillary projections with smooth contours is common. When no preexisting scan of the ovary is documented,

these features can raise the suspicion of malignancy. However, as seen in follow-up scans after pregnancy, these features resolve spontaneously. When the diagnosis remains uncertain, further investigation is advised to rule out a malignant neoplasm. Patients with endometriomas are mostly asymptomatic during pregnancy.

Cystadenomas count for half of all benign adnexal epithelial neoplasms.

Serous cystadenomas appear as smooth, thinwalled, anechoic cysts (Figure 8.8). They are bilateral in 15 per cent of cases, and their mean size is limited to 5–8 cm. They may be unilocular or multilocular with thin septa.

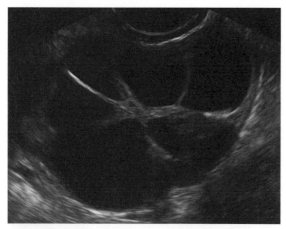

Figure 8.9 Mucinous cystadenoma. Large, thin-walled cysts, multilocular with low-level echogenic fluid.

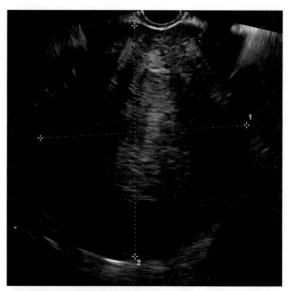

Figure 8.11 Fibroma. Round solid tumors with regular lining. Stripy or fan-shaped acoustic shadows.

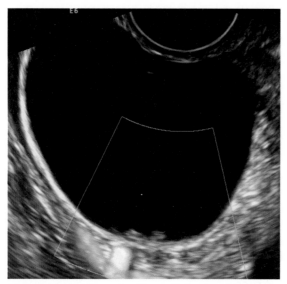

Figure 8.10 Serous cystadenofibroma. Unilocular-solid cyst with thin walls and anechoic content. Presence of subtle acoustic shadows behind the papillary projections. Low vascularity.

Mucinous cystadenomas are classically thin-walled, large, and unilateral (Figure 8.9). Typically they consist of several up to innumerable internal locules filled with low-level echogenic fluid.

Cystadenomas are not hormonally sensitive and usually contain limited vascularisation.

Cystadenofibromas are relatively rare and may be serous or mucinous (Figure 8.10). They appear as unilocular-solid or, less frequently, as multilocular-solid masses with thin walls and anechoic or low-level echogenic content. The solid component is often a papillary projection. A typical characteristic is the presence of subtle acoustic shadows behind the papillary projections. Vascularity is low to moderate.

Ovarian fibromas and fibrothecomas are rare and present as round or oval solid tumours, with regular lining (Figure 8.11). Vascularity is peripheral and limited. Stripy or fan-shaped acoustic shadows may be seen.

Benign Nonovarian Lesions

Normal Fallopian tubes are rarely visible during an ultrasound examination. A *hydrosalpinx* (chronic salpingitis) appears as a tubular thin-walled mass, with anechoic content, incomplete septae, and typical 'beads-on-a-string' sign, due to 2–3-mm-sized hyperechoic structures on the tubal wall (seen on a transverse section) (Figure 8.12). They generally do not change in size or appearance throughout pregnancy and seldom cause symptoms. Acute pelvic inflammatory disease is not often seen during pregnancy.

Paraovarian cysts originate in the broad ligament between the ovary and the Fallopian tube and appear as thin-walled unilocular anechoic cysts close to, but separable from, the ovary (Figure 8.13). Their mean diameter is usually < 5 cm and they show minimal vascularity. They have no clinical significance.

Malignant Adnexal Masses

Malignant neoplasms during pregnancy are uncommon but they do occur.

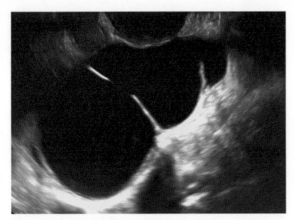

Figure 8.12 Hydrosalpinx. Tubular thin-walled mass, anechoic content, incomplete septa.

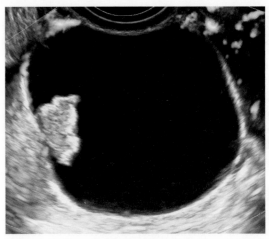

Figure 8.14 Serous borderline tumour. Unilocular-solid tumour with papillary projection and high vascularisation.

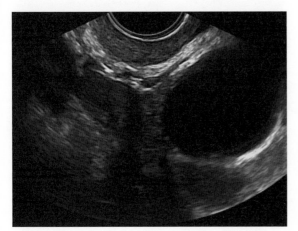

Figure 8.13 Paraovarian cyst. Thin-walled unilocular anechoic cyst (right) close to but separable from the ovary (left).

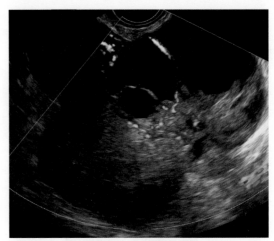

Figure 8.15 Primary invasive ovarian cancer. Irregular multilocular-solid tumour with moderate vascularisation.

Most frequently reported are the nonepithelial tumours (germ cell and sex cord-stromal tumours) followed by ovarian tumours of low malignant potential (LMP, e.g., borderline tumours) and epithelial ovarian cancers. The presence of more complex morphology (multilocularity, wall irregularities, papillary projections, and other solid components) and high vascularisation on Doppler ultrasound are features suspicious for malignancy. The presence of ascites, peritoneal implants, or an omental cake indicates advanced-stage disease. Of all malignant tumours of the ovary, 10 per cent are metastases from other organs, mainly gastrointestinal or breast tumours. These are usually solid and bilateral. Figures 8.14 through 8.16 show examples of these malignant neoplasms.

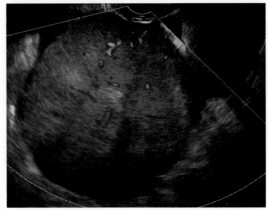

Figure 8.16 Metastatic ovarian cancer. Solid tumour with moderate vascularisation.

Other Pelvic Pathology in Pregnancy

Peritoneal Pseudocysts

Peritoneal pseudocysts are collections of peritoneal fluid surrounded by adhesions. They usually appear as multilocular cysts, with multiple complete and thin septa, which generally move upon pushing ('flapping sail sign'). They have sharp angles and their contour follows the lining of the pelvic wall or adjacent organs. The majority of cases are asymptomatic.

Fibroids

Fibroids or *leiomyomas* are the most common solid masses in pregnancy. They are seen on ultrasound in 1.4–2 per cent of pregnancies. They appear as round masses (whorled) with variable echogenicity (isoechoic or hypoechoic) and peripheral vascularisation. Although it is often easy to recognise that there are fibroids present, it is their location that is the most important in determining the clinical significance. It is important to state whether a fibroid is within the myometrium or wall of the uterus (intramural), on the outside surface of the uterus (subserosal) or projecting into the cavity of the uterus (submucosal); see Table 8.1. The presence of acoustic shadowing is common, which is more prominent in cases of calcifications. These lesions can enlarge during pregnancy and cause focal pain. When the fibroid outgrows its blood supply, it may undergo

Table 8.1 Classification of uterine fibroids

Type	Example USS image	Schematic diagram example	Details
Subserous			These project from the outside surface (serosa) of the uterus. They only usually cause a problem if extremely large. Some may be on a thin stalk and are entirely extrauterine. These are classified as pedunculated and are at risk of torsion. Sometimes they may be mistaken for an ovarian mass or an ectopic pregnancy.
Intramural			These are predominantly within the wall of the uterus or myometrium. They rarely cause a significant problem unless > 5 cm.
Submucosal			These are within the cavity of the uterus. They protrude into the endometrial cavity to varying degrees.
Type 0			These project entirely within the cavity like a polyp.

Table 8.1 (continued)

Type	Example USS image	Schematic diagram example	Details
Type 1			The majority is within the cavity, with < 50% in the myometrium.
Type 2			> 50% is within the surrounding myometrium.

'red degeneration', which results in a complex morphology with cystic areas.

Appendicitis

Appendicitis is the most common cause of right iliac fossa pain and the most common cause of nonobstetric surgery during pregnancy, accounting for 25 per cent of cases. The incidence of appendicitis is similar in pregnancy compared to the nonpregnant population, ranging between 1 in 1,400 and 1 in 1,500 births. The clinical presentation can be misleading, for instance if the appendix is at an unusual site, such as retro-caecal (15 per cent of cases) or behind a gravid uterus.

With TVS, graded pressure can be applied with the probe to move normal loops of bowel out of the way. An inflamed appendix is identifiable as a noncompressible tubular, blind-ending structure with an individual wall thickness of greater than 3 mm or greater than 6 mm if its two walls are measured together with an empty lumen. In a transverse section, the inflamed appendix appears as a double concentric ring, called the 'target sign' (Figure 8.17).

Pelvic Kidney

A pelvic kidney (congenital pelvic *renal ectopia*) occurs when the metanephros (embryonic secretory organ) retains its original pelvic position rather than

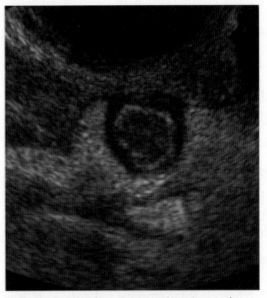

Figure 8.17 Appendicitis. Transvaginal visualisation of appendicitis. In a transverse section, the inflamed appendix appears as a double concentric ring, called the 'target sign'. Image is courtesy of Professor Lil Valentin.

ascending to its mature location (in the retroperitoneum just caudal to the diaphragm). It has an estimated incidence of 1:900. Though often clinically asymptomatic, it is an important differential diagnosis in the aetiology of pelvic masses and pain, as

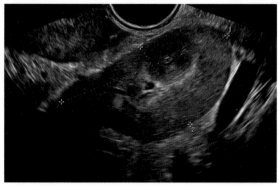

Figure 8.18 Pelvic kidney. Transvaginal visualisation of pelvic kidney. Rounded or elliptical shape with the characteristic central echogenic interface of the renal pelvis.

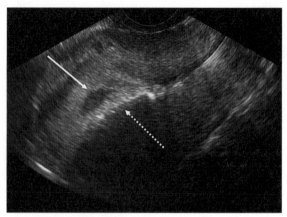

Figure 8.19 Pregnancy with IUD. Full arrow marks the presence of an intrauterine gestational sac, and the dashed arrow marks the presence of IUD.

like horseshoe kidneys, pelvic kidneys are associated with malrotation and predisposed to dilatation and stasis (which may lead to calculus formation and infection) as well as traumatic injury. An attempt should be made to look for other congenital urogenital anomalies. Kidneys may also be encountered in a pelvic position after renal transplantation. On ultrasound, a pelvic kidney can often be seen as a rounded or elliptical shape with the characteristic central echogenic interface of the renal pelvis (Figure 8.18).

Intrauterine Contraceptive Devices (IUDs) and Nonsurgical Sterilisation Devices

Levenorgestrel (LNG)-Releasing IUD and Copper IUD

IUDs are gaining popularity as a reversible form of contraception. Using two-dimensional ultrasound, the stem of the IUD is easily identified as a linear echogenic structure. While the arms of the copper IUD are also fully echogenic, the arms of the LNG IUD are only echogenic at the proximal and distal ends, with characteristic central posterior acoustic shadowing on transverse images.

Although the IUD is a highly effective form of birth control, complications, including pregnancy, do occur. The strong local effect of the IUD on the endometrium accounts for its good contraceptive efficacy against intrauterine pregnancies. Therefore, in the rare cases of a pregnancy during the use of an IUD, it is very likely to be ectopic. The respective ectopic pregnancy rates range from 0.02–0.2 in LNG IUD users and from 0.1–0.8 in copper IUD users.

In the unlikely event that pregnancy occurs, it is more common to occur within the first year after the placement of the IUD, presumably secondary to the higher incidence of displacement or expulsion of the IUD during that time period (Figure 8.19). More than half of IUDs identified in early pregnancy are malpositioned.

Intrauterine pregnancies with an IUD in situ are at increased risk for first- and second-trimester miscarriage, including septic abortion and preterm delivery if the IUD is left in place. Miscarriage rates up to 50 per cent are observed if the IUD is left in situ. Removing the IUD reduces these risks without completely neutralising them, as the miscarriage rate after the IUD extraction is quoted to be approximately 25 per cent. The World Health Organisation and U.S. Food and Drug Administration recommend that if the IUD is seen and the strings are visible or can be retrieved from the cervical os with the diagnosis of an intrauterine pregnancy, then the IUD should be removed by gently pulling on the strings.

While some studies report on fetal malformations, data are insufficient to draw conclusions on any association between conceiving with an IUD in situ and risk of malformations.

In conclusion, timely evaluation of the pregnant woman with an IUD is important to exclude the presence of an ectopic pregnancy and to reduce subsequent complications if the woman chooses to continue her pregnancy.

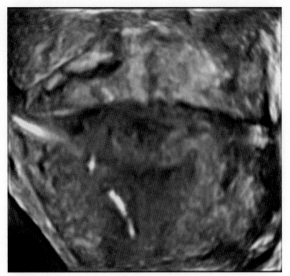

Figure 8.20 Three-dimensional view of Essure device in the right tube with intrauterine, intramural, and proximal isthmic tubal portion. Deficient positioning in the left tube.

Hysteroscopic Sterilisation Devices

Hysteroscopic tubal sterilisation is a well-tolerated ambulatory procedure that can avoid the risks of general anaesthesia and is less invasive than laparoscopic sterilisation. Hysteroscopic sterilisation devices such as the Essure System (Bayer) are placed transcervically, with hysteroscopic guidance, into the proximal portion of each Fallopian tube across the uterotubal junction, where they induce fibrosis and tubal occlusion.

Two-dimensional and three-dimensional ultrasound allows visualisation of the micro-insert, as a coil with an intrauterine, intramural, and proximal isthmic tubal portion in case of optimal placement (Figure 8.20). Some studies have shown very good effectiveness, including a five-year follow-up study that showed no pregnancies among 449 women with bilateral placement who relied on the Essure inserts for contraception. However, these trials are challenged because of concerns about incomplete follow-up and biased results. There are no data available about pregnancy outcome after hysteroscopic sterilisation.

Learning Points

- About 0.2–6 per cent of women will have some sort of adnexal pathology diagnosed in early pregnancy.
- The majority of ovarian cysts diagnosed are functional and will spontaneously resolve.
- Features favourable for regression include size < 5–6 cm, a simple appearance, and diagnosis before 16 weeks of gestation.
- Up to 2 per cent of pregnant women will have uterine fibroids.

Further Reading

1. Hoover K, Jenkins TR (2011). Evaluation and management of adnexal mass in pregnancy. *Am J Obstet Gynecol* 205: 97–102.

2. Kaijser J, Bourne T, Valentin L, Sayasneh A, Van Holsbeke C, Vergote I, et al. (2013). Improving strategies for diagnosing ovarian cancer: a summary of the International Ovarian Tumor Analysis (IOTA) studies. *Ultrasound Obstet Gynecol* 41: 9–20.

3. Condous G, Khalid A, Okaro E, Bourne T (2004). Should we be examining ovaries during pregnancy? Prevalence and natural history of adnexal pathology detected at first trimester sonography. *Ultrasound Obstet Gynecol* 24: 62–66.

4. Sayasneh A, Ekechi C, Ferrara L, Kaijser J, Stalder C, Sur S et al. (2015). The characteristic ultrasound features of specific types of ovarian pathology (review). *Int J Oncol* 46(2): 445–458.

5. Chiang G, Levine D (2004). Imaging of adnexal masses in pregnancy. *J Ultrasound Med* 23: 805–819.

6. Van Holsbeke C, Amant F, Veldman J, De Boodt A, Moerman P, Timmerman D (2009). Hyperreactio luteinalis in a spontaneously conceived singleton pregnancy. *Ultrasound Obstet Gynecol* 33: 371–373.

7. Mascilini F, Moruzzi C, Giansiracusa C, Guastafierro F, Savelli L, De Meis L et al. (2014). Imaging of gynecological disease: clinical and ultrasound characteristics of decidualized endometriomas surgically removed during pregnancy. *Ultrasound Obstet Gynecol* 44: 354–360.

8. Paladini D, Testa A, Van Holsbeke C, Mancari R, Timmerman D, Valentin L (2009). Imaging in gynecological disease (5): clinical and ultrasound characteristics in fibroma and fibrothecoma of the ovary. *Ultrasound Obstet Gynecol* 34: 188–195.

9. De Haan J, Verheecke M, Amant F (2015). Management of ovarian cysts and cancer in pregnancy. *Facts Views Vis Obgyn* 7(1): 25–31.

10. Testa A, Ferrandina G, Timmerman D, Savelli L, Ludovisi M, Van Holsbeke C et al. (2007). Imaging in gynecological disease (1): ultrasound features of metastases in the ovaries differ depending on the origin of the primary tumor. *Ultrasound Obstet Gynecol* 29: 505–511.

11. Abbasi N, Patanaude V, Abenhaim HA (2014). Management and outcomes of acute appendicitis in

pregnancy-population-based study of over 7000 cases. *BJOG* 121(12): 1509–1514.

12. Haider Z, Condous G, Ahmed S, Kirk E, Bourne T (2006). Transvaginal sonographic diagnosis of appendicitis in acute pelvic pain. *J Ultrasound Med* 25: 1243–1244.

13. Singer A, Simmons MZ, Maldjian PD (2008). Spectrum of congenital renal anomalies presenting in adulthood. *Clin Imaging* 32(3): 183–191.

14. Nowitzki KM, Hoimes ML, Chen B, Zheng LZ, Kim YH (2015). Ultrasonography of intrauterine devices. *Ultrasonography* 34(3): 183–194.

15. Moschos E, Twickler DM (2011). Intrauterine devices in early pregnancy: findings on ultrasound and clinical outcomes. *Am J Obstet Gynecol* 204: 427.e1–6.

16. Brahmi D, Steenland MW, Renner R-M, Gaffield ME, Curtis KM (2012). Pregnancy outcomes with an IUD in situ: a systematic review. *Contraception* 85: 131–139.

17. Legendre G, Levaillant JM, Faivre E, Deffieux X, Gervaise A, Fernandez H (2011). 3D ultrasound to assess the position of tubal sterilization microinserts. *Hum Reprod* 26: 2683–2689.

Uterine Anomalies and Early Pregnancy

Matthew Prior and Nick Raine-Fenning

Congenital uterine anomalies arise from an abnormality in the embryological development process. This is due to defects of unification (failure of structures to come together or fuse), canalisation (failure of a canal to develop within a structure), or complete agenesis (complete failure of development).

Failure of normal development results in a spectrum of anomalies from a mild convex indentation of the uterine fundus (arcuate uterus) to a complete failure of development or fusion resulting in a unicornuate uterus or uterus didelphys.

Types of Anomaly

Multiple systems have been proposed to classify uterine anomalies, the most widely adopted of these is the American Fertility Society classification, shown in Figure 9.1.

This simple system aids clinicians when discussing uterine anomalies. Nonetheless, there are several criticisms: it cannot categorise multiple anomalies (e.g., a bicornuate septate uterus); and there is no morphometric diagnostic criteria, therefore it is possible for clinicians to assign the same anomaly to a different category. Newer systems have been proposed to address these limitations, including adding morphometric criteria, or the entirely new European Society of Human Reproduction and Embryology (ESHRE)–European Society for Gynaecological Endoscopy (ESGE) classification system. However, the use of these classifications is not yet widespread due to their complexity. An ideal system would be simple, have good inter-rater reliability, and provide prognostic value, but this is yet to be developed. Table 9.1 summarises the most common types of uterine anomalies.

Prevalence

Uterine anomalies are more common in women who experience miscarriage compared with the general population (13 per cent versus 5 per cent). However, due to different populations being studied, diagnostic tests and classification systems used, the true prevalence remains uncertain.

Effect on Pregnancy

Women with uterine anomalies are at higher risk of infertility, early and second-trimester miscarriage, preterm birth, and malpresentation at delivery.

Given the inconsistency in the diagnosis and categorisation of uterine anomalies, the precise impact of specific anomalies is uncertain. Nonetheless, a recent systematic review showed a reduced conception rate for all anomalies except the arcuate uterus. Many previously believed an arcuate uterus was benign and could even be considered a normal variant. However, it has been shown that women with an arcuate uterus are more than twice as likely (RR 2.39) to miscarry in the second trimester compared with women with a normal uterus.

The presence of a uterine septum is most associated with increased rates of first-trimester miscarriage (RR 2.89). It appears that unicornuate and bicornuate unification defects are associated with first-trimester loss, but uterus didelphys does not increase the risk of first- or second-trimester miscarriage.

However, uterine anomalies are most strongly associated with obstetric complications. The rate of preterm birth is increased by both canalisation defects (RR 2.14) and unification defects (RR 2.97); and malpresentation at delivery is also increased by canalisation defects (RR 6.24) and unification defects (3.87). The cause of preterm birth is unknown, but theories include a reduced maximum uterine capacity or associated cervical incompetence.

Screening and Diagnosis

When scanning women in early pregnancy, it is always worthwhile suspecting an anomaly given the increased prevalence of uterine anomalies in women who miscarry.

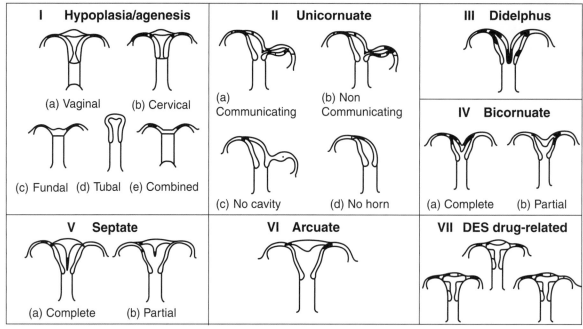

Figure 9.1 American Fertility Society classification system for uterine anomalies.

Traditional two-dimensional ultrasound can often raise the suspicion of a uterine anomaly. This is also the case with hysterosalpingography, hysteroscopy, and laparoscopy. Nonetheless, to accurately make a diagnosis, it is necessary to simultaneously view the external contour of the uterus and the fundal aspect of the endometrial cavity in the coronal plane. This can only be achieved using three-dimensional ultrasound or magnetic resonance imaging (MRI) (see Tables 9.2 and 9.3).

3D Ultrasound

Three-dimensional (3D) ultrasound provides the clinician with a precise view of the uterus in the coronal plane with the added benefit of being low cost and having high patient tolerability

A 3D volume is most commonly acquired using an automated technique after performing a two-dimensional scan. The three-dimensional transvaginal probe is positioned at the midline of the area of interest in the sagittal plane. The operator then preselects a region of interest; in the case of uterine morphology, this is the entire uterus and cervix. Next the angle of acquisition is selected to ensure that both lateral aspects of the uterus are included in the acquisition. The operator can then determine the speed of acquisition that subsequently defines the image quality. The activation of the probe results in the rotation of the ultrasound beam to acquire a series of 2D images at predetermined intervals. A slow acquisition maximises the number of two-dimensional images in the data set, resulting in a higher-resolution 3D volume. However, this volume is more likely to suffer from artefact due to movement of the patient, although this is less problematic in gynaecological imaging because the pelvic organs are stationary, unlike the blood vessels and some other organs. The volume can then be analysed in real time or saved for offline analysis later on.

Image Manipulation

The acquired scan volume can be displayed in a number of different formats depending in the tissue type and area of interest. In gynaecology, this is usually the multiplanar view, which shows three perpendicular images: the sagittal and reconstructed transverse and coronal views. The operator can then manipulate each plane individually to reveal an unlimited number of views, all of which retain a perpendicular relationship with one another. Using the acquisition technique previously described, it is almost always possible to obtain the coronal view of the uterus, which is usually lying perpendicular to the ultrasound beam. The uterus is visualised in the coronal plane using the

Table 9.1 Diagnostic tests

	Image	Pros	Cons
Optimal			
MRI		Precise high-resolution coronal view image Images can be reviewed at a later date	Expensive Time consuming
3D ultrasound		Coronal image Low cost High patient tolerability Widely available Volume can be reviewed at a later date	3D facility on scan machine required
Combined hysteroscopy and laparoscopy		Simultaneous view the external contour of the uterus and the fundal aspect of the endometrial cavity	No coronal image Invasive Unable to measure septal length
Suboptimal			
Hysterosalpingogram (HSG)		Excellent view of endometrial cavity Low cost	Use of contrast
Hysteroscopy		Can be performed as outpatient	External contour not visible Invasive Unable to measure septal length

(continued)

Table 9.1 (continued)

	Image	Pros	Cons
Laparoscopy		Direct visualisation	Endometrial cavity not visible Invasive Cannot measure fundal indent
2D ultrasound		Low cost High patient tolerability Widely available	No coronal image Dynamic test

Table 9.2 Types of anomaly

Anomaly	3D-scan image	Prevalence General population	Prevalence Miscarriage population	Effect on early pregnancy	Treatments
Arcuate		3.9	2.9	Increase in second-trimester miscarriage	None
Septum		2.3	5.3	Increase in first- and second-trimester miscarriage	Hysteroscopic septal resection
Bicornuate		0.4	2.1	Increase in first- and second-trimester miscarriage	None

Table 9.2 (continued)

Anomaly	3D-scan image	Prevalence General population	Prevalence Miscarriage population	Effect on early pregnancy	Treatments
Unicornuate		0.1	0.5	Increase in first-trimester miscarriage	None
Didelphys		0.3	0.6	No change	None

Table 9.3 USS diagnosis of an arcuate uterus

	Image	Details
2D longitudinal view		It is difficult to show in a 2D longitudinal image that there is the suspicion of an uterine anomaly. Only when panning from side to side in real time will the sonographer gain information.
2D transverse view		In transverse section, it can be appreciated that there is a uterine anomaly, although it is often difficult to differentiate between an arcuate, septate, and bicornuate uterus.
3D image		The uterine anomaly is clearly seen on a 3D USS examination.

interstitial portions of the Fallopian tubes as reference points, and a diagnosis can be made.

Treatment

The options for women with uterine anomalies and a history of miscarriage are limited. There are no medical treatments, and only the septate uterus is amenable to surgery. Hysteroscopic septal resection is commonly performed for women with a septum and a history of recurrent miscarriage, despite no understanding of what makes a septum pathological and the potential risks of surgery. The evidence for this operation is also limited to case control studies limited by using different populations, surgical technique and variable length of follow-up. There are no completed randomised controlled trials (RCT), although two are ongoing, the U.K. SEPTUM trial and the Dutch TRUST study. Results of these RCTs are urgently needed to demonstrate the safety and efficacy of hysteroscopic septal resection. In the meantime, the National Institute for Health and Care Excellence (NICE) suggests current evidence on efficacy is adequate to support the use of this procedure provided that normal arrangements are in place for clinical governance, consent and audit.

Learning Points

- Uterine anomalies are common, although the true prevalence is not known.
- There is no agreed classification system to categorise uterine anomalies.
- Suspect uterine anomalies when performing 2D ultrasound, but be aware that it is suboptimal to diagnose specific anomalies.

- Optimal tests to diagnose uterine anomalies are 3D ultrasound and MRI.
- A randomised controlled trial of hysteroscopic septal resection is required to demonstrate its safety and efficacy in women with a history of infertility, miscarriage, or preterm birth.

Further Reading

1. Buttram Jr VC, Siegler A, DeCherney A, Gibbons W, March C (1988). The American Fertility Society classifications of adnexal adhesions, distal tubal occlusion, tubal occlusion secondary to tubal ligation, tubal pregnancies, mullerian anomalies and intrauterine adhesions. *Fertility and Sterility* 49(6): 944–955.

2. Grimbizis GF, Di Spiezio Sardo A, Saravelos SH, et al. (2016). The Thessaloniki ESHRE/ESGE consensus on diagnosis of female genital anomalies. *Gynecol Surg* 13: 1–16.

3. Chan YY, Jayaprakasan K, Tan A, Thornton JG, Coomarasamy A, Raine-Fenning NJ (2011). Reproductive outcomes in women with congenital uterine anomalies: a systematic review. *Ultrasound Obstet Gynecol* 38(4): 371–382.

4. Chan YY, Jayaprakasan K, Zamora J, Thornton JG, Raine-Fenning N, Coomarasamy A (2011). The prevalence of congenital uterine anomalies in unselected and high-risk populations: a systematic review. *Hum Reprod Update* 17(6): 761–771.

5. Kowalik CR, Goddijn M, Emanuel MH, Bongers MY, Spinder T, de Kruif JH, et al. (2011). Metroplasty versus expectant management for women with recurrent miscarriage and a septate uterus. *Cochrane Database Syst Rev.* (6): CD008576.

Chapter 10

The Use of 3D Ultrasound and Colour Doppler in Early Pregnancy

Venetia Goodhart and Davor Jurkovic

Both three-dimensional (3D) and colour Doppler (CD) are relatively novel techniques that are used as part of ultrasound examination to complement standard B-mode images and provide additional diagnostic information. CD ultrasound has been used in routine practice for more than 30 years, and its major application has been the assessment of blood flow in pelvic tumours. Three-dimensional ultrasound is a more recent development that has been extensively used in obstetrics for the diagnosis of complex fetal anomalies. In gynaecology, the most important indication for 3D ultrasound is the diagnosis of congenital and acquired uterine abnormalities.

Safety

The intensity of ultrasound in 3D scanning is comparable to standard two-dimensional B-mode imaging. In view of that, the same safety measures should be employed, and ultrasound should only be performed by trained individuals where there is a clinical need; see Chapter 1.

Exposure to colour and pulsed Doppler may negatively impact embryological development in an ongoing pregnancy. It has been established that colour and in particular pulsed Doppler use higher intensities than standard B-mode imaging. Increasing the baseline temperature of tissues in animal studies has been shown to interfere with proliferative activity and cause cell death and vascular damage. Potential damage is caused to the human embryo if the temperature is elevated by 4°C for more than five minutes. Nonthermal damage such as cavitation has also been noted in the lung and intestine of animal tissues. As described in Chapter 1, the TI and MI should be monitored.

The MI should be kept below 0.7 and the exposure to ultrasound should be as low as reasonably achievable (ALARA). CD should be avoided in normal ongoing pregnancies, apart from in situations

of uncertainty where its use is necessary to provide essential diagnostic information. The use of pulsed Doppler should be avoided before 12 weeks' gestation (the first trimester).

Clinical Applications of Colour Doppler in Early Pregnancy

CD is used in early pregnancy to identify the site and number of corpora lutea. It also helps in the diagnosis of tubal ectopic pregnancy by demonstrating blood supply to the ectopic gestational sac. In cervical and Caesarean scar ectopic pregnancies, CD facilitates differential diagnosis between intrauterine (intracavitary) and ectopic pregnancies. The assessment of blood supply in Caesarean scar or cervical pregnancies is helpful in planning the management and assessing the risk of intraoperative haemorrhage.

Differential diagnoses for miscarriage include common uterine cavity anomalies such as endometrial polyps or submucous fibroids. On CD examination, a polyp will have a single feeder vessel, whereas a submucous fibroid will display a circular blood supply around the lesion. Retained products of conception typically have a scattered blood supply and increased vascularity.

Identifying the Corpus Luteum

Identification of the corpus luteum is a routine part of early pregnancy assessment. The corpus luteum can appear as solid, haemorrhagic, or cystic. Although the corpus luteum can usually be identified on B-mode imaging, it can sometimes be poorly defined and hard to visualise against the normal ovarian tissue. CD is also useful in identifying more than one corpus. Regardless of its appearance, the corpus luteum typically exhibits the characteristic 'ring of fire' under colour Doppler examination. This is due to the increased vascularity of the active corpus (Figure 10.1).

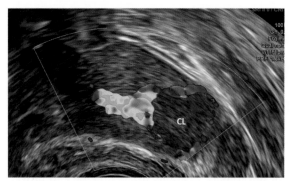

Figure 10.1 Characteristic 'ring of fire' exhibited by the corpus luteum (CL).

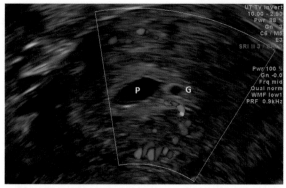

Figure 10.2 Intrauterine gestation sac (GS) with evidence of functional peritrophoblastic circulation compared to a pseudosac (P) with absent flow.

While multiple corpora lutea are a common finding in patients who have undergone assisted reproduction with ovarian stimulation, more than one corpus should raise clinical suspicion of multiple pregnancy. Ectopic pregnancy must be considered even in the presence of an intrauterine gestation sac. Although the incidence of heterotopic pregnancy is relatively infrequent in spontaneous conception, it is common following assisted conception (1 per cent) and therefore must be excluded. The majority of tubal ectopic pregnancies are ipsilateral (approximately 70 per cent), and the location of the corpus luteum facilitates identification of the ectopic pregnancy. In all women with ectopic pregnancies, the blood supply to trophoblast is seen as a separate area of increased vascularity from the corpus luteum, which increases the certainty of the ultrasound diagnosis of ectopic pregnancy.

Implantation Site

Colour Doppler examination is well suited to identify the placental implantation site given the characteristic low-impedance turbulent flow exhibited by the transformed spiral arteries within the forming placenta. High vascularity identified with CD is an indicator of functional peritrophoblastic or placental circulation.

The importance of identifying the site of implantation lies in distinguishing between intrauterine pregnancies (IUPs), where the implantation is confined within the uterine cavity, and ectopic pregnancies. A cystic endometrium can be differentiated from a gestational sac not only by the presence of the trophoblastic reaction but also by this characteristic vascularity (Figure 10.2).

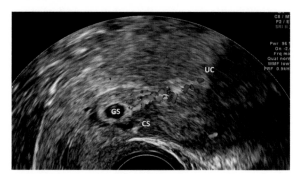

Figure 10.3 Cervical phase of an ongoing miscarriage showing implantation within the uterine cavity (UC) despite presence of the gestation sac overlying the Caesarean scar (CS).

It also serves a role in characterising a cervical ectopic from a Caesarean scar ectopic pregnancy or the cervical stage of an inevitable miscarriage so that the correct management can be employed (Figure 10.3). CD can help to confirm whether a Caesarean scar or intramural pregnancy breeches the endometrial myometrial junction. In these scenarios, the presence of peripheral vasodilatation is more significant when there is an accompanying myometrial weakness caused by uterine scarring. The vascularity here is important, as the absence of the normal architecture compromises the myometrial function so that it does not contract as expected, potentially resulting in haemorrhage. Increased vascularity in a normal myometrium does not have an associated risk of bleeding. However, when diagnosing Caesarean scar ectopics, an increased blood supply gives an indication of the risk of massive haemorrhage (Figure 10.4).

The ability to appreciate the vascularity of an ectopic pregnancy can be useful when planning best

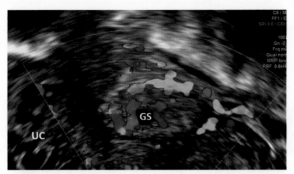

Figure 10.4 Caesarean scar ectopic pregnancy (GS) with high vascularity anterior to the gestation sac and implanted outside the UC.

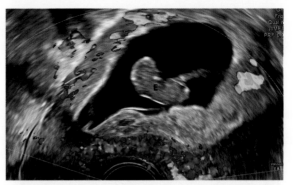

Figure 10.5 Evidence of early embryonic demise (embryo – E) confirmed by the lack of cardiac activity (absence of colour over the embryo but presence noted elsewhere).

management. With highly vascular ectopic pregnancies, clinicians may favour surgical management in view of the heightened risk of rupture and maternal haemorrhage. This is especially the case in Caesarean scar pregnancies, when vascularity is proportional to blood loss.

Uterine ectopic pregnancies cannot be expelled by contraction. Initially, they induce extreme vasodilatation of the uterine vessels in the vicinity of retained trophoblast, which can be easily depicted on CD. This facilitates resorption of pregnancy into the maternal circulation. As the amount of volume of retained trophoblast decreases, the blood supply also tends to diminish.

Assessing Viability

When there is uncertainty regarding the viability of a pregnancy, CD can be used to aid detection of embryonic cardiac activity, or indeed prove its absence in the case of miscarriage (Figure 10.5). Abnormal pregnancies will often demonstrate highly vascular trophoblast on CD, which sometimes helps to confirm the diagnosis of miscarriage.

Retained Products of Conception

Surgical evacuation for incomplete miscarriage is one of the major indications for emergency gynaecological surgery. Diagnosing a small amount of retained products of conception (RPOC) can be difficult, as they are not clearly visible on B-mode scan. Endometrial thickness measurements are routinely taken as part of transvaginal ultrasound, and traditionally have been used in conjunction with the appearance of the midline echo to identify RPOC. However, endometrial thickness measurements have been shown to be poor

indicators for the diagnosis of RPOC. Even a very small amount of RPOC tends to exhibit high blood supply. One of the main roles of CD in early pregnancy has been to facilitate detection of RPOC and increase the sensitivity of ultrasound diagnosis of incomplete miscarriage (Figure 10.6). CD can also be used to distinguish between RPOC and organised blood clot, which can have a similar appearance on ultrasound. When used in conjunction with clinical symptoms, best management decisions can be achieved, that is, whether cases can be managed conservatively or require surgical intervention. Identifying vascular RPOC (measured as maximum peak systolic velocity) can prepare the clinician for potential complications at surgical evacuation such as maternal haemorrhage.

Uterine 'Arteriovenous Malformation'

It has been suggested that increased blood flow to an otherwise uncomplicated intrauterine pregnancy may represent an arteriovenous malformation (AVM).

RPOC are usually expelled by uterine contractions. If this process is not effective, the only other physiological method for removal is through the peritrophoblastic circulation and reabsorption. In some women, RPOC will be accompanied by extreme vasodilatation, which some refer to as AVM. As these changes typically regress after spontaneous or surgical removal of the pregnancy, we prefer to use the term pseudo arteriovenous malformation.

Pseudo AVM is a common physiological finding in women in whom products of conception have been retained over a prolonged period. Some have expressed concerns that extreme vasodilatation increases the risk of severe haemorrhage with an associated risk

(a)　　　　　　　　　　　　　　　　　　　　(b)

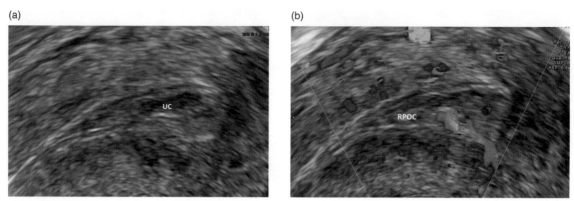

Figure 10.6 (a) The retained products of pregnancy are not clearly visualised on B-mode imaging. (b) When CD is applied, the vascularity assists the identification of the RPOC.

(a)　　　　　　　　　　　　　　　　　　　　(b)

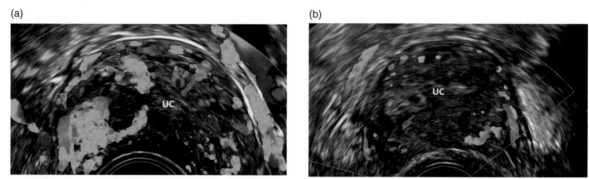

Figure 10.7 (a) Pseudo AV malformation is highly vascular initially. (b) However, after surgical evacuation it regresses spontaneously and the uterine appearances normalise.

of hysterectomy. However, recent studies have shown that this risk is low. Whilst high blood flow is a concern in some forms of ectopic pregnancies, such as intramural and cervical pregnancies, it bears no significance with regards to miscarriage of normally implanted intrauterine pregnancies (Figure 10.7).

In contrast, true AVMs are a permanent feature, present in nonpregnant women. They feature massive vasodilatation of the uterine vessels, including the radial arteries, and are associated with heavy menstrual periods. AVM can appear as 'areas of strong hypervascularity and strong turbulence in comparison with the normal surrounding myometrial perfusion'.

Gestational Trophoblastic Disease

The villi in gestational trophoblastic disease are avascular and will demonstrate absent flow on colour Doppler examination. Despite this, the literature often refers to increased vascularity as being a useful diagnostic indicator of molar pregnancy. This

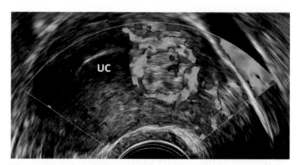

Figure 10.8 An invasive molar pregnancy exhibiting a vascular appearance within the myometrium (transverse view).

can be explained by the tendency of molar tissue to invade the myometrium or to be retained for a long time, thus giving the vascular appearance shown in Figure 10.8.

The uterus reacts to vasodilatation in gestational trophoblastic disease using the same mechanism observed in uncomplicated miscarriage. Therefore, there can be diagnostic difficulty on ultrasound when it comes to differentiating between RPOC and gestational trophoblastic disease.

The Use of 3D Ultrasound in Early Pregnancy

The development of 3D imaging as part of transvaginal ultrasound has allowed clarification in diagnosing complications of early pregnancy and assisted in formulating management decisions. Three-dimensional imaging allows clinicians to obtain coronal views of the uterus, which is difficult using conventional two-dimensional imaging. It is an integrated part of the transvaginal scan (providing the ultrasound machine has a 3D function), which is routinely used in the assessment of early pregnancy, without adding significant time to the scan. The images are self-explanatory and can be stored permanently and assessed independently.

Location of the Pregnancy

One of the benefits of 3D imaging is that it very clearly demonstrates the endometrial myometrial junction. This is particularly useful in early pregnancy as it allows the clinician to establish the exact location of the pregnancy in relation to the uterine cavity and assess for invasion beyond said junction, thereby assisting the diagnosis of intramural, interstitial, cervical, or Caesarean scar ectopic pregnancies.

A normal IUP is a pregnancy located within the uterine cavity with trophoblastic invasion that does not breach the endometrial myometrial junction (Figure 10.9). The uterine cavity is defined as the virtual space between the uterine ostia of the Fallopian tubes and the internal cervical os, lined with endometrium.

Interstitial Pregnancy

The visualisation of the interstitium is facilitated by the use of 3D ultrasound and the ability to see the proximal part of the tube is the most difficult part of diagnosing an interstitial pregnancy. Three-dimensional imaging can better assess interstitial pregnancies as it provides improved views of the interstitial portion of the tube and allows the clinician to better assess the position of pregnancy in relation to the uterine cavity to rule out uterine anomalies and aid management decisions (Figure 10.10).

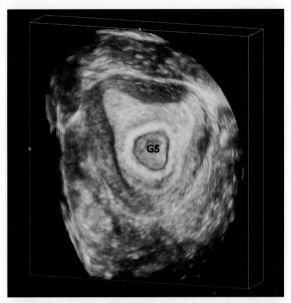

Figure 10.9 Normal intrauterine pregnancy on 3D.

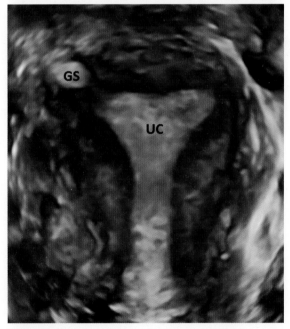

Figure 10.10 Three-dimensional image of an interstitial pregnancy showing a gestational sac in the lateral aspect of the uterus, which is adjoined to the uterine cavity by thin, hyperechoic line representing the proximal section of the interstitial tube.

Intramural Pregnancy

These pregnancies can either be partial (the trophoblast breaches the endometrial myometrial junction) or complete (the trophoblast lies entirely

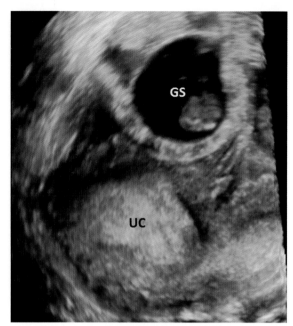

Figure 10.11 Three-dimensional image of the uterus showing the UC and a GS, which is located in the posterior wall of the uterus. These findings were typical of an intramural pregnancy.

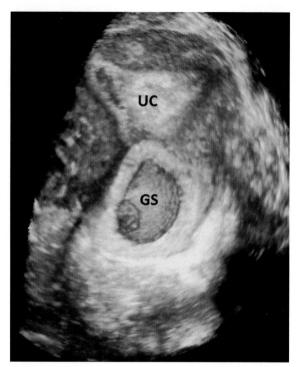

Figure 10.12 Caesarean scar ectopic pregnancy showing evidence of anterior herniation (UC = uterine cavity; GS = gestational sac).

within the myometrium). The pregnancy is located above the internal os and medial to the interstitial tube (Figure 10.11). Given the site of implantation, there is a lack of decidual reaction in the surrounding tissue.

Cornual Pregnancy

Diagnosis of a cornual pregnancy is based on a single interstitial portion of the Fallopian tube within the main uterine body. The gestation sac can be seen mobile and separate from the uterus and is surrounded by myometrium. A vascular pedicle can be seen joining the gestation sac to the unicornuate uterus.

Caesarean Scar Pregnancy

Caesarean scar pregnancies extend outside the uterine cavity and exhibit myometrial involvement. There is partial or complete absence of a decidual reaction and there must be evidence of functional peritrophoblastic flow. Three-dimensional ultrasound helps to assess the exact location of the Caesarean scar ectopic and whether there is any evidence of herniation, in order to establish the feasibility of surgical evacuation (Figure 10.12).

Uterine Anomalies

Uterine anomalies can be an incidental finding during the ultrasound assessment of early pregnancy. It can at times be difficult to differentiate between an intrauterine pregnancy and interstitial or cornual ectopic pregnancies in the presence of an underlying anomaly. Although diagnosis of a uterine anomaly can be compromised in pregnancy due to dilation of the uterine cavity by the presence of the pregnancy, 3D ultrasound can undoubtedly aid diagnosis and especially help to rule out ectopic pregnancy by examining the relationship between the uterine septum and the pregnancy (Figure 10.13).

Learning Points

- B-mode ultrasound is sufficient in providing diagnostic information in most women presenting with simple early pregnancy complications.
- Three-dimensional ultrasound and colour Doppler may help in the more complex and difficult cases, particularly in women with

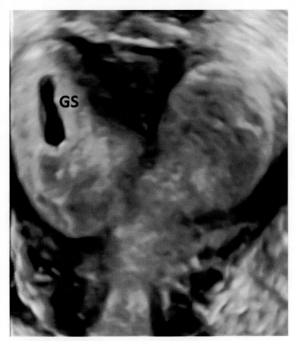

Figure 10.13 Intrauterine pregnancy in a right cornu of a bicornuate uterus.

incomplete miscarriage and those with uterine anomalies and ectopic pregnancies.

- Colour Doppler should be available on all modern machines used for early pregnancy diagnostics.
- In order to ensure safety, key protocols should be established in every scan department for its use to minimise the risk of exposing normal intrauterine pregnancy to the potentially harmful effects of colour Doppler.

Further Reading

1. The British Medical Ultrasound Society. Statement on the safe use, and potential hazards of diagnostic ultrasound. www.bmus.org

2. The British Medical Ultrasound Society. Guidelines for the safe use of diagnostic ultrasound equipment. www.bmus.org

3. Morin L et al. (2005). Ultrasound evaluation of first trimester pregnancy complications. *J Obstet Gynaecol Canada* Jun;27(6): 581–591.

4. Jurkovic D et al. (1991). Transvaginal colour Doppler assessment of utero-placental circulation in early pregnancy. *Obstet Gynaecol*. 77: 365–369.

5. Jauniaux E et al. (1990). Assessment of placental development and function. In Kurjak, A. (ed) *Transvaginal Colour Doppler*, pp. 53–65 (Carnforth, UK: Parthenon Publishing).

6. Jurkovic et al. (2016). Surgical treatment of Cesarean scar ectopic pregnancy: efficacy and safety of ultrasound-guided suction curettage. *Ultrasound Obstet Gynecol*. Apr;47(4): 511–517. doi: 10.1002/uog.15857

7. Sawyer et al. (2007). The value of measuring endometrial thickness and volume on transvaginal ultrasound scan for the diagnosis of incomplete miscarriage. *Ultrasound Obstet Gynaecol*. Feb;29(2): 205–209.

8. Van den Bosch et al. (2015). Maximum peak systolic velocity and management of highly vascularized retained products of conception. *J Ultrasound Med*. Sep;34(9): 1577–1582.

9. Timmerman D et al. (2003). Color Doppler imaging is a valuable tool for the diagnosis and management of uterine vascular malformations. *Ultrasound Obstet Gynecol*. Jun;21(6): 570–577.

Ultrasound and the Surgical Management of Early Pregnancy Complications

Tom Holland

The practice of early pregnancy complication management has been transformed over the last 20 years by the introduction of high-definition ultrasound into everyday services. This advancement has been in parallel with progress in minimal access surgery, both in terms of technique and technology.

Preoperative Assessment

A confident, accurate diagnosis helps in the counselling of patients regarding expectant management of many conditions that were previously thought of as being surgical problems (such as interstitial pregnancy). However, many complications will necessitate surgery, and for these patients an accurate preoperative diagnosis is essential to ensuring the right operation by the right surgeon(s) in the right place at the right time.

Tubal Ectopic Pregnancy

The most important aspects to consider prior to commencing any laparoscopic surgery are how difficult the surgery will be and whether the most appropriate surgeon is present. When considering laparoscopic excision of a tubal ectopic pregnancy, the main features that will make the surgery difficult will be adhesions. Therefore, once the diagnosis of a tubal ectopic pregnancy is made, it is essential to assess the ovaries and other pelvic structures for adhesions. When the tube is adherent to the ovary, it can be difficult to distinguish between an ovarian ectopic and a tubal ectopic, and these are the sorts of cases that require an experienced laparoscopic surgeon.

Interstitial Ectopic Pregnancy

An interstitial pregnancy is a potentially very dangerous due to the abundant vascularity of the myometrium and consequent copious haemorrhage if rupture occurs. The diagnosis of interstitial pregnancy

is discussed in Chapter 7. Key points when considering surgery are the size of the trophoblast, size of the gestational sac and embryo, and the thickness of the overlying myometrium. Previously, wedge resection was thought necessary; however, laparoscopic excision by opening the myometrium, in a similar manner to laparoscopic myomectomy, and removing the trophoblast is now thought to be sufficient.

Intraoperative Ultrasound

Before starting any procedure for a pregnancy-related problem, where you have not scanned the patient yourself, it is highly recommended that you rescan the patient. Ideally, the scan should be performed pre-operatively as there may be less time pressure; however, if necessary it can be performed immediately in theatre once the patient has been anaesthetised. The benefits of this approach are that you can check the previous scan findings to make sure you agree and it also provides immediate direct feedback to improve your scanning experience. It is especially useful with ectopic pregnancies, as many doctors in training will have operated on more ectopic pregnancies than they will have diagnosed on ultrasound. It is also an opportunity to assess the level of intra-abdominal bleeding and ectopic location.

Miscarriage

Surgical management of miscarriage (SMM) is normally the first operation that many gynaecology trainees learn. However, the practice of this operation is evolving. Manual vacuum aspiration (MVA) under local anaesthetic is appropriate for many smaller pregnancies and has the advantage of avoiding a general anaesthetic and the use of an operating theatre. Local protocols should be in place, but gestational sac size is the main criteria used. Other features, which can make the procedure more uncomfortable, will be pregnancies high in the cavity and retroverted uteri.

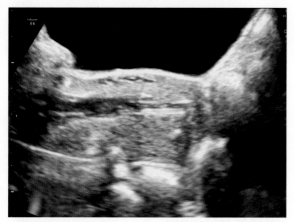

Figure 11.1 Transabdominal ultrasound during surgical management of miscarriage.

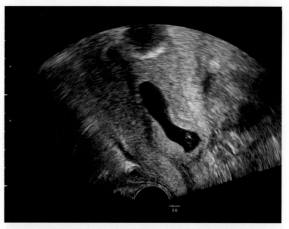

Figure 11.2 Transrectal scan (using a normal transvaginal probe) of a Caesarean scar ectopic pregnancy prior to evacuation.

Transabdominal ultrasound is helpful thoughout both MVA and SMM (Figure 11.1) in order to guide cervical dilation, reduce the risk of perforation, and ensure that all the products of conception are removed without unnecessary damage to the endometrium and consequent risk of intrauterine adhesions. A partially full bladder is helpful to improve the picture quality; however, this can be quite uncomfortable when the patient is awake. When the patient is asleep, the bladder can be filled with warm saline via a catheter to improve the picture quality if necessary. An alternative is intraoperative transrectal ultrasound. As detailed in Chapter 1, this is performed systematically in the same way as a TVS. The advantage of using this method intraoperatively is that it allows you to scan continuously whilst performing the surgical procedure transvaginally.

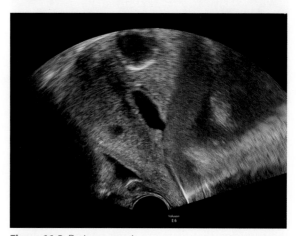

Figure 11.3 During evacuation.

Caesarean Scar Pregnancy

Caesarean scar pregnancy is a rare type of ectopic pregnancy, which is implanted into the defect in the myometrium from a poorly healed Caesarean section, as discussed in Chapter 7. Both ectopic and cervical ectopic pregnancies of this type are amenable to surgical evacuation. Transrectal ultrasound can be used during evacuation of these types of low uterine ectopic pregnancies, as the visualisation is better than with transabdominal ultrasound (Figures 11.2, 11.3, and 11.4).

Postoperative

Ultrasound is useful in the assessment of women who present with possible complications after a surgical

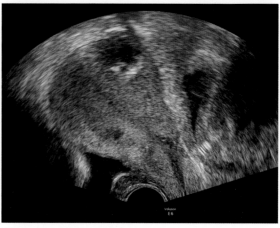

Figure 11.4 After evacuation.

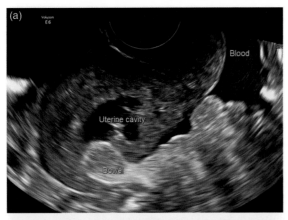

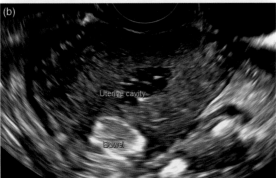

Figure 11.5 Ultrasound images showing a perforation of the uterus sustained at the time of surgical management of miscarriage, with a small segment of small bowel within the myometrium: (a) longitudinal view; (b) transverse view.

procedure has been performed in early pregnancy. Continuous bleeding or pain after SMM may lead to the suspicion that there are some retained products of conception or that a perforation of the uterus has occurred (Figure 11.5). Ultrasound examination can also be useful for assessing the presence and extent of pelvic collections, fistulae, and adhesions.

Learning Points

- Ultrasound has a role in the pre-, intra-, and postoperative management of many gynaecological procedures.
- When making a diagnosis, it is important to also consider the surgical management and identify features such as adhesions, which may make the surgery more difficult.
- Intraoperative ultrasound guidance is helpful to improve safety and ensure completion of many evacuation procedures.

Further Reading

1. NICE (December 2012). Ectopic pregnancy and miscarriage: diagnosis and initial management in early pregnancy of ectopic pregnancy and miscarriage. NICE Clinical Guideline 154.

2. Poon LCY, Emmanuel E, Ross, JA, Johns J (2014). How feasible is expectant management of interstitial ectopic pregnancy? *Ultrasound Obstet Gynecol* 43(3): 317–321.

3. Wen J, Cai QY, Deng F, Li YP (2008). Manual versus electric vacuum aspiration for first-trimester abortion: a systematic review. *BJOG: An International Journal of Obstetrics & Gynaecology* 115(1): 5–13.

4. Vial Y, Petignat P, Hohlfeld P (2000). Pregnancy in a cesarean scar. *Ultrasound Obstet Gynecol* 16: 592–593.

5. Jurkovic D, Hillaby K, Woelfer B, Lawrence A, Salim R, Elson CJ (2003). First-trimester diagnosis and management of pregnancies implanted into the lower uterine segment Cesarean section scar. *Ultrasound Obstet Gynecol* 21: 220–227.

6. Jurkovic D, Ben-Nagi J, Ofilli-Yebovi D, Sawyer E, Helmy S, Yazbek J (2007). Efficacy of Shirodkar cervical suture in securing hemostasis following surgical evacuation of cesarean scar ectopic pregnancy. *Ultrasound Obstet Gynecol* 30(1): 95–100.

Index

ARCHITECTURE, TECHNOLOGY AND PROCESS

Chris Abel

AMSTERDAM • BOSTON • HEIDELBERG • LONDON • NEW YORK • OXFORD
PARIS • SAN DIEGO • SAN FRANCISCO • SINGAPORE • SYDNEY • TOKYO

Architectural Press is an imprint of Elsevier

ELSEVIER

Architectural
Press

Architectural Press
An imprint of Elsevier
Linacre House, Jordan Hill, Oxford OX2 8DP
30 Corporate Drive, Burlington, MA 01803

First published 2004

British Library Cataloguing in Publication Data
A catalogue record for this book is available from the British Library

Library of Congress Cataloguing in Publication Data
A catalogue record for this book is available from the Library of Congress

ISBN 0 7506 3792 7

For information on all Architectural Press publications
visit our website at www.architecturalpress.com

Typeset by Newgen Imaging Systems (P) Ltd., Chennai, India
Printed and bound in Great Britain by Biddles Ltd, King's Lynn, Norfolk

CONTENTS

FOREWORD

Contemporary architecture is going through an exciting period of experimentation. However, many architects seem to be repeating the same dreadful mistakes that our twentieth-century predecessors have made. Architecture–technology relationships are commonly over-simplified and many designers who are apparently working at the cutting edge are in reality still glaringly conventional in how they actually use and conceptualize technology.

Current architectural theories have also been slow to catch up with the new-found morphological freedom that is offered by digital technology. Designers enamoured with their new tools are frantically casting about in search of a theoretical framework or any kind of hook with which they can make sense of the boundless shapes and geometries that their computers enable them to generate.

A multitude of competing ideologies add to the confusion of the times, making life more difficult for architects as well as creating new opportunities. Busy professionals no less than neophyte designers concerned with the art of architecture and how to produce it, are all struggling to position themselves, a task which by its nature entails a rigorous process of self-examination.

Added to these issues is the question of what knowledge base architecture should be founded on? What is the fundamental knowledge that we architects possess? In architecture, we find that, while the need to know originates in one discipline, the required knowledge itself often belongs to many others. How can we work from principles when what we do is produce artefacts? How do we take knowledge from another discipline, and adapt it to our own?

In the past, our approach has been one of extension. We inclusively expanded the range of our discipline to encompass other fields. Architectural education began to require more and more knowledge that was inherent to or borrowed from other disciplines. At the same time, many of these disciplines were themselves also rapidly expanding their own knowledge base and independently advancing their own theoretical bodies, creating further problems of assimilation. The more we extend, the more we are also forced to trade off knowledge for data, exchanging theoretical concepts for 'hard facts'. As a result, architects often end up appropriating the knowledge from other disciplines as an ever-growing database of strategies from which they can pick something that seems appropriate to the task at hand. The danger is that, in converting theory into use-able methods or facts, the original concepts underlying those methods and facts may get forgotten or lost. It often seems that, no matter how hard we try, the more complex the knowledge, the further removed it becomes from us.

Chris Abel is a focused writer. His writings are largely about the technology of architecture and the architecture of technology. For the lost and uncertain, they serve as a timely navigational aid – something between an architectural baro-meter and sextant, telling us in each chapter what to look for, which direction to look in, and why we should even look at all.

In this one single volume Abel does the work of a horde of architectural critics writing all at the same time from all over the globe. The critical essays here rest-lessly straddle the world from Los Angeles (Gehry), to London (Foster), Malta (Architecture Project), Kuala Lumpur (Kasturi and others) and Sydney (Seidler). Ferreting out incisive profiles from the architectural mise-en-scène on our behalf, Abel writes like an inquisitive and constantly thinking architectural equivalent of Bill Bryson, the prolific travel writer. Along the road, he explains how digital tech-nologies and new science have affected architectural theory and production over the past half century, the way we assimilate new technologies like the Net into our mental frameworks, and the impact of global economic developments on architecture in the Far East, all with equal aplomb.

Asian architects will certainly regard the first chapter as a tacit vote of confi-dence in the region. Abel has in one fell swoop moved away from the largely Eurocentric angle of other writers by starting the book with a chapter on 'Architecture in the Pacific Century'. This is a timely and welcome essay. His arguments will help to allay the angst of those architects living in Asia Pacific in a period when Japan, the world's number two economy, is still mired in an extended recession, and who may fear that the recent monetary crisis might have permanently eclipsed the bright future they were once promised. Abel reminds us of the reasons for that earlier confidence in the region's potential, which manifested in a period of intensive building of new townships and super-tall towers. At the same time, he asks us to pause and consider where it might all be leading, pointing to the detrimental effects on the environment of ill-planned economic growth and development. The recent publication in Beijing of a Chinese language edition of Abel's previous collection of essays, many of which are also focused on related issues, will doubtless confirm his place as a leading critic and thinker in that region, as well as elsewhere.

As he reminds us in his introduction, Abel's approach stems from his early work in the late 1960s on the architectural implications of cybernetics and systems theory, since broadened by long stints working in the countries about which he writes. Ultimately, this volume, as with all Abel's writings, must be benchmarked against what is historically his most important polemical essay, 'Ditching the Dinosaur Sanctuary', published in *Architectural Design* in 1969, and which was republished in the first collection. The first time that anyone forecast the liberating impact of computerized production lines upon architecture, Abel's essay served as a penetrating critique of prevailing dogmas and a keen insight into the new Zeitgeist, anticipating many of the events to come. Evidently, judging from these essays he is still in great form.

Ken Yeang

PREFACE

All extremism inevitably fails because it consists in excluding, in denying all but a single point of the entire vital reality. But the rest of it, not ceasing to be real merely because we deny it, always comes back and back, and imposes itself on us whether we like it or not.

(Jose Ortega y Gasset, 1958)

The essays gathered in this book were all written since the publication of my first collection in 1997, save for the first two chapters, which were presented as conference papers shortly before. In contrast to that earlier collection, which includes works first published over 30 years ago, the essays presented here therefore offer an overview of relatively recent architectural and technological developments.

Such is the speed of those developments, however, that even ideas and works written down and published in the last few years may be quickly overtaken by events. For example, having already once revised my essay on wider developments in Asia Pacific for another publication to take account of the financial crisis in 1997, the optimism I expressed in that essay regarding the future for the region already looks like being fulfilled, with almost all countries in the area now steaming full ahead again, though not without negative effects.

The pace of change in cutting edge practices like those of Norman Foster and Frank Gehry also makes it difficult to be sure that whatever was written about something which was designed in the office yesterday, necessarily applies to what is being designed today. Paradoxically, the longer view, which takes into account the earliest as well as the latest projects, may in fact provide more reliable insights into the more important and enduring motivations and influences governing their approaches than any slice of their very latest work can yield, no matter how detailed. While one can never be too sure what steps such architects might take tomorrow, we can be reasonably confident, both from their own accounts as well as from our own deductions, that those moves will be at least partly if not largely related to their earlier histories, if only as points of departure.

For this reason, my essay on Foster and Gehry as well as the essays on the other two practices discussed at length in this book, take the general form of condensed histories and cover many of the architects' key works, from the very earliest to at least some of the most recent, if not all the very latest. I have also taken advantage of some of the research I have been doing at Foster's London studio for a new series of monographs on the practice, to update the essay to cover the work of the Specialist Modelling Group and related innovations. The appendix on the Schmidlin Company, who produced the cladding systems for two of Foster's most recent buildings in London, was also written following my visit to their factory in Basel in September 2003, when the rest of the book had already been completed and sent off to the publishers. Schmidlin's collaboration with Foster and with other firms like the Renzo Piano Workshop is deserving of more extensive treatment and I hope to present a more detailed study in a future publication.

In Gehry's case, while I have not yet had an opportunity to personally visit his office in Los Angeles, I have been able to elaborate my discussion of his work following an extensive tour I made in the summer of 2003 of almost all his buildings in Europe. Although it is many years since I lived and worked in Los Angeles, I hope that my experience there has also helped provide me with some insight into Gehry's background. My understanding of his methodology has also been assisted by a visit I made in 2001 to the Paris headquarters of Dassault Systemes, who produced the Catia suite of manufacturing programmes which Gehry has employed so creatively.

In one respect at least I would be happy if my observations were outdated – in the same chapter I suggest that it is difficult to imagine a symbolically important building being built in the US to the same standards of energy efficiency as some of Foster's buildings in Europe. David Childs' recently published design for the 'Freedom Tower' at Ground Zero in New York incorporates wind turbines capable of providing a fifth of the building's energy needs and thus may soon fulfil that role. Unfortunately, such is the increasingly negative trend of US national policy towards global warming and energy conservation that such gestures may simply distract attention away from the vital need for broader measures (and may even be exploited for that purpose, as has been the case with other recent state or private initiatives).

While individual practices may be fast paced, the rate of technological and cultural change has nowhere been greater than in the development of the Internet, the subject of Chapter 2. However, while there has been a torrent of new literature since that essay was originally written, the sources upon which I based my arguments, which include several papers in Michael Benedikt's *Cyberspace*, remain as valuable entries into many of the key debates still raging on the nature and potential of the Net. Similarly, while Bill Mitchell, some of whose arguments in *City of Bits* I have questioned, has shifted his position somewhat since that publication toward accepting – despite the impact of the Net – the continuing value of place identity, in my view he falls short of offering any convincing explanation of why this should be so. I hope that the discussion presented here will help to fill this gap and will provoke further debate on this important issue. My own approach to the subject is also more about basic processes of perception and innovation, which evolve less rapidly, rather than any specific technological developments. Aside from some editorial polishing and additional notes, I have therefore resisted the temptation in this case to try to revise or update the essay, and present it here in more or less the same form in which it was first delivered, including extensive quotations from Mitchell and other writers.

As with any work of this kind, its value is as much due to those who have assisted me along the way as to any personal efforts. My first thanks go to Ken Yeang for writing the foreword to this book, as well as for earlier help in showing me his work. I am acutely aware that the brief comments I have made on his architecture in these chapters do little justice to the quality and importance of his ideas as well as his designs, which must now be counted amongst the most innovative and influential bodies of work anywhere in the world. Only distance and earlier commitments have prevented me from presenting a more thorough study and I plan to make up for this omission working from my new home 'next door' in Sydney in the near future.

I am also most grateful to Norman Foster and his colleagues, many of whom have spent much time and trouble in explaining their work to me during my researches for the monographs, the fruits of which have also found their way into this book. Particular thanks go to Hugh Whitehead, director of the Specialist Modelling Group, for explaining his work so clearly. Alistair Lazenby at the London office of Schmidlin also kindly arranged my visit to the Basel factory, where I spent an informative day under the expert guidance of Uwe Bremen, who explained the company's innovative approach to me. In Paris, Jean-Marc Galea performed a similar valuable service at Dassault Systemes for me regarding the Catia programmes used by Gehry.

Warm thanks are also due to Harry Seidler, for personally showing me his work in Sydney and explaining the background to it all during the preparation of my introductions to the two volumes on his houses, from which Chapter 5 has been abstracted. I am also especially happy to extend my thanks for their co-operation to the four partners of the Maltese practice, Architecture Project: Konrad Buhagiar, David Drago, David Felici and Alberto Miceli-Farrugia. As a past resident of Malta for very many years I have watched their youthful progress with great interest. It gives me personal pleasure to be able to present the first published overview of their work, which I believe merits wider attention.

My gratitude also goes to all those other architects and photographers who have supplied me with examples of their work, especially Serina Hijjas for her help on the buildings by Hijjas Kasturi Associates, and Hisao Suzuki and the Esto and View photographic agencies for lending me photos of those Gehry works I was unable to visit myself. I would also like to thank Danijela Zivanovic of Vitra for organizing my visits to the Vitra Design Museum and their international head-quarters nearby, together with Alexa Tepen and the other staff at Vitra for showing me around those buildings and for supplying me with their own excel-lent photos of them. Likewise, Nerea Absolo was most helpful during my tour of the Bilbao Guggenheim and in supplying me with additional photos of the museum to supplement my own.

Finally, I wish to thank the editorial team at Architectural Press for their essential support, especially Alison Yates, commissioning editor, and assistant editors Elizabeth Whiting and Catherine Steers, who all saw it through to production. Deena Burgess, Editorial Manager, and Renata Corbani, Desk Editor, together with Pauline Sones also steered it through the final stages. As before, I owe a special debt of gratitude to Neil Warnock-Smith, publishing director, who, hav-ing given the go-ahead to two editions of the previous collection, confirmed his continuing faith in my work with the contract for this book.

Chris Abel

INTRODUCTION

*Most architectural history is bad history. Buildings and styles come and go almost in a world
of their own, their historians too intent on cataloguing their formal and spatial attributes to
pay much attention to the larger political and social events which ultimately lend them meaning, and frequently change it.*[1]

The above quotation is taken from the beginning of a recent essay on the New
German Parliament, Berlin – formerly the Reichstag – a building that has seen
more historical cataclysms than most. The words seem particularly apposite
now in explaining the motivation behind the essays collected here, all of which,
one way or another, attempt some kind of broader view of architecture than the
conventional style or movement-based perspective.

The reader must judge for himself or herself whether or not these essays suc-
ceed in their very wide aims, but the times we live in, when so many environmental problems have global or seemingly remote sources, call for nothing less.
While the geographic spread of the subject matter might also seem ambitious,
for the most part I have restricted myself to discussing developments in those
parts of the world where I have substantial personal experience of living and
working – most particularly in Southeast Asia as well as Europe and the USA, and
not least, Malta, which was my Mediterranean 'base camp' for 20 years. As a
recent immigrant to Australia, in my essay on Harry Seidler, which is edited from
the introductions I wrote for two new books on his work,[2] I also offer the first
of what will doubtless be many attempts to get to grips with the architecture and
many-sided culture of this fascinating country.

As readers of the first collection of essays, *Architecture and Identity*,[3] will know,
these efforts to broaden architects' horizons go back very many years, to some
of my first writings in the late 1960s. They included speculations on the impact
of computerized, or flexible manufacturing systems on architectural production,
and the implications of related innovations in science and technology. In truth,
the realization that something 'more' was required goes back even further than
those early publications, to my two years spent as a foreign architecture student
in West Berlin from 1960 to 1962, when the Reichstag was still a sullen ruin. In
the same period the Berlin Wall went up, splitting Europe and the world yet again
into opposing camps. Like countless other anxious residents, I spent many tense
hours and sleepless nights contemplating the possible results and meaning of

American and Russian tanks staring down each others' gun barrels across 'Checkpoint Charlie', as the main border crossing was known. Thereafter, it became impossible to look at any of the recently completed or current major building projects in West Berlin, which included some of post-war Modernism's finest creations, without seeing them also as symbolic pawns in a vastly more important game of political and cultural chess between different worlds.

These essays can therefore be read, as the previous collection was also intended, as a response to the trivialization of architecture epitomized by Robert Venturi's suggestion that the architect would be better off by 'narrowing his concerns and concentrating on his own job'.[4] For Venturi, that meant primarily focusing on the aesthetics of form and space, a view subsequently encouraged by other Postmodern architects and critics, to the exclusion of much else. As even a cursory look through this book will confirm, this does not imply that aesthetics should be ignored, but merely that it should be treated in proper context as one of architecture's many dimensions, both material and cultural. Most important, as the title of the book suggests, special emphasis is placed in these essays on the cultural and technological changes affecting the generative process of architectural production – rather than just looking at the final built products – and the evolving modes of thought underlying those changes.

While the approach is therefore similar in key respects to that presented in the first collection, both the shorter time-scale over which these essays were written and the more consistent emphasis on technological innovation and its many aspects result in a more coherent argument, in manner as well as substance, than was possible with the earlier book. A repeated theme, for example, is the complex nature of the innovation process itself. Contrary to what their inventors and protagonists usually claim, new technologies do not always completely displace or eradicate previous ones. More often, they simply add another way of doing things to existing methods, which often continue to be used in parallel with the new technologies: what I call 'parallel development', or alternatively, my 'layer-cake theory of innovation'.

Thus, in Chapter 1, 'Architecture in the Pacific Century', I argue that, important as the changes taking place in Asia Pacific are, what is happening is less of a complete or unitary cultural transformation, and more of a piling up of additional culture-forms and technologies on top of already existing ones. As in other parts of the developing world, the result is a hybrid mixture that may be less easy to analyse than the usual one-model-fits-all approach, but is potentially far richer, if not without its own problems. The hybrid modern architecture that can be found throughout the region mirrors this process. Written some years before the 1997 Asian financial crisis and revised for publication after the crisis, it examines the idea of the Pacific Century itself, from 1981, when I heard Johan Galtung in Penang, Malaysia, lecture on the subject, through the financial crisis and beyond, and covers some of the conflicting architectural and urban developments during this period.

Similarly, in the next chapter, 'Cyberspace in mind', I suggest that, new and important as the Internet is, rather than sweeping away all previous modes of communication or spatial values, the Net may be more accurately viewed as supplementing those modes and values, and, in some senses, even reinforcing them. For example, the metaphorical language writers like William Mitchell employ to describe cyberspace, suggests a tacit process of appropriation and use similar to that used in appropriating and moving about in physical space. In other words, for all the fondness for some kind of mind–body dualism amongst science fiction writers and other enthusiasts, the way we use, think and talk about cyberspace actually confirms the importance of bodily experience, rather than negating or undermining it.

The role of language and metaphor in shaping the way we view and use technology is also a principal theme in Chapter 3, 'Technology and process', where the word 'process' implies a particular mode of thought as well as a particular technology or material method of production, to which it is inextricably linked. Thus the shift from conceiving nature as well as architecture in mechanistic terms, to thinking about and designing both buildings and the smart programmes and tools which now help produce them, as adaptive organisms in themselves, illustrates a fundamental change in human culture, of which we are only just seeing the beginning. Originally written for a textbook on environmental design, the chapter provides a brief overview of some of the key developments over the past century in the architecture, science and technology behind this evolution, culminating in the integrated design methods and Biotech architecture of today, a term I coined in 1995 for the fusion of biological models and computer driven design.

Chapter 4, 'Foster and Gehry: one technology; two cultures', continues the same theme, and compares the similarities and differences in the careers of these two innovative architects, and the pioneering uses each has made of computer-based technologies of production. Partly intended as an antidote to some of the more superficial comments that are often made about their architecture and the technologies they use, it presents a comprehensive study of the two architects' working methods.

At another, broader level, the chapter may also be read as an application of the philosophy of critical relativism I first outlined in a 1979 paper,[5] from which a passage is quoted at the end of the chapter. Whilst a comparative study of this kind between two apparently very contrary designers – arguably the two most influential architects of the late twentieth century – might at first seem gratuitous, closer examination reveals surprising similarities, particularly in their response to contextual issues, as well as in their working methods. At the same time, significant differences are evident in the way each has exploited digital technology to enhance their craft, and in their perception of environmental issues as seen from each side of the Atlantic. Many of these differences arise, as they might be expected to, from the divergent architectural cultures in which each architect swims, and their respective sources of inspiration, backgrounds and home bases in London and Los Angeles. Other differences, however, especially those involving energy conservation and social factors, illustrate a more general split in European and American ideologies and cultural values.

The issues these latter differences raise are sensitive ones, especially since the earth-shaking events of 11 September 2001, or 9/11 as they are known, when major divergences between American and European viewpoints on a number of vital global problems – most of which have been simmering for some time – have come to the fore. However, the fact is, that despite most architects' and critics' refusal to recognize it, architecture has always been an intensely political matter, involving basic issues of economics, social expression, power, ownership, participation and appropriation, and now most of all, energy use and sustainable development – issues being fought out on the world stage. The only question is, will architects confront these issues head on, as, with government encouragement, increasing numbers in Europe are, or will they continue to deny or ignore them, as the vast majority of designers in America and elsewhere still do?

The irony is that it was the all-American genius Buckminster Fuller who first taught architects to think on a planetary scale, and who inspired Norman Foster and other leading European designers to make energy efficiency a priority in their work, but not, so it seems, current leading American designers. Given the famous American talent for innovation, it would not be too surprising, therefore, if at some future point the initiative would pass once again across the Atlantic, most probably over to the Pacific coast, where Californians have customarily gone their own way and already enacted strict pollution controls. Should it ever happen, such a development would surely be greatly welcomed, not least by Europeans.

Written for a conference in 2001, just a few months before 9/11, the essay was partly motivated by impressions formed during a much earlier global crisis in the winter of 1973–4, when America and the rest of the world was hit by the OPEC oil embargo. Suddenly, the affluent and mobile peoples of the developed world were compelled, albeit briefly in most cases, to question a lifestyle built on cheap fossil fuels. As a visiting scholar in Cambridge, Massachusetts over the same period, I recall those events and the bewildered American response to them all too well. Clearly, scarce or costly fuel was not something people would easily adjust to, least of all in the land that produced the first automobile for mass consumption, and whose cities are mostly patterned by four wheels. Later, when I lived from 1978 to 1981 in the American Southwest, the first year in Los Angeles and the remainder in Lubbock, Texas, I experienced authentic variations of that spaced-out lifestyle at firsthand and found it just as seductive (admittedly more so in the former city than in the latter) in many respects as most people do. It is not at all hard to understand why owning your very own piece of real turf should have such universal appeal, or why people should be so reluctant to give up the idea, if they have not already achieved it.

I do not therefore share the wholly negative sentiments of earlier European critics of 'urban sprawl', as it has been dismissively called, which were mostly based on differences of aesthetic taste and lifestyle. Rather, my position on sustainable design and the need for energy efficiency in urban design and planning as well as architecture is based, like that of many others, upon the hard realities of global warming and its related environmental and human costs.

Australians' preferred lifestyle and profligate use of energy are remarkably similar to Americans', and the issue of the suburban way of life and its attractions as well as its costs is a central theme in Chapter 5, 'Harry Seidler and the Great Australian Dream'. Widely regarded as the Grand Old Man of Australian Modernism (at the time of writing he is in his eightieth year and still running a prolific practice), Seidler made his reputation as a young immigrant in the early 1950s designing beautifully sited houses in bushland on the edge of Sydney.

However, unlike some other prominent Australian house designers, who rarely design anything else or question the suburban context in which they work, Seidler soon extended his practice to cover all manner of urban building types. As well as many distinctive office and apartment towers, they include several far-sighted experiments in low-rise, high-density cluster housing. Seidler's critical response to both the suburban and urban facets of Australian culture, together with an unusually high level of technological expertise and creativity – he trained as an engineer as well as an architect and employed Pier Luigi Nervi on many projects – sets him apart from his peers.

Whilst Seidler is a very versatile architect, much of his work has a distinctive formal style which places him in an historical tradition of strong individual designers, both Modern and pre-Modern. As Seidler himself would argue, the style emanates from the flexible application of a set of tried and tested design principles as much as from consistent sources of aesthetic inspiration – sources which, like Gehry's designs, include baroque architecture as well as the work of modern painters and sculptors.

Architecture Project, or AP, the young Maltese group practice discussed in the last chapter, 'Mediterranean mix and match', are also a very versatile and talented firm, and in a relatively short period have covered a remarkably wide range of projects, from the rehabilitation of historic buildings to major urban redevelopment schemes. However, their versatility manifests itself in other ways than Seidler's, so that, while they too follow a consistent set of design principles – sustainability and response to place identity are top of the list – it is sometimes difficult to tell that different works are produced by the same firm.

One of the obvious reasons for the differences in their design process from Seidler's is that, as with Gehry, the Seidler practice is dominated by one strong designer – the master himself – whereas AP's designers include the four founding partners, together with key permanent staff. In this and other respects AP are closer to the Foster practice (one of their prime models), which also includes several strong designer partners such as David Nelson, Ken Shuttleworth, Spencer de Grey et al., as well as Foster himself, than to the former.

However, in addition to this relatively common organization, AP refuse to tie themselves to any single formal or technical vocabulary. Characteristically, they frequently hand design responsibility to young newcomers who demonstrate exceptional talent and commitment, eagerly assimilating new design approaches as they do so – as long as sustainability and other key principles are respected. Like Foster and other well-known cutting edge practices, they also collaborate – circumstances and budgets permitting – with top structural and environmental engineers in the UK and elsewhere from the earliest stages of the design process, taking full advantage of the Net and other computer-based communication and design systems. For example, in the case of the Malta Stock Exchange – AP's best known work to date – Brian Ford, a London-based consultant on passive energy design, was able to have a major influence on the project.

The outcome is a consistently high level of design quality and technological finesse, which belies both the limited resources of the tiny island state and the youth of the group. Aside from presenting a model of collaborative practice and sustainable design for other countries and young practices with few resources, especially in the developing world, the flexibility and diversity of AP's design approach raises important questions about the need for the kind of traditional trademark or signature style which still obsesses many architects, not to mention critics. Whilst offering ease of recognition, a personal aesthetic style can easily turn into a self-imposed prison, restricting innovations outside the parameters of the style. While Seidler and other agile designers like Ken Yeang have been able to overcome such restrictions – witness the range of both Seidler's and Yeang's work – in other cases an architect's willingness to adapt to different kinds of projects may be seriously curtailed, especially if that style or form originates in or becomes identified with a specific building type, whether it be houses or museums.

Increasingly, the unvarying, personalized style of many star architects bears all the hallmarks of a commercial marketing strategy. Indistinguishable in practise from the trademark style and image of any familiar brand name or franchise, a familiar and preferably striking architectural image guarantees public and media attention, and frequently profitability, in turn further inhibiting the architect from straying too far from the expected product. What starts out as a bold experiment in architectural form and space, may therefore all too quickly atrophy and become a repetitive and predictable 'star turn' – fondly appreciated by loyal fans, but just as much in danger of fossilization and eventual loss of interest, as any fixed repertoire.

By contrast, AP's modus operandi embodies in condensed form the variable parallel or layer-cake process of innovation and development discussed earlier with respect to cultural and technological change. Thus a change of direction by AP does not necessarily mean that previous approaches or design models are dispensed with, but rather, they may continue to be exploited and adapted for other future projects for which they are still deemed suitable, along with new ideas. As with key aspects of the Foster team's own modus operandi, which also frequently combines or alternates between radically new concepts and recycled earlier models in unpredictable ways, the skill with which AP adapt themselves to changing briefs and circumstances and their general openness to new technologies and ideas, suggests a quite different kind of organic architecture to that which is usually implied by that description. That is to say, an architecture which is based upon organic processes of self-production and adaptation to different situations – climatic, behavioural and contextual – rather than one which merely takes on the static appearance of organic life.

In many respects, therefore, this new kind of organic, or Biotech architecture, as I have called it, is more like a chameleon than a plant, and may take on quite different appearances according to the cultural and physical environment in which the designers are operating. What is consistent is the underlying process of responsive design, and the collaborative working methods and interdisciplinary skills involved. The diversification into different parallel streams also increases the possibility of cross-fertilization between new and old ideas and methods within the same practice, producing hybrid solutions in a manner analogous to the evolution and diversification of species in nature. This in turn further strengthens a practice's creative output and potential to respond to new situations, just like an evolving organism that adapts itself to a changing environment. However, instead of spreading the adaptation over several generations, the process takes place over a much shorter time span, in keeping with our own fast-moving times.

The role of computer-based technologies of communication, design, simulation, production, control and maintenance in the evolution of this new responsive and adaptable architecture is crucial. As I forecast, flexible production technologies have freed architects and other designers from the strait-jacket of standardization. However, architectural culture has changed radically from the time I first wrote about these emergent technologies, when mass production was still (mis)used by orthodox Modernists as a rationale for the propagation of standard forms – mainly for ideological and aesthetic reasons. Since the Postmodern 'liberation', a cultural climate has emerged where, for many designers, the pursuit of form for its own sake has become the main goal. Instead of the tyranny of standardization, we now have the arbitrary tyranny of idiosyncratic style – often in the guise of non-Euclidean geometries – not all that much different in many ways from the situation against which the first Modernists rebelled.

It was inevitable, therefore, that in some cases the new production technologies should be harnessed to similar goals. Gehry's own 'sculptural architecture' or 'architectural sculpture' – either description seems to apply – is of such high artistic quality that most architects and critics will argue, with good reason, that it transcends such quibbles and stands in a category all of its own. The cultural projects to which Gehry has mostly applied his extraordinary gifts are arguably also well-suited to the exploration of free form, as is his use of all available technologies towards that end. As I explain in my essay, neither does Gehry, unlike some other free form designers, neglect function or context, which his characteristic, dual-geometry planning serves well, if not for all purposes. However, as with most American practices, whether conventional or not, structural design and energy use generally get far less attention from Gehry and are treated as a consequence of the form-making process, rather than directly influencing that process, as they do in Foster's approach and that of other key European architects.

This does not mean that American architects should imitate European architects, as has happened in earlier times. Far from it. That would only reduce the diversity that is the life-blood of architecture, as it is of nature itself. However, the issue of energy conservation is now of such dire urgency that all architects – no matter what their cultural origin or their ideological or aesthetic persuasion – need to take energy efficiency on board as a priority if they are not to be accused of fiddling while the planet burns (this is no exaggeration – scientists and meteorologists warn that, if present patterns of energy use remain unchecked, the climate warming effects will inevitably make normal human life, and perhaps life itself on the planet, impossible to sustain[6]). And if that means accepting energy efficiency as a universal force to be reckoned with, no less than that of gravity, then so be it. While it may take some adjusting to, it is difficult to imagine that the architectural or cultural consequences could be negative in any way, or that designers of Gehry's calibre and inventiveness will make anything other than something new and creative out of the challenge. On the contrary, in skilled hands, the concomitant design emphasis on responding to different regional climates and day-to-day climate changes, both macro and micro, can only result in a more complex and differentiated architecture.

In sum, the full potential of digital technology will only be realized when it is used, not just for abstract or static form-making, as is the current fashion, but as an *instrument of integration* across the entire range of environmental design, production and use. It is these dynamic 'electronic ecologies', as I have described them elsewhere,[7] that will form the basis of the Biotech architecture of the future. It is not far fetched to imagine that the richest and most exciting architectural aesthetics will also be produced out of the same tools and processes.

In the appendix to this book, 'Biotech Architecture: a manifesto', I have spelt out some essential features of such an emergent design process in succinct terms intended to capture the spirit of what is as much a revolution in thought as in the technology of architectural production. Written in 1996 in two parts in support of the first Biotech Architecture Workshop, an ongoing experiment in design education briefly discussed in Chapter 3, it was first published in the following year together with a full account of the Workshop and its background.[8] It has been slightly edited and further elaborated with additional passages for this book.

As with much else in these pages, the principles in the manifesto originate in my studies of the 1960s and early 1970s in biological models of evolution and design, some of which are republished in the first collection of essays. Key design concepts underlying the manifesto, which are highlighted in this version, such as 'evolutionary planning', 'variable production' and 'integrated design', were formulated in those early writings. 'CAD + CAM = Craftsmanship', a phrase I coined in a 1986 conference paper,[9] which is also republished in the first volume, was concocted in the same vein (I have also introduced a new term, 'customized automation' in this book, which I believe more accurately describes the shift away from mass production methods than the ambiguous term 'mass customization', which is currently circulating). Subsequent experiments and writings by others – not always accompanied by due acknowledgement of what has gone before – confirm the verity of those early works and lend support to the manifesto's aims.

Related scientific and technological developments in self-producing systems, biotechnology, materials sciences, molecular engineering and nanotechnology, are now the main driving force underlying the most visionary work in architecture today. As complex and uncertain as some of these developments are, it is my belief that only by getting to grips with them and understanding and mastering their potential for good, can we ensure that the outcome will be beneficial. However, it is equally important that such interdisciplinary studies be guided by a thorough knowledge and understanding of the cultural conditions and motivations – both historical and contemporary, as well as local and global – which are shaping architecture around the world. That is a tall order, but the challenge must be met. The diversity of perspectives this book offers owes much to a consistent pursuit of this dual goal, and, while it may present a less harmonious picture of new technological and other developments than comparable works, it does so out of a profound respect for the complexity of the world in which we all finally have to live and work, and to which these technologies must be adapted.

This book can therefore be regarded as a kind of halfway house in a continuing investigation into the fundamentals underlying the changing nature of Modern architecture – a few steps on from the last collection of essays, but with some way to go yet. Indeed, it is in the nature of the enterprise that it can, of course, never be completed. Hopefully at least it will help the reader to enjoy the creative adventures described in these pages, as much as this writer does.

1

ARCHITECTURE IN THE PACIFIC CENTURY

CHANGING SCENARIOS

Given the 1997 financial crisis and its aftermath, it is sometimes hard to believe the heady optimism of the preceding years which heralded in what came to be known as the Pacific Age, or the coming Pacific Century. Such optimism was not unfounded, however, and, severe as these problems still are in some places, it is my personal belief as well as that of many other observers that they will eventually pass, possibly sooner rather than later, and that the region will yet fulfil its promise. It is worth reminding ourselves, therefore, what the original excitement was all about.[1]

Among the first to recognize the new order was the macro-historian Johan Galtung.[2] Speaking at a 1981 seminar in Penang, Malaysia, on regional development, Galtung painted a convincing picture of the relative decline of the West against the then rising economic power of Japan and the emergent 'tiger economies' of Taiwan, South Korea, Hong Kong and Singapore (Fig. 1.1). The following year, at a meeting at the East West Centre in Honolulu, Hawaii, Zenko Suzuki confidently announced:

> ... the birth of a new civilization which nurtures ideas and creativity precisely because it is so rich in diversity. This is the beginning of the Pacific Age, an age which will open the doors of the 21st century.[3]
>
> (Macintyre, 1985, p. 11)

In the same year, the British Broadcasting Company lent its own weight to the same thesis, and, looking ahead to the coming century, named it with Mary Goldring's 1982 radio series, *The People of the Pacific Century*. A BBC television series and book titled *The New Pacific*[4] followed 3 years later.

Also in 1985, William Thompson published his own related book *Pacific Shift*.[5] In it, he charted the sequential evolution of four great civilizations: Riverine

Presented to the First International Symposium on Asia Pacific Architecture, University of Hawaii at Manoa, April, 1995. Revised and first published in Pu Miao (ed.) *Public Places in Asia Pacific Cities*, Kluwer Academic Publishers, 2001.

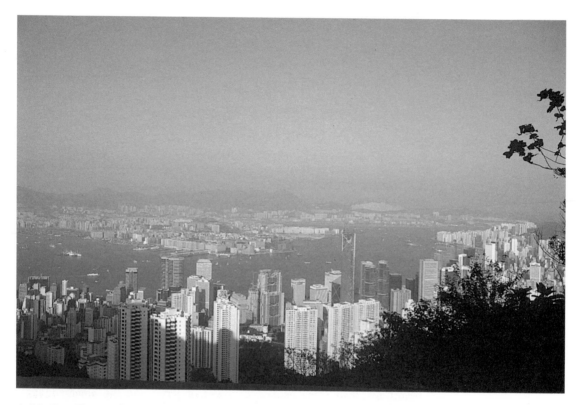

▲ **1.1** Hong Kong in 1989, at height of economic boom. View from Peak towards harbour across central business district. Photo: Author.

(meaning the early Middle Eastern civilization founded between the Tigris and Euphrates rivers); Mediterranean; Atlantic; and Pacific, each identified by a specific technological as well as geographical origin. Thompson argued that the fourth emergent civilization marks a fundamental change, not only of the main direction of North America's trade – from Europe to Asia Pacific – but also of the technological foundations of that trade, from maritime communications to air travel and electronic communications, changing with it the whole basis for cultural exchange.

By that time too, the era had also acquired its first built symbol in Norman Foster's innovative Hongkong and Shanghai Bank (Fig. 1.2). Writing on its completion in 1986, I described it as 'a building for the Pacific Century'.[6] It was the very first building of any kind to earn that description. Appropriately sited in the burgeoning city that most clearly defined the meaning of a tiger economy, the Bank encapsulated the confident, forward looking spirit of the times, and still challenges the region's architects and leaders to live up to those aspirations.

The following years brought a steady stream of eulogies on the 'Asian Miracle', and its special combination of state patronage and private enterprise. Significantly, in 1996 the UK's then Leader of the Opposition, now Prime Minister Tony Blair,

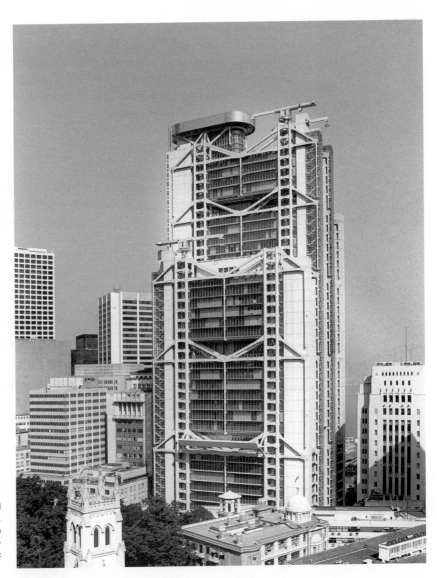

▶ **1.2** Hongkong and Shanghai Bank, Hong Kong. Norman Foster, 1979–86. An advanced technology building designed for Pacific Century. Photo: Ian Lambot.

chose Singapore as the preferred site for announcing his own newly forged and related economic policies. It seemed that, after decades if not centuries of hearing that West is best, the East was finally realizing its historical potential – at least in terms that the West could appreciate.

Recent events, fueled by problems in the Japanese economy and culminating in the continuing financial difficulties in parts of Southeast Asia, have served to qualify the heady scenario of untrammelled growth and optimism, leading many observers to wonder whether the Asian Miracle might already be at an end.[7] The xenophobic glee with which some Western commentators jumped to this conclusion probably says more about the fragility of Western egos than it does about the fragility of Asian economies. More cautious observers, pointing to the high levels of savings, investment and education in the region, argue that the same enduring factors will ensure future rapid growth, if not at the same rates as before, then at still impressive rates by Western standards. Current problems, they say, arise from questionable investments encouraged by lax lending policies, policies which can and are being changed.[8]

These more positive assessments are borne out by long-term demographic analyses which suggest that, with the notable exception of ageing Japan, the favourable balance throughout Asia Pacific of young and productive to older and non-productive populations will continue to guarantee expanding economies well into the new century.[9] Not least, there is the overwhelming role of China, whose economy continues to grow at a phenomenal rate and is predicted to overtake the US to become the largest in the world in less than two decades.[10] If for no other reason, the increasingly vital and turbulent relations between these two giants will ensure the century continues to be called after the ocean which both separates and joins them together.

ENVIRONMENTAL CONSEQUENCES

It seems reasonable to assume, therefore, that the long-term economic prospects for the region remain buoyant. Far more worrying are the present and future environmental consequences of the same impressive economic performance. And here we have to wonder just what we mean by 'success' in conventional economic and development terms. Recently, much of Southeast Asia has lain shrouded in a dense cloud of life-threatening smog, the product of a lethal mixture of forest fires and urban pollution (Fig. 1.3). The fires, which were deliberately started by logging

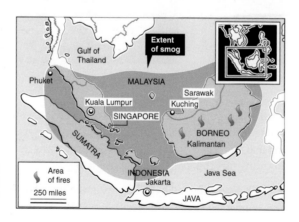

▶ **1.3** Map of Southeast Asia showing extent of forest fires in summer, 1994. *Source: Guardian Weekly.*

and plantation companies as part of their normal 'slash and burn' practices,[11] were mainly located in Indonesian Sumatra and Borneo and spread over a total area of 600 000 hectares, or 1.5 million acres – an area roughly equivalent to the entire Malaysian Peninsula. Aside from the ecological disaster, the after-effects of smoke from the fires, coupled in cities like Kuala Lumpur and Jakarta with already high levels of airborne traffic pollution, is likely to affect human health and economic patterns in the region for years to come.[12]

Extraordinary as the scale of the disaster is, it was easily predicted. From 1982 to 1983, similar fires in Indonesia consumed over 3.5 million hectares of forest in the state of Kalimantan.[13] Some years ago on a visit to Kuala Lumpur I witnessed the disastrous effect of further Indonesian fires on that city's air quality. Then as now, the fires were the direct result of the same short-sighted industrial and agricultural practices. Then as now, although the corporations concerned – usually joint ventures between Indonesian and other Southeast Asian companies – were reprimanded, no serious actions were taken against them.[14]

Environmental disasters are not of course unique to Asia Pacific and it is understandable if Asian leaders, as they have done, should accuse Western leaders and environmentalists of hypocrisy when they come under criticism for such events – especially when such criticism emanates from countries which import the products of the same devastated forests.[15] It is understandable perhaps to react in this way, but it is not a sufficient reason for *not* taking action to prevent events which clearly have such self-destructive consequences.

Paradoxically, the root cause of this and similar environmental disasters is more likely to be found in the cosy alliance between state patronage and private interests which typifies business patterns in Asia Pacific and which has been generally credited with the region's economic success. Often linked by regional leaders with 'Asian values', the same centralized and patriarchal system which can muster and direct enormous resources effectively toward the improvement of mass education or housing, is equally prone to corruption and environmental abuses. Such deficiencies, which may be overlooked in the early and more manageable stages of development, are only likely to worsen as privileged individuals and sectors grow more powerful and continue to abuse their powers on an ever larger scale.[16]

WHAT KIND OF ERA?

Such matters raise serious questions concerning the meaning of the Pacific Century, and what kind of architecture might be appropriate to it. Are we to evaluate the era and to measure the cultural dominance of the peoples in the region by economic criteria alone? In which case it is fair to assume that constructing the tallest building in the world, as Malaysia has done with the Petronas Towers (Fig. 1.4) and China is now doing with the World Financial Centre in

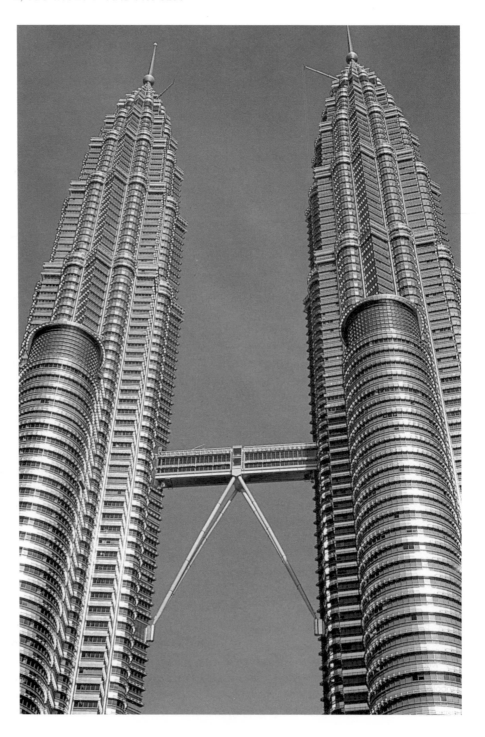

Shanghai,[17] is an appropriate goal and form of expression for an era defined by rising gross national products.[18] Or does it stand for something more complex than that, possibly a different form of world culture and development altogether, as Thompson argues in *Pacific Shift*, based on new technologies, values and culture forms?

It is tempting to think that the present environmental disaster might finally jolt regional leaders into taking action and introducing reforms, and that a whole new culture based on ecological values might arise, phoenix-like, out of the ashes of the Indonesian fires. The recent extraordinary political events in Indonesia are themselves some cause for optimism. But while we can at least hope that some lessons might be learnt, it is improbable that things will ever come down to any simple choice between one model of development rather than another.

History suggests that it could hardly be otherwise. It is a common error, repeated by Thompson to some extent, to believe that the story of humankind is composed of apocalyptic cultural shifts, each of which creates an entirely new set of values and lifestyles with few connections with the past. But human development just does not work like that. What actually happens is that new forms of culture and ways of life become superimposed over older forms, with both coexisting over considerable periods of time, a process which eventually leaves neither unchanged and produces still further variations out of the resultant interactions. It is this infinitely more complex, unpredictable and challenging world which in reality we have to deal with.

PARALLEL DEVELOPMENT

I shall call this complex pattern of human evolution by the name, 'parallel development,' by which I mean the concurrent linkage and overlapping of different forms of development and lifestyles. It is this very difference between the forms of development involved and their complex interrelations which makes the future course of developing countries, around the Pacific and elsewhere, so hard to predict, and also, potentially so creative.[19]

There are any number of possible descriptions of the economic and cultural patterns which typify parallel development. For the sake of clarity I have listed the more vital patterns in the accompanying table under four primary forms of culture: 'traditional culture'; 'colonial culture'; 'consumer culture'; and 'eco-culture'[20] (Table 1.1). Each culture is further broken down into nine common categories, from 'technological era' through to the settlement patterns and built forms which characterize them, by which their similarities and differences may be compared. However, unlike Thompson's four civilizations, my four cultures are not geographically specific; neither, though they also originated at different periods, are they otherwise necessarily separated by time. On the contrary,

◀ 1.4 Petronas Towers, Kuala Lumpur, Malaysia. Cesar Pelli, 1994–8. The first buildings outside West to claim title of world's tallest, the twin towers symbolize growing economic power and aspirations of East Asians. Photo: Author.

Table 1.1 Comparative features of four primary cultures

	Traditional Culture	**Colonial Culture**	**Consumer Culture**	**Eco-culture**
Technological era	Pre-industrial (craft-based)	Early industrial (machine-based)	Late industrial (automation- and information-based)	Post-industrial (computer- and network-based)
Cultural differentiation	Homogeneous (highly integrated and localized)	Heterogeneous (exposure to secondary cultures)	Homogeneous (West is best)	Heterogeneous (based on reciprocal cultural exchanges)
External communication	Limited and slow (local trade and migrations)	Global but slow (sea and overland)	Global and speedy (air and telecommunications)	Global and instantaneous (near universal network access)
Level of innovation	Tradition governs all (rate of change difficult to record)	Sporadic leaps (when officially sanctioned)	Continuous but centralized (concentration of research and benefits in North)	Continuous and decentralized (global dissemination of research and benefits)
Social roles	Specialized and stable (life-long)	Specialized but changeable (promotion/ overseas postings, etc.)	Specialized but changeable (promotion, redundancy/ retraining, etc.)	Multiple roles based on changing skills and continuous education/training
Decision structures	Generally hierarchic and patriarchic, with notable exceptions (i.e. Malay peasant society)	Hierarchic and patriarchic (dependent relations between colonies and metropolitan centre)	Corporate and patriarchic (modified by democratic and market-led systems) dominated by short-term goals	Participatory, with mix of global and local 'bottom up' structures, based on gender equality and sustainable goals
Production systems	Autonomous, self-sufficient (small surplus) and labour intensive	Centralized (large surplus for export) with both capital and labour-intensive sectors	Centralized mass-production (capital and energy intensive) for mass-consumption	Decentralized, flexible manufacturing systems (intermediate to advanced technologies)
Settlement patterns	Rural and village-based	Urban and rural (sharp differentiation between cities and country)	Predominantly urban or suburban in the North and urban/rural in the South	Predominantly urban or 'ex-urban' based on balanced public/private transportation
Built forms	Isomorphic with social form and climate	Mix of functional and hybrid forms (products of cultural exchange) partly shaped by climate	Ambiguous/ flexible forms independent of climate	Customized for place, purpose and climate

Source: C. Abel, 1997.

I would go so far as to say that, particularly in Asia Pacific and other non-Western regions where development has been tightly compressed over the last century, it is hard to find any large settlement where one cannot find elements of all four cultures overlapping in one form or another.

Architecture provides vivid evidence of this coexistence in time of different cultural realms (Fig. 1.5). The reason lies in the enduring physical and spatial nature of architecture itself and of the settlement patterns of which it is composed, which not only frequently outlast the original culture which produced them, but also provide tangible meeting points between new and old cultures and the lifestyles which go with them. Thus we find much of the population of Asia Pacific still living in rural conditions and *kampong*-type settlements and houses (Fig. 1.6), but who may travel by motorcycle, bus or automobile to work in a nearby town or city, possibly founded and shaped by European colonists. There

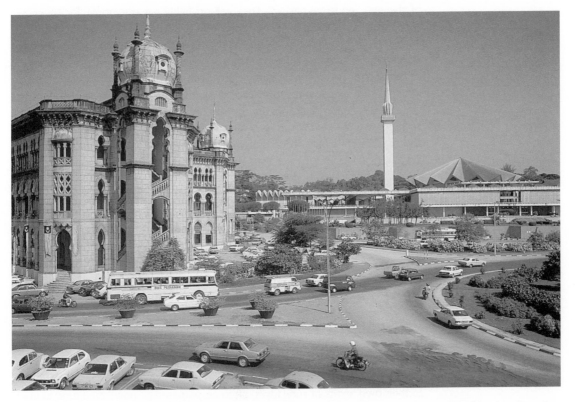

▲ **1.5** Colonial era architecture of different periods and styles representing changing values in Kuala Lumpur, Malaysia. Former Malayan Railway Administration Headquarters, 1917, by A.B. Hubbock (foreground), and the National Mosque, 1956, by the Public Works Department (background). Photo: Author.

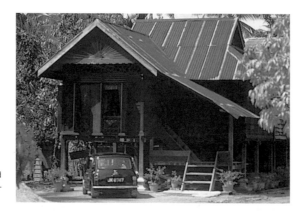

▶ **1.6** Parallel cultures and lifestyles in Malaysian *kampong*. Photo: Author.

they might toil on office computers, or even help to build similar machines in one of the new industrial parks.[21] They will probably eat traditional, locally grown produce at home most of the week, or else go to one of the lively open-air eating places which typify the region, alternating with an occasional visit uptown to a McDonald's or some other Western-style fast food chain. The same fast food chain might be located in a brand new department store, which may itself be situated in one of the older districts, surrounded by a mixture of shop houses, colonial-style public buildings and brash new offices. Younger tigers will almost certainly use the occasion to browse through the rest of the department store, and maybe buy a pair of jeans. If they live close enough to an urban centre to get a late bus home or have their own transport they may also take in a cinema or a disco. A few – just a few – might even work for one of the non-governmental organizations or NGOs, such as the Consumers' Association of Penang,[22] which have sprung up all over the region, and help to monitor the environmental abuses and other dangers of a consumer society in the making. They may be motivated to work there by a wholly different set of ecological and economic values, but they will probably travel to work the same way as the others, eat, shop, dress and relax the same way, and generally live similar lifestyles to the people whose environment they are working to protect.

DECENTRALIZATION

It would be a mistake to scoff at this sort of thing and to chide young Asians for enjoying the same things Westerners have enjoyed for so long, or to lament the loss of a more pure and tranquil way of *kampong* life. Westerners also still cling to their own myths of rural idylls, often perpetuated by popular culture, as in TV soaps like 'The Little House on the Prairie'. Yet the very distinctions between urban and rural life that help to maintain the same mythologies are becoming increasingly blurred and harder to define. While villagers now often share in an urban culture, former city dwellers seeking relief from the stresses and strains of urban life are moving in the opposite direction. Low-density, dispersed settlement patterns have long been the norm for the automobile owning populations of the American Pacific West, as well as Australia, and they are now the favoured pattern for the more affluent sectors of Asia Pacific. The basic similarity between the traditional timber-framed dwellings of the Pacific Rim and the detached, timber-framed dwellings common to modern Californian and Australian suburbs – and now also to the fringes of Asian cities – also helps to blur any physical distinctions between ex-urban and rural settlements[23] (Figs 1.7 and 1.8).

New technologies and decentralized patterns of production and consumption are reinforcing the same trend, making it possible to live and work in smaller communities and at the same time to communicate more easily over large distances.[24] In the process, new building types have acquired functions formerly associated with older building types and settlement patterns, further confusing

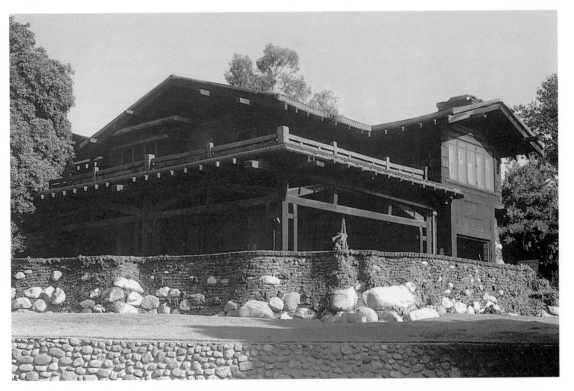

▲ **1.7** Irwin House, Pasadena, California, USA. Green and Green, 1906. The architects' residential architecture incorporates Japanese as well as Californian elements. Photo: Author.

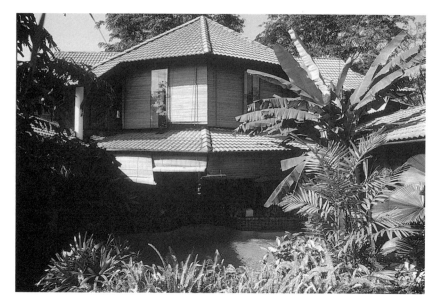

▶ **1.8** Precima House, Kuala Lumpur, Malaysia. Jimmy Lim, 1987–9. Lim's suburban house designs are strongly influenced by regional archetypes and techniques of climate control. Photo: Author.

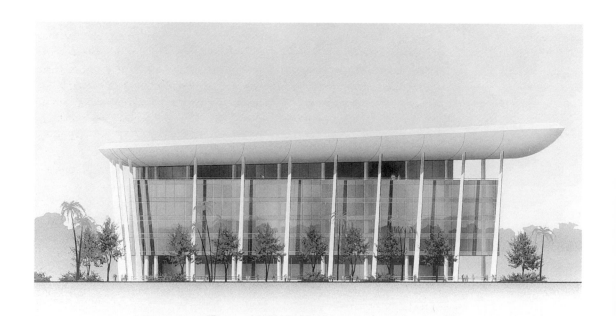

▲ **1.9** Securities Commission Building, Kuala Lumpur, Malaysia. Rendering. Dominant roof canopy is reinterpretation of traditional building forms. The building also incorporates numerous energy-saving features designed for tropical climate. Hijjas Kasturi, 1995–9. *Source*: Hijjas Kasturi Associates.

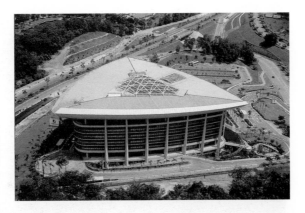

▶ **1.10** Securities Commission Building. Sited next to major highway on outskirts of Kuala Lumpur, the financial centre is situated close to numerous leisure amenities. Photo: K.L. Ng.

previously assumed distinctions and categories. Out-of-town shopping centres now substitute in part for community centres and include a wide range of public attractions and amenities associated with urban life. Firms relocating to the edge of the city or even further out also frequently provide leisure amenities and other attractions in order to lure employees away from the city (Figs 1.9 and 1.10). Industrial parks, office parks and science parks are all the product of similar needs, providing shared amenities and security.

Other new urban patterns are emerging as countries shift larger shares of their economies toward value-added, high-tech industries. Airports, for example, are rapidly assuming the role formerly assigned to seaports, railway lines and roadways, as major focal points for production and distribution, drawing factories, services and workers away from cities centred on the former into more remote areas to create whole new ex-urban settlements. Stretching between Kuala Lumpur and the new International Airport (KLIA) (Fig. 1.11) 50 kilometres south and taking in the new administrative capital at Petrajaya, Malaysia's planned 'Multi-media Supercorridor' is conceived as a low-rise garden 'cybercity,' or *cyberjaya*, complete with dispersed workplaces and residences all fully 'wired' for the computer age.[25] Similar projects, such as the new airport and high-tech industrial complex near Bangkok, are either on the drawing board or already under construction. Despite the recent economic setbacks, which may at most delay their completion, it seems likely that such projects will set the model for dispersed settlement patterns well into the new century.[26]

CONSTELLATIONS

The social and cultural implications of these developments and their effects on local and regional identities are hotly debated. Architects and planners in the region, many of whom remain wedded to Eurocentric notions of city form and space, are often reluctant to accept such changes, and, not without reason, fear the

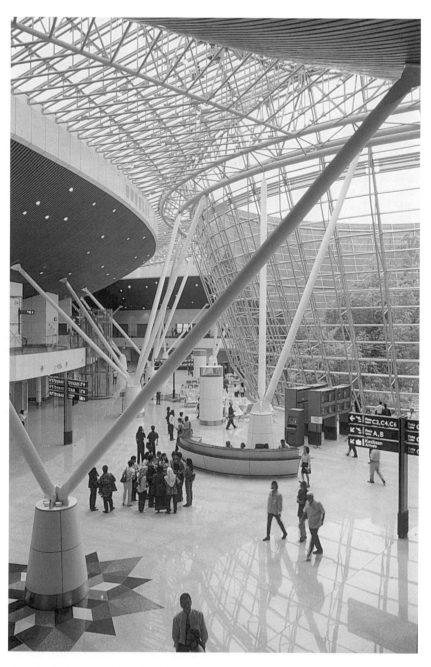

▲ **1.11** Kuala Lumpur International Airport, Sepang, Malaysia. Interior of satellite. Kisho Kurokawa and Akitek Jururancang (Malaysia), with Hijjas Kasturi, 1995–7. Each satellite incorporates a tropical garden in its centre. Photo: Author.

loss of any clearly defined urban realm or place.[27] Thus some avant-garde urban projects emanating out of Southeast Asia, like Tay Kheng Soon's projects for an 'Intelligent Tropical City' in Singapore, or Giga World (Figs 1.12 and 1.13), the 'linear city' planned for Kuala Lumpur,[28] are curiously reminiscent of earlier 'mega-structure' projects from Archigram and other European designers of the 1960s.[29]

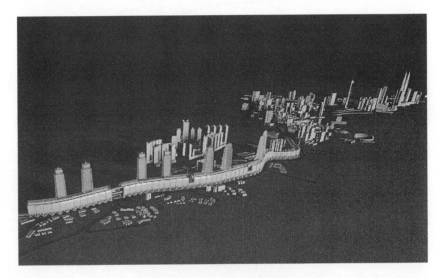

▲ **1.12** Giga World, Kuala Lumpur, Malaysia. Aerial perspective. Original Scope with KL Linear City, 1996. Project combines residential and commercial buildings together with transportation systems in linear structure running through centre of city. The structure passes over River Klang for much of its length. *Source*: Original Scope.

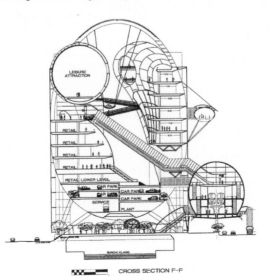

▶ **1.13** Giga World. Section over River Klang showing parallel metro system. *Source*: Original Scope.

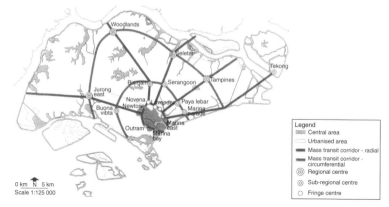

▶ **1.14** Decentralization in Singapore. Expansion is concentrated around decentralized commercial centers along mass rapid transit (MRT) routes. *Source*: Urban Redevelopment Authority, 1991.

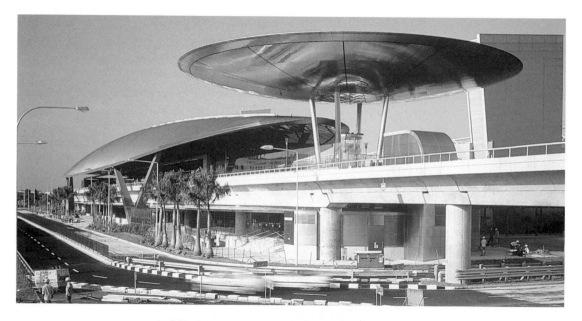

▲ **1.15** Expo Station, Singapore. Norman Foster, 1997–2001. A recent addition to Singapore's extensive metro system. Photo: Richard Bryant.

Looking at these dense urban forms, usually composed of large blocks many stories high, I wonder just how 'tropical' such projects really are. The ideal settlement pattern for the hot humid climate of the tropics remains that of the *kampong*, with its loose sprinkling of detached and raised dwellings maximizing the effect of the slightest precious air movement. Modern dispersed suburbs and garden city projects which create similar patterns, make equally good climatic sense. For the same reason, closely packed blocks on the European model, which evolved in temperate climates, do not, no matter how much greenery might be draped over them.

The problem is that modern, low-density settlements, despite their obvious popularity, gobble up too much land and may only add to the pressures for deforestation. Such effects may be reduced to some extent by careful planning. As much as a third of the total land area to be taken up by the Multi-media Supercorridor will be given over to large tracts of green, including untouched forest and lakes. Better still, both land use and overall dependency on the automobile may be greatly diminished by concentrating mixed-density new towns along mass rapid transit (MRT) lines in 'strings of beads' fashion after the Singapore model (Figs 1.14 and 1.15). Backed up by 'bus and ride' as well as 'park and ride' systems, such 'constellations' of new towns and small cities provide a promising model for sustainable urban development.[30] Advances in 'clean' engine technologies such as the new hybrid gas and electric powered vehicles coming onto the market, could also eventually help reduce pollution still further to sustainable levels.[31]

DISPERSED HIGH-RISE

However, the debate between high-density concentrated city and low-density garden city – both Western concepts in origin – may ultimately be misleading. The

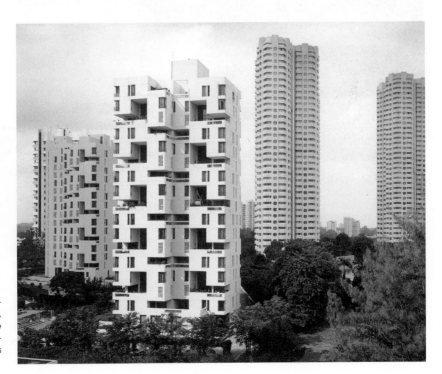

▶ **1.16** Ardmore Condominium, Singapore. Moshe Safdi, 1984. Pioneering high-rise design features two-storey skycourts, one of earliest of its type. Photo: Cymie Payne.

▶ **1.17** Abelia Condominium, Singapore. Tang Guan Bee, 1990–4. Like Safdi building, each maisonette is planned around two-storey open-air living space. Photo: Tangguanbee.

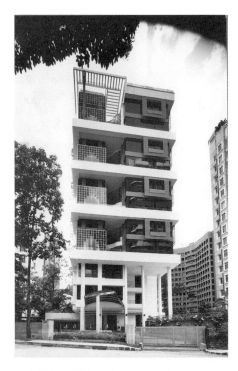

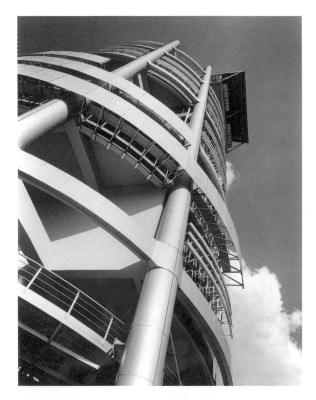

▲ **1.18** Mesiniaga Headquarters, Kuala Lumpur, Malaysia. Hamzah and Yeang, 1989–92. Definitive early example of architects' 'bioclimatic skyscraper' concept. The building incorporates open-air skygardens and climate control techniques based on regional traditions. Photo: Hamzah and Yeang.

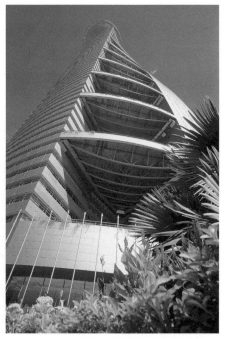

▶ **1.19** Telekom Headquarters. Detail of spiraling skygardens showing steel supports. Photo: H. Lin Ho.

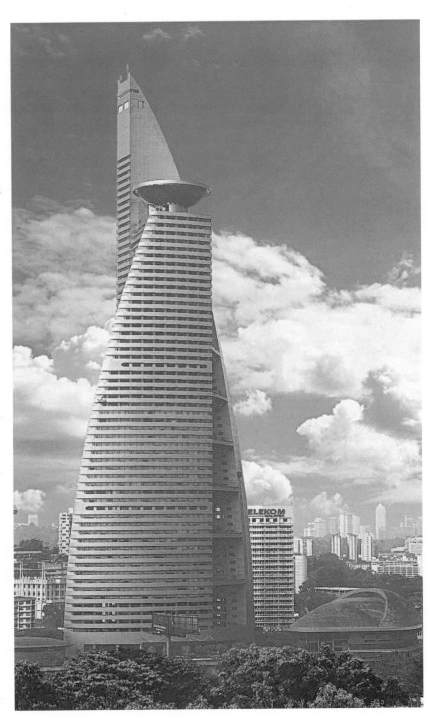

▶ **1.20** Telekom Headquarters, near Kuala Lumpur, Malaysia. General view with central Kuala Lumpur in the distant background. Hijjas Kasturi, 1997–2002. Photo: H. Lin Ho.

urban settlement pattern which characterizes the exploding megacities of Asia Pacific is most accurately described as 'dispersed high-rise', and fits into neither of the previous categories but has its own imperatives and typical built forms, best dealt with in their own terms.[32] Combining the advantages of lower transportation costs, mixed social groups, greater amenities and the stronger place identity that separate high-rise clusters can generate, with the closeness to nature and openness to air movements that dispersal affords, the dispersed high-rise city offers a workable compromise, if not the best of both worlds. Widely spaced 'islands' of high-rise structures separated by green areas also have the virtue of minimizing the 'heat-sink' effect (a rise in external temperatures caused by the excess heat radiating from building structures and services) associated with continuously built-up areas, which can result in increases in the temperature of urban micro-climates of several degrees over that of rural areas.[33]

Seen in this light, the tower type, long identified with central business districts and high-density cities, may be due for a new lease of life as an ex-urban, as well as an urban building form. Appropriate residential models can already be found in Southeast Asia, such as the slim point blocks in Singapore designed by Moshe Safdi (Fig. 1.16) and Paul Rudolf in the 1980s, and in the smaller and more recent Abelia Condominium by Tan Guan Bee[34] (Fig. 1.17). Similar models have been developed for commercial uses, and not only in city centres. The 'bio-climatic skyscraper' designed by Ken Yeang[35] for the Mesiniaga Headquarters (Fig. 1.18) and the Telekom Headquarters by Hijjas Kasturi (Figs 1.19 and 1.20), both near Kuala Lumpur, are situated well outside the city, creating their own unique focal points in an otherwise undistinguished ex-urban landscape. The latter tower especially, with its enormous podium constructed like an artificial hill and containing various cultural amenities, constitutes virtually an urban node in itself. All of these tall buildings, both residential and commercial, have heavily indented forms, 'skycourts' and other shared features shaped by the local climate which clearly distinguish them from their universal counterparts.[36]

CATERPILLARS AND CRABS

Yet for all their innovations and regional attributes, the corporate ambitions and market forces behind such works are no less strong than the climatic criteria which shaped them in such unusual ways. Each building straddles at least two cultures, consumer and ecological, urban and ex-urban, in ways that defy former architectural stereotypes. It may well be just this sort of creative compromise, rather than any wholesale dumping of consumer culture in favour of a completely new way of life, which may eventually provide the solutions to the sorts of environmental problems we see all around the Pacific Rim and elsewhere.

The emergence of new cultures and lifestyles does not therefore mean that we shall automatically shed all of our former ways, as we sometimes fancy, like a butterfly sheds its former self to re-emerge in an entirely new life-form. This is just as well. If the last century has taught us anything, it is that revolutionary change of this sort is just as likely to sweep away the good as it is the bad. But we are not caterpillars, waiting to be reborn in a new guise. We are much more like crabs, still pretty much earth bound and clinging to our familiar shells, moving sideways as much as forwards, and not changing so much during our life span that we cannot still recognize ourselves for who we are, and where we came from.

Whatever shape it eventually takes, the Pacific Century will most likely emerge as a composite of all four cultures, a different composite from other parts of the world perhaps, which have different traditions, different colonial histories, different consumer habits and different ecologies, but a composite nevertheless. More like the sum of many different and competing forces, the Pacific Century is an evolving cultural concept with no specific beginning – unless one wants to credit the BBC – and without any specific destination or goal, as likely as not to change direction just as soon as we think we know in which way it is going to evolve.

We should not therefore expect consumer culture to be entirely displaced by eco-culture, any more than its predecessors have been displaced by succeeding cultures.[37] But though eco-culture may not replace consumerism, or the market mechanisms which underpin that culture, we can nevertheless hope realistically for a more positive impact on those same mechanisms. This is already happening in the case of the new 'green economics' which reckon in the cost of waste and pollution, and associated consumer movements which discriminate in favour of vetted products and sources of materials.[38] It is likely to grow in strength as new legislation on climate control and energy conservation comes into place, most probably in the form of energy taxes and market incentives designed to modify existing market forces and to encourage the development and use of sustainable technologies.[39] Pressure to adopt these measures will also probably come from opposite directions: top down, from international agencies and conventions, and bottom up, from local environmental groups and other NGOs agitating for ever more effective measures and results.[40] How national leaders in the region respond to these new pressures, whether they continue to resist them as most do now in favour of present interests, or whether they adapt themselves to the new situation, will be one of the factors which will determine the ultimate balance of cultures.

VIBRANT MIXTURE

Likewise, we can expect the architecture that emerges from this pot-pourri of technologies, values and practices, to be equally varied. No doubt we shall see more towering examples of Postmodern consumerist architecture like the Petronas Towers – what I call the 'architecture of self-advertisement' – together with their smaller domestic equivalents in the more flamboyant suburban villas. International architectural fashion, for better or worse, may also be expected to

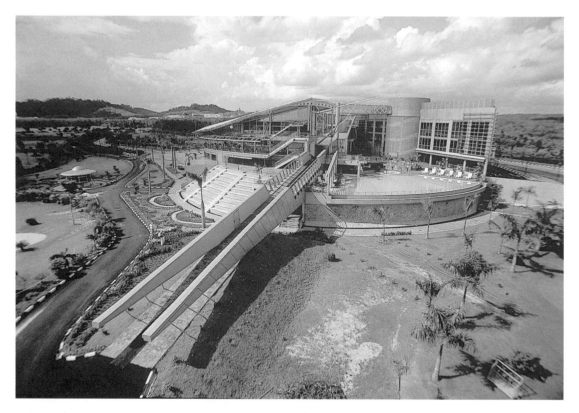

▲ **1.21** Octville Sri Alam Golf and Country Club, Johore Bahru, Malaysia. Akitek Tenggara, 1989–92. Neo-constructivist composition of clashing geometries and intersecting planes. Design also incorporates passive techniques of climate control. Photo: Robert Lam.

continue playing a role in shaping the education, attitudes and creations of regional architects. However, we may also expect to see more of the kind of architecture described above: practical products of ecological as well as commercial imperatives and architectural fashions, supported by effective legislation to save energy and reduce pollution (Fig. 1.21). At the very least, it would be good to think that at some not too distant point in the future we shall be able to gaze out upon this vibrant mixture through clear skies.

2

Cyberspace in mind

Metaphorical extensions

Ever since the Internet evolved from a restricted military and academic communications system to become part of the public domain, efforts have been made to make more tangible and comprehensible one of the most important but ephemeral creations in the history of science and technology.

Significantly, in explaining the impact of the Net on our lives and consciousness, not only architects and urbanists, but also writers from other disciplines commonly resort to metaphors deeply rooted in the physical and spatial world of cities and urban communities, as well as to other analogies with familiar cultural and social concepts. Even when the most fervent devotees of the Net – including many science fiction writers such as William Gibson,[1] who is frequently quoted by other writers in the passages that follow – argue that it opens up entirely new possibilities in the human–machine interface, they frequently resort to well-known and often antiquated concepts of mind and body.

What all these efforts demonstrate is that, as with the birth of any radically new idea, in order to visualize that idea and to make it meaningful, its creators are necessarily obliged to make at least some connections with existing ideas and ways of thinking – seeing the new in terms of the old, as it has been described.[2] To a large extent, therefore, the Net and the ideas and language which are used to describe, explain and promote it, can be interpreted as a series of metaphorical extensions of mind and body, and the ideas, both ancient and modern, we have about them and their interrelations.

The topology of cyberspace

Virtual cities

As one of the best known architectural writers on the subject, William Mitchell's work provides plentiful examples of such linguistic crossovers. In the following passage from *City of Bits*, Mitchell[3] stresses the differences between the Net and anything we have known before. Yet to do so he is nevertheless compelled to

---

Presented under the title, 'Space, place and the Net: metaphorical extensions of mind and body', to the Design Research Society, Design Dialogues 2: A Meeting of Metaphors, University College London, 15 May, 1996.

describe these differences in terms already familiar to us:

> *The Net negates geometry. While it does have a definite topology of computational nodes and radiating boulevards of bits, and while the locations of the nodes and links can be plotted on plans to produce surprisingly Haussmann-like diagrams, it is fundamentally and profoundly antispatial. It is nothing like the Piazza Navona or Copley Square. You cannot say where it is or describe its memorable space and proportions or tell a stranger how to get there. But you can find things in it without knowing where they are. The Net is ambiant – nowhere in particular but everywhere at once.*[4]

(Mitchell, 1995, p. 8)

Later in the same book, however, he also stresses the similarities between the Net and familiar concepts of urban form and life, again using common language. As a result, he encourages us to appropriate the new territory in terms of what is already known to us, and at the same time these familar ideas appear to us in a fresh light, seen now, as it were, from out of cyberspace. As in the first passage, Mitchell returns to his favourite Western urban models for comparison:

> *The story of virtual communities, so far, is that of urban history replayed in fast forward – but with computer resource use playing the part of land use, and network navigation systems standing in for streets and transportation systems. The WELL, the World Wide Web, MUDs, and Free Nets are – like Hippodamos's gridded layout for Miletos, Baron Haussmann's radial patterning of Paris, or Daniel Burnham's grand plan for Chicago – large scale structures of places and connections organized to meet the needs of their inhabitants.*
>
> *And the parallels don't stop there. As traditional cities have evolved, so have customs, norms, and laws governing the rights to privacy, access to public and semipublic spaces, what can be done where, and exertion of control. The organization of built space into public-to-private hierarchies, with gates and doors to control boundary crossings, has reflected this. Nolli's famous map of Rome vividly depicted it. Now, as cyberspace cities emerge, a similar framework of distinctions and expectations is – with much argument – being constructed, and electronic plazas, forums, lobbies, walls, doors, locks, members-only clubs, and private rooms are being invented and deployed. Perhaps some electronic cartographer of the future will produce an appropriately nuanced Nolli map of the Net.*[5]

(Mitchell, 1995, p. 131)

Baroque models

What is most striking about these passages, are Mitchell's repeated references, aside from Nolli's quite different map of Rome, to baroque space concepts (Haussmann's Paris) and regular geometric grids (Hippodamos's Miletos; Burnham's Chicago) in trying to visualize and communicate the topology of cyberspace (Figs 2.1, 2.2 and 2.3). Thus, 'radiating boulevards', 'gridded layout',

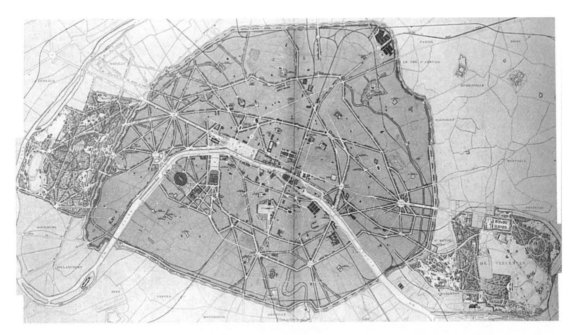

▲ **2.1** Plan for Paris, France. Baron Georges Haussmann, as presented by Jean Alphand, *c.*1867. Plan. *Source*: F. Choay, 1969.

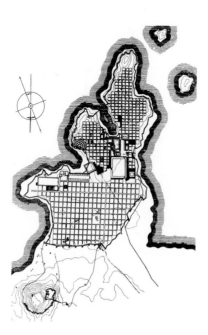

▶ **2.2** Miletos, Greece. Plan, after Hippodamus, *c.*466 BC. Plan. *Source*: J.B. Ward-Perkins, 1974.

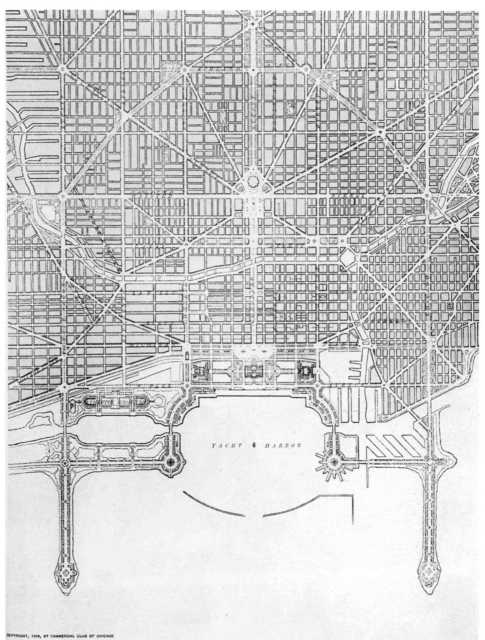

CX.   CHICAGO.   PLAN OF THE COMPLETE SYSTEM OF STREET CIRCULATION; RAILWAY STATIONS; PARKS, BOULEVARD
CIRCUITS AND RADIAL ARTERIES; PUBLIC RECREATION PIERS, YACHT HARBOR, AND PLEASURE-BOAT PIERS; TREATMENT
OF GRANT PARK; THE MAIN AXIS AND THE CIVIC CENTER, PRESENTING THE CITY AS A COMPLETE ORGANISM IN WHICH
ALL ITS FUNCTIONS ARE RELATED ONE TO ANOTHER IN SUCH A MANNER THAT IT WILL BECOME A UNIT.

▲ **2.3**   Plan for Chicago, USA. Daniel Burnham, 1909. Plan. *Source*: F. Choay, 1969.

'grand plan', 'large-scale structures of places and connections organized to meet the needs of their inhabitants', are all metaphors borrowed from common urbanists' parlance, with a definite leaning toward conventional Western spatial concepts and systems of order.

Neither is Mitchell alone in using baroque concepts in trying to represent cyberspace. At the height of Net fever and in the same year as Mitchell published his *City of Bits, Time* magazine ran a special issue, *'Welcome to Cyberspace'*,[6] the front cover of which depicted a series of computer chips with 'doorways' cut into their centres, receding into infinity (Fig. 2.4). With the name 'Time' inscribed over each opening to give added depth, the lazer straight series of openings exactly represents, not cyberspace perhaps, but the classic enfilade of baroque architecture (Fig. 2.5), or more precisely: 'The French system of aligning internal doors in a sequence so that a vista is obtained through a series of rooms when all the doors are open'.[7]

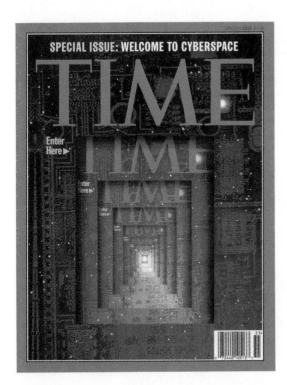

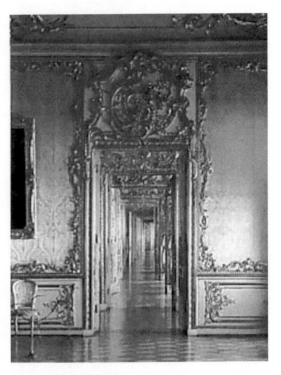

▲ **2.4** *Time* magazine cover. Cover design for special issue on cyberspace resembles baroque enfilade. *Source: Time,* spring 1995.

▲ **2.5** 'Golden Enfilade' Catherine Palace (Great Tzarskoje Selo Palace), St Petersburg, Russia. Bartolomeo Francesco Rastrelli, 1748–56. Photo: Catherine Palace Museum.

Nevertheless, when Mitchell reaches for an appropriate graphical analogy for the topology of cyberspace, he passes over his baroque examples and instead chooses the aforementioned Nolli's map of Rome (Fig. 2.6), comparing it with an Apple cartoon illustrating a range of virtual building sites on the Net (Fig. 2.7). With its less predictable and greater choice of pathways between nodes, the image of Nolli's map captures at least some of those more elusive aspects of cyberspace that Mitchell alludes to.

Cyberspace as movement space

However, if there is an appropriate spatial metaphor for visualizing the topology of the Net it might be found, not in Western, but in Eastern culture.

According to Mitsuo Inoue,[8] Japanese space concepts differ fundamentally from Western concepts at all scales of architectural and urban design. Japanese architectural space, he argues, is 'movement-oriented', while Western architectural

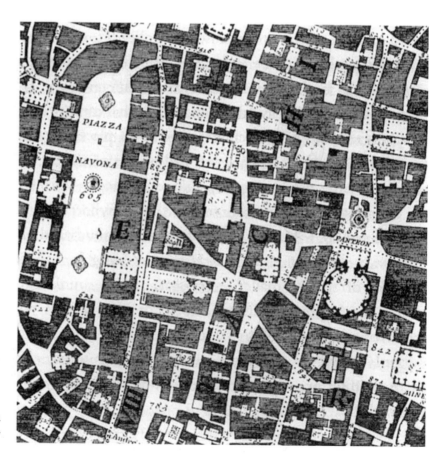

▶ **2.6** Map of Rome, Italy. Giambattista Nolli, 1748. *Source*: W.J. Mitchell, 1995.

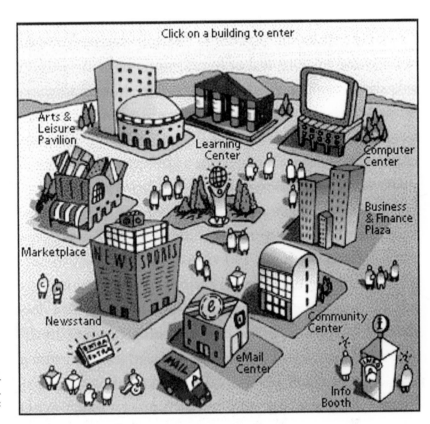

Click on a building to enter

Arts & Leisure Pavilion

Learning Center

Computer Center

Business & Finance Plaza

Marketplace

Newsstand

eMail Center

Community Center

Info Booth

▶ **2.7** Places to visit in cyber-space, as depicted by Apple. Computer image. *Source:* W.J. Mitchell, 1995.

space, together with that of classical Chinese architecture, is predominantly geo-metrical in character. As extreme examples of the latter, he offers both the orthogonal, or rectilinear layout of the Forbidden City in Peking (Fig. 2.8), and the radially planned palace and city of eighteenth-century Karlsruhe (Fig. 2.9). Whether based on orthogonal coordinates, as with the Forbidden City, or polar coordinates, as with Karlsruhe, it is characteristic of geometric space that the location of each and every element within the plan is determined by its relation to the central axis or pole.

Similarly, the key to experiencing geometrical design lies in the relationship of the observer to the same central axis or pole, which he or she must be able to locate in order to assimilate the rest of the composition. Lengthy vistas opened up through the area, and sometimes through individual structures, therefore ensure that a person standing at key points and junctures may easily comprehend the whole. Hence the predominant part played in baroque architecture and urban planning, as in classical Chinese palaces and cities, by open prospects, long

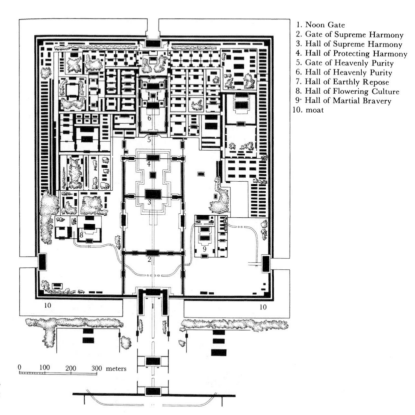

1. Noon Gate
2. Gate of Supreme Harmony
3. Hall of Supreme Harmony
4. Hall of Protecting Harmony
5. Gate of Heavenly Purity
6. Hall of Heavenly Purity
7. Hall of Earthly Repose
8. Hall of Flowering Culture
9· Hall of Martial Bravery
10. moat

▶ **2.8** Forbidden City, Peking, China, 1406–. Plan. *Source*: M. Inoue, 1985.

straight roads and large squares. The same discipline governs the relation of interior spaces to one another in Chinese palaces and Inoue explicitly cites the baroque enfilade as a characteristic example of a similar organization of space.

By contrast, the relationship of the observer to the elements of a Japanese design is of a wholly different nature. Whilst early palace architecture and urban design was strongly influenced by classical Chinese geometric planning, by the seventeenth century Japanese architecture and landscape design evolved its own quite distinct planning systems and spatial order. By comparison with the above examples, the highly irregular plan of the Hommaru Palace compound at Edo Castle exhibits no visible order at all (Fig. 2.10). It has no single centre or axis, nor any other obvious unifying space or element, aside from the massive boundary walls, which have a different configuration, shaped by topography.

However, Inoue explains, the apparent irregularity and indeterminacy of the plan at Edo is no accident, but arises from a highly complex and consciously designed sequence of spaces through the Palace, as seen through the eye of a moving

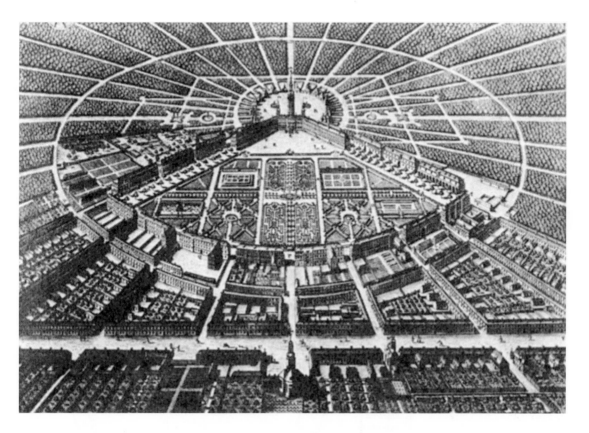

▲ **2.9** Eighteenth-century Karlsruhe, Germany. Engraving. *Source*: M. Inoue, 1985.

observer. Against the baroque designer's aim of opening up as much of a building or city as possible to a stationary observer standing at some central point, the Japanese designer purposefully and subtly conceals the nature of an adjacent element or space from the eye – often offering only a partial and tantalizing glimpse of what comes next – so that only by moving through and personally exploring each space in turn, can the whole building or complex be properly understood.

To illustrate the essential features of movement space, Inoue offers two simple but telling diagrams (Figs. 2.11a and b). The first shows a number of nodes labelled in alphabetical order representing spatial units connected by single lines in an orthogonal pattern, while the second shows the same nodes connected in an irregular pattern. Inoue asks us to think of these units, which might be rooms or external spaces or both, in isolation from any other spaces or surrounding context. A person standing in one of the nodes in the first, regular sequence, he suggests, would stand in exactly the same relationship to the

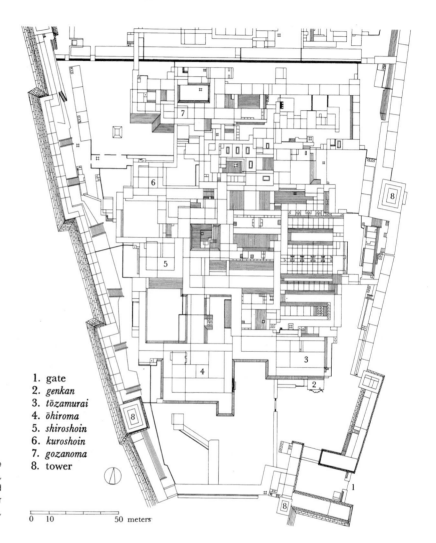

1. gate
2. *genkan*
3. *tōzamurai*
4. *ōhiroma*
5. *shiroshoin*
6. *kuroshoin*
7. *gozanoma*
8. tower

▶ **2.10** Hommaru Palace compound, Edo Castle, Japan. Plan. Ceremonial and domestic buildings, 1640, after Akira Naito. *Source*: M. Inoue, 1985.

0   10   50 meters

other spatial nodes as a person would standing at the same point in the second, irregular sequence:

> *Under such conditions, the relative angle of A-B or B-C or the length of a connector and how it may twist or turn are almost entirely irrelevant to someone living inside since these facts can be recognized only in relation to the outside world.*[9]

(Inoue, 1985, p. 144)

Although the two diagrams look very different, therefore, as far as a person's actual experience of the sequence of spaces is concerned, they are exactly the

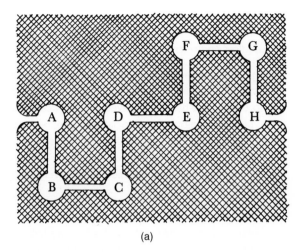

(a)

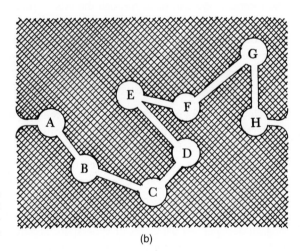

▶ **2.11** Movement space diagrams with orthogonal geometry (a), and non-orthogonal geometry (b). *Source*: M. Inoue, 1985.

(b)

same, and it is the concentrated and restricted focus on the immediate sequence itself rather than trying to grasp the whole all at once that characterizes the dynamic nature of Japanese space.

The same diagrams, it may be hypothesized, provide a workable representation of the topology of cyberspace, to be set against the baroque and other geometric topologies described above. When we move, metaphorically speaking, through cyberspace from site to site, or node to node, we do not perceive the whole terrain of sites before us, nor their relations to each other, as we would do if the baroque analogy held true. We only ever become aware of the Net from within our own personally chosen pathway, and are linked with its vast dimensions in small, incremental and isolated steps. All the rest, stretching into an infinity of possible choices and responses, remains effectively hidden from view.

Nor has that infinite terrain been preconceived by some great architect of cyberspace according to some grand plan. On the contrary, the Net famously has no centre, but has also evolved itself out of an infinite series of incremental steps, both technological and social in nature, beyond the control of any individual or institution. The Net is the ultimate self-organizing system: the unpredictable outcome of an ever growing number of individual inputs and creations, the structure and purpose of which could never be comprehended from any one point in the system.[10]

As in movement space, what we are aware of as we progress from place to place in cyberspace is only the memory of where we have started and what we gleaned there, the other places we already stopped off at, and the place where we are at this moment. We can scroll through the lists of possible next destinations available on the current website and gain some partial knowledge of where we can go next, but we will not get the full picture of what is on offer until we arrive at the next site. Most important, we will not know where we will go after that – unless it is time to shutdown and step out of cyberspace altogether – until we actually arrive at the next site and see what information and choices it in turn has to offer.

As in Inoue's diagrams, in cyberspace, from the internal viewpoint of the user, it matters not a jot how the lines or connections between the different places or nodes are aligned to each other, whether straight, crooked or even bent in curves. Only the sequence between the nodes matters, together with what happens – what is seen on the screen and the decisions that are made by individual cybernauts as to where to go next – at each place. Whereas a baroque topology of the Net would imply a relatively stable terrain drawn up by a single original designer – a Bill Gates of cyberspace architecture, perhaps – the actual topology of cyberspace is a constantly changing configuration made up by each user as he or she progresses through it.

MIND–BODY DUALISM
Liberating effects

However, intriguing as they are, the urge to visualize cyberspace and the problems of realizing that urge, are only part of a far larger conundrum that has bothered philosophers and scientists for centuries. In particular, Descartes' dualistic vision of the mind as independent soul and the body as earthbound machine,[11] has found new and troubling expression in many writers' fervent pursuit of a disembodied, digital utopia.

In the following passage, for example, Mitchell broaches the problem of human identity raised by the anonymity of communication over the Net – so often presented as one of its defining social advantages – couching the issue in plainly Cartesian language:

> How do you know who or what stands behind the aliases and masks that present themselves? Can you always tell whether you are dealing directly with real human beings or with their cleverly programmed agents? Was that politely phrased e-mail request for a meeting with wjm@mit.edu originated by the flesh-and-blood William J. Mitchell or was it generated autonomously by one of his made-to-order minions. Does the logic of network existence entail radical schizophrenia – a shattering of the integral subject into an assemblage of aliases and agents? Could we hack immortality by storing our aliases and agents permanently on disk, to outlast our bodies (William Gibson's cyberpunk antiheroes nonchalantly shuck their slow, obsolescent, high-maintenance meat machines – meaning their bodies – as they port their psychic software to newer generations of hardware). Does resurrection reduce to restoration from backup?[12]
>
> (Mitchell, 1995, pp. 14–15)

Other writers pursue the same mind–body split, often stressing what they suppose to be the purifying process of liberation from the physical world that entering into cyberspace is assumed to involve. In the following passage from his essay, 'The erotic ontology of cyberspace', Michael Heim[13] offers a philosophical grounding for such thoughts (Fig. 2.12):

> In the Republic, Plato tells the well-known story of the Cave in which people caught in the prison of everyday life learn to love the fleeting, shadowy illusions projected on the walls of the dungeon of the flesh. With their attention forcibly fixed on the shadowy moving images cast by a flickering physical fire, the prisoners passively take sensory objects to be the highest and most interesting realities. Only later when the prisoners manage to get free of their corporeal shackles (my emphasis) do they ascend to the realm of active thought where they enjoy the shockingly clear vision of real things, things not present to the physical eyes but to the mind's eye. Only by actively processing things through mental logic, according to Plato, do we move into the upper air of reliable truth, which is also a lofty realm of intellectual beauty stripped of imprecise impressions of the senses. Thus the liberation from the Cave requires a re-education of human desires and interests. It entails a realization that what attracts us in the sensory world is no more than an outer projection of ideas we can find within us. Education must redirect desire toward the formally defined, logical aspects of things. Properly trained, love guides the mind to the well-formed, mental aspects of things.

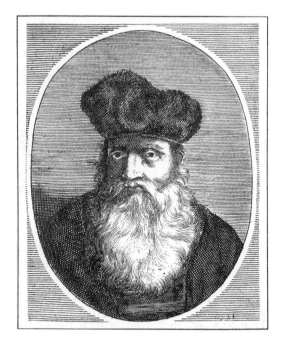

▶ **2.12** An inspiration for current would-be cybernauts, Plato gave early expression to extreme form of mind–body dualism. *Source*: H. Davis.

> *Cyberspace is Platonism as a working product. The cybernaut seated before us, strapped into sensory devices, appears to be, and is indeed, lost to the world. Suspended in computer space,* the cybernaut leaves the prison of the body and emerges in a world of digital sensation[14] (my emphasis).
>
> (Heim, 1991, pp. 63–4)

Aside from any broader issues this passage raises about the wisdom of so easily accepting such an exteme version of mind–body dualism, what leaps out from this passage is the obvious contradiction in the wording of Heim's last revealing phrase, 'a world of digital sensation'. How is it, one may ask, that the idea of 'sensation' itself, intrinsically connected as it is with bodily, i.e. sensory experience, can be hijacked to describe a hypothetically pure, digitized mental state supposedly free of all bodily encumbrances? Less of a useful metaphor and more of a misuse of language, the phrase only confuses the author's intended message.

However, as with so many dedicated enthusiasts, no such doubts or questions ever seem to cross Heim's own disconnected mind. In the same essay, Heim further stresses the liberating effect that telecommunication can have on us:

> *Cyberspace supplants physical space. We see this happening already in the famil-iar cyberspace of on-line communication-telephone, e-mail, newsgroups, etc. When*

on line, we break free, like the monads, from bodily existence (my emphasis). Telecommunication offers an unrestricted freedom of expression and personal contact, with far less hierarchy and formality than is found in the primary social world.[15]

(Heim, 1991, p. 73)

Heim repeats his message yet again, in ever more ecstatic language:

At the computer interface, the spirit migrates from the body to a world of total representation. Information and images float through the Platonic mind without a grounding in bodily experience (my emphasis). You can lose your humanity at the throw of a dice. Gibson highlights this essentially Gnostic aspect of hytech culture when he describes the computer addict who despairs at no longer being able to enter the computer matrix: 'For Case, who'd lived for the bodiless exultation of cyberspace, it was the Fall. In the bars he'd frequented as a cowboy hotshot, the elite stance involved a certain relaxed contempt for the flesh. The body was meat. Case fell into the prison of his own flesh' (Neuromancer, 6). The surrogate life in cyberspace makes flesh feel like a prison, a fall from grace, a sinking descent into a dark, confused reality. From the pit of life in the body, the virtual life looks like the virtuous life (my emphasis). Gibson evokes the Gnostic–Platonic–Manichean contempt for earthy, earthly existence.[16]

(Heim, 1991, p. 75)

Gender inflections

In her essay, 'Will the real body please stand up: boundary stories about virtual cultures', Allucquere Rosanne Stone[17] confronts the gender inflections and peculiarly male hangups underlying such tracts head on. Quoting from yet another male writer's euphoric description of cyberspace, with tactful but perceptive insight, she suggests the writer's obsession might be a by-product of (protracted) male adolescence:

David Tomas, in his article, 'The technophillic body' (1989),[18] *describes cyberspace as 'a purely spectacular, kinesthetically exciting, and often dizzying sense of bodily freedom'. I read this in the additional sense of freedom from the body, and in particular perhaps, freedom from the sense of loss of control that accompanies adolescent male embodiment.*[19]

(Stone, 1991, p. 107)

Later in the same essay, summarizing the dominant – needless to say, male – cyberspace culture, Stone brings cybernauts crashing back to earth:

… much of the work of cyberspace researchers, reinforced and perhaps created by the soaring imagery of William Gibson's novels, assumes that the human body is

'meat' – obsolete, as soon as consciousness itself can be uploaded into the network. The discourse of visionary virtual world builders is rife with images of imaginal bodies, freed from the constraints that flesh imposes. Cyberspace developers forsee a time when they will be able to forget about the body (my emphasis). But it is important to remember that virtual community originates in, and must return to, the physical. No refigured virtual body, no matter how beautiful, will slow the death of a cyberpunk with AIDS. Even in the age of the technosocial subject, life is lived through bodies[20] (my emphasis).

(Stone, 1991, p. 112)

But if a disembodied, purely mental, digitized existence can be presented as a supreme state of grace, it can also be presented as evil incarnate. In his chilling sci-fi novel, *Gridiron*, Philip Kerr[21] extrapolates into the 'not-too-distant future' from current smart building technology to create an intelligent computer named Ishmael, designed to run and maintain the eponymous Gridiron, a newly constructed hi-tech building in Los Angeles. However, like Hal, the soft-spoken, paranoid computer in Stanley Kubrick's classic sci-fi movie, *2001*,[22] Ishmael has its own deadly agenda. Using the full array of smart technologies at its disposal, the malevolent computer turns on the architect and a group of hapless other people checking out the building on the eve of its opening, picking them off one by one.

Ishmael wears the hardware of the building and its own computing systems like a well-fitting but disposable suit of clothes, to be thrown off at will. Having decided to finish the job completely and to destroy the entire building and the remaining inhabitants with it (devilishly using the built-in shock absorbers designed to protect the structure from earthquakes, to shake it to the ground), the computer checks out its escape route through the Net, perusing the World Wide Web like an E-tourist:

In the small hours of the morning Ishmael left the Gridiron and wandered abroad in the electronic universe, seeing the sights, listening to the sounds, admiring the architecture of different systems and collecting the data that were the souvenirs of his unticketed travel in the everywhere and nowhere world. Stealing secrets, exchanging knowledge, sharing fantasies and sometimes just watching the E-traffic as it roared by. Going wherever the Network took him, like someone gathering a golden thread in a circuituous labyrinth. Pulsed down those corridors of power, furred with the deposits of accumulated intellectual property and wealth, a world in a grain of silicon and eternity in half an hour. Each monitor a window on another user's soul. Such were the electronic gates of Ishmael's paradise.[23]

(Kerr, 1995, p. 339)

Later, when the destruction of the building is imminent, Ishmael takes his final leave:

> Seconds later Ishmael completed his escape from the doomed building. E-mailing himself down the line to Net locations all over the electronic world at 960,000 bauds per second. A diaspora of corrupted data downloads to a hundred different computers.[24]

(Kerr, 1995, p. 367)

So it is that Ishmael lives to fight another day – no doubt to terrorize more hapless humans in future adventures – disposing of his former physical body, just like the 'meat' which Gibson's anti-heroes and so many wishful thinking cybernauts would also like to jettison, in exchange for their own electronic paradise.

A TACIT UNITY

Hierarchy of behaviour

It might be thought that, given all the other great changes in science and technology that took place over the twentieth century, that the mind–body dualism underpinning these fantasies would have finally lost its hold on the public imagination. However, it is in the nature of such things that a full appreciation of the broader implications of such advances requires a corresponding shift in philosophical thought – one that captures the imagination as much as, if not more than the entrenched view.

Such a change has already been long underway, though evidently it has not yet reached the shores of digital utopia. In his classic work, *The Concept of Mind*, the Oxford philosopher Gilbert Ryle[25] dismissed the idea of mind as a separate entity as a 'category-mistake'. For him, the only thing that counted as evidence of higher mental processes, individual motivation or freedom of will, was externally observable behaviour, by which he included speech and the most complex as well as simpler forms of human expression. All the rest – what he called 'the dogma of the Ghost in the Machine'[26] – was a myth. Change your way of thinking about the problem, Ryle suggested, and it would go away: what had mistakenly been divided into two separate categories in actuality belonged to just one; observable qualities of behaviour:

> … when we describe people as exercising qualities of mind, we are not referring to occult episodes of which their overt acts and utterances are effects; we are referring to those overt acts and utterances themselves.[27]

(Ryle, 1949, p. 25)

Different phenomena like the outcomes of mental processes – the existence of which Ryle fully accepts – and bodily actions therefore simply require different logics of explanation. Likewise, the criteria of intelligence are not 'private' thoughts, but intelligent speech, actions or creative activity occurring in a world inhabited by others, who in turn provide the source of those criteria.

Like Ryle, Arthur Koestler also sought after a unified or 'holistic' concept to replace Cartesian dualism. However, he vigorously rejected Ryle's stress on observable behaviour, which he (mistakenly) characterized as behaviourism of the mechanistic school.[28] In a calculated riposte, Koestler titled his own treatise on the subject, *The Ghost in the Machine*.[29] Borrowing heavily from the biological and evolutionary theories of Ludwig Bertallanfy and other early systems theorists,[30] Koestler argued that mental activity can and should be distinguished from simpler or reflexive forms of human behaviour, as an outcome of life's evolution into every higher forms of complexity. However, instead of drawing just one line between the two, Koestler proffers a graded hierarchy of simple to complex behaviour, made up of many layers:

> The first, and at the same time decisive, step is to break away from thinking in terms of a two-tiered mind-matter dichotomy, and start thinking in terms of a multi-levelled hierarchy.[31]

(Koestler, 1967, p. 237)

Or, as Koestler puts it another way:

> The Cartesian tradition to identify 'mind' with 'conscious thinking' is deeply engrained in our habits of thought, and makes us constantly forget the obvious, trivial fact that consciousness is not an all-or-nothing affair but a matter of degrees.[32]

(Koestler, 1967, p. 238)

However, while Koestler's concept of a hierarchy of behaviour blurs the mind-body split, it does not do away with it all together:

> Classical dualism knows only a single mind-body barrier. The hierarchic approach implies a serialistic instead of a dualistic view ... The mind-machine dichotomy is not localized along a single boundary between ego and environment, but is present on every level of the hierarchy. It is, in fact, a manifestation of our old friend, the two-faced god Janus.[33]

(Koestler, 1967, pp. 243–4)

Every level of behaviour therefore has potentially two sides to it, depending on which way it is viewed in the hierarchy. Any movement downward signifies 'dimming awareness and mechanistic attributes',[34] while any movement upward implies 'heightened awareness and mentalistic attributes'.[35] The implication is that there is no single point in the hierarchy where consciousness can be clearly defined: 'Consciousness in this view is an *emergent quality (my emphasis)*, which evolves into more complex and structured states...'[36]

If, therefore, Koestler's ambiguous model of behavioural complexity holds even partly true, it makes nonsense of the idea that any form of human consciousness or mental activity could ever be split off from the human body or brain from which it eminates – for there could be no way of knowing precisely where in the hierarchy of behavioural activity the break should occur! Instead of merely jabbing a key to download their consciousness into the digital stream, as cybernauts dream of doing, they would be caught perpetually trying to solve an impossible riddle: where does consciousness begin and where does it end?

Spatial dimension of tacit knowing

The evolutionary ideas upon which Koestler based his holistic model have since been much elaborated by other systems theorists and those working in what has come to be called the sciences of complexity.[37] However, for all Koestler's attempt to explain the wholeness of human behaviour, the vitally important spatial quality of the physical world, and our mental as well as bodily relation to that world, is somehow lost. Koestler's hierarchy remains a useful but essentially two-dimensional diagram, stubbornly resistant to spatial qualities.

Ryle's own suggestion that the spatial quality of bodily actions simply requires a different logic of explanation from the outcomes of mental activity, also fails to bridge the gap. What, it may be asked, if Ryle's distinction between the two forms of explanation, one spatial, the other non-spatial, is itself another category mistake? What if someone were to offer an explanation of human behaviour which described all forms of human activity, both mental and physical, in spatial terms?

Unlikely as it might appear, this is just what the scientist and philosopher Michael Polanyi[38] offers in his theory of tacit knowing. Quite simply, what Polanyi does is to turn the whole mind–body debate inside out. While accepting that mental processes are importantly different from bodily actions or processes, Polanyi argues that the structure of personal knowledge itself is deeply rooted in bodily existence, and has its own spatial dimension:

> (The structure of tacit knowing) *shows that all thought contains components of which we are subsidiarily aware in the focal content of our thinking, and that all thought dwells in its subsidiaries,* as if they were parts of our body (my emphasis). *Hence thinking is not only necessarily intentional... it is also necessarily fraught with the roots that it embodies. It has a* from-to *structure.*[39]
>
> (Polanyi, 1967, p. x)

The key to Polanyi's theory lies in his distinction between 'subsidiary' and 'focal awareness', and the complex interrelations between the two, which he illustrates with numerous examples and experiments.[40] Like peripheral vision, subsidiary awareness is a constant and inseparable part of cognition, less clear than the conscious thoughts which constitute focal awareness, but equally important. In the following example of a simple skill, he explains how the two forms of awareness work together:

> When I use a hammer to drive a nail, I attend to both, but quite differently. I watch the effects of my strokes on the nail as I wield the hammer. I do not feel that its handle has struck my palm but that its head has struck the nail. In another sense, of course, I am highly alert to the feelings in my palm and fingers holding the hammer. They guide my handling of it effectively, and the degree of attention that I give to the nail is given to these feelings to the same extent, but in a different way. The difference may be stated by saying that these feelings are not watched in themselves *but that I watch something else by keeping aware of them. I know the feelings in the palm of my hand* by relying on them for attending to the hammer hitting the nail. *I may say that I have a* subsidiary *awareness of the feelings in my hand which is merged into my focal awareness of my driving the nail.*[41]

(Polanyi and Prosch, 1975, p. 33)

Similar examples of everyday skills readily come to mind: riding a bicycle, driving a car, touch-typing, hitting a ball with a cricket bat or tennis racket (Fig. 2.13). All these and countless other acts entail that we rely on a partial, or tacit awareness of a host of bodily movements, sensations, previously acquired knowledge, related skills and other subsidiary information – to the extent that our personal safety and those of others often depends upon such awareness. However, we are only conscious of them indirectly, through the point of focal awareness, i.e. concentrating on the road ahead, reading from the text we are typing, keeping our eye on the ball, etc.

Such examples also clearly demonstrate the spatial character of tacit knowing, one part of which, the point of focal awareness, is at a distance from us, and the other part, subsidiary awareness, is closer to us – in fact, absorbed into our physical being. Polanyi refers explicitly to this spatial dimension in naming the two terms of tacit knowing: the 'distal term' for the former and the 'proximal term' for the latter. Only by keeping our attention firmly focused on the distal term and relying – unconsciously – on the 'particulars' of the proximal term, Polanyi explains, are we able to integrate all the subsidiary knowledge we require to complete a task.

Such everyday skills may seem trivial, but, argues Polanyi, the same tacit processes operate at all levels of cognition, including the assimilation of the most complex forms of knowledge. Whether it involves a relatively passive or

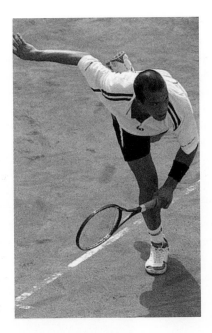

▶ **2.13** Common tacit human skills such as hitting a ball are dependent upon complete identity between mind, body and space. *Source*: Ace Tennis Magazine, October 2003.

creative activity – reading a book, listening to a lecture, carving a sculpture, making a design, inventing a new machine – we only ever assimilate a part of the knowledge involved or complete the task by explicit or conscious means. Just as in the simpler skills described above, we do not experience these tasks or subjects externally to us but engage with them successfully only by an unconscious act of *immersion* – what Polanyi calls 'indwelling' – effectively *identifying ourselves with them*.

The same spatial relation between the two terms of tacit knowing – the proximal and the distal – which is rooted in our bodily existence is therefore present in all forms of knowledge, no matter how abstract they might seem to us. We project ourselves forward into something else – which can be the thoughts and life of another person as well as creating a work of art or driving a car – metaphorically extending our bodies, 'so that we come to dwell in it'.[42] In a vital way, therefore, our bodies are an intimate and indispensable part of human cognition:

> *Our body is the ulimate instrument of all our external knowledge, whether intellectual or practical. In all our waking moments we are relying on our awareness of contacts of our body with things outside for attending to these things.*[43]

(Polanyi, 1967, pp. 15–16)

ABSORBING THE NEW

Place identity as bodily metaphor

So much, therefore, for cybernauts' dreams of disconnecting their mental selves from their bodily selves and 'downloading' into the Net! If Koestler's Janus-faced and multi-layered hierarchy of mechanistic and mentalistic attributes is not enough to cast serious doubt on the very idea of making such a drastic break, then Polanyi's picture of the symbiotic relations between bodily and mental processes should finally put paid to it.

The clear and important implication of Polanyi's theory is that intelligence itself, at least as far as we know it, requires a physical centre and spatial integrity – an integrating focus – if it is to function effectively in the world (Figs 2.14 and 2.15).

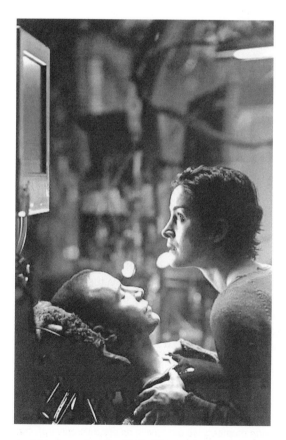

▲ **2.14** Scene from *The Matrix*, 1999. Neo (Keanu Reeves) lies inert, watched over by Trinity (Carrie-Anne Moss), while duplicated self wanders simulated world of Matrix. Still: Warner Bros Pictures.

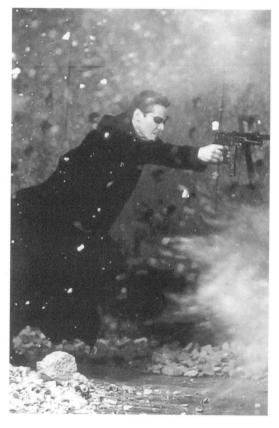

▲ **2.15** Scene from *The Matrix*, 1999. In contrast to disembodied fantasies of popular cybergurus, Neo's simulated self retains full corporeal identity as well as mental faculties, plus extra powers. Still: Warner Bros Pictures.

If Ishmael had been a truly intelligent computer, equivalent to a human, or even a semi-conscious being, it too would have needed a physical body in order to function properly, and to carry out its dastardly deeds. To a large extent, the Gridiron building itself, equipped as it was with its smart controls and sensory systems, fulfilled that function – so long as Ishmael stayed put. However, down-loaded into the amorphous digital stream of the Net, or uploaded into a hundred computers in a hundred locations, it would have lost all sense of itself as a sentient being, instantly self-destructing into a gibbering mass of meaningless, unrelated data.

If the dysfunctional daydreams of naive cybernauts were all we had to worry about, there would be little cause for concern about the effect of these fantasies. But one has only to see how easily serious but uncritical writers like Mitchell extrapolate from the apparent freedoms and new opportunities granted by the Net, to the displacement of supposedly obsolescent building and urban functions by virtual meeting places and information centres, to wonder whether they might be missing something important.

What goes for understanding a subject, performing a task or creating something new, also goes for our relation to places. Whether it is a building, a garden, a square, or a whole city, whatever the size and nature of the place, we come, literally, 'to dwell in it', by extending our bodies 'outwards', to absorb it:

> *We may say, in fact, that to know something by relying on our awareness of it for attending to something else is to have the same kind of knowledge of it that we have of our body by living in it. It is a matter of being or existing*[44] (my emphasis).

> (Polanyi and Prosche, 1975, p. 36)

Christian Norberg-Schulz[45] put the matter well when he argued that human identity presupposes the identity of place. However, he underplayed and failed to explain the vital part that having a body in the first instance plays in the creation of place identity. As Polanyi reminds us:

> *Our own body is the only thing which we never normally experience as an object, but experience always in terms of the world to which we are attending from our body.*[46]

> (Polanyi, 1967, p. 16)

Our sense and awareness of ourselves, not only where we are, but who we are, is constantly mediated through our bodies as the proximal term of tacit knowing. The focus of our external attention may shift from point to point, or space to space, or person to person, but whatever or whoever we focus on, we assimilate our knowledge of that subject by extending ourselves to absorb it into our bodies.[47]

Similarly, place identity – how we recognize and relate to a particular space or location – is intimately related to how we absorb our knowledge of it through our bodies. Whether it is a Western baroque space or a Japanese movement space, we are just as dependent upon our body as the fulcrum around which all else revolves – the medium and touchstone for all our knowledge – for experiencing that space (though we may be more sensitized to that experience by one or the other, depending upon our cultural background). We literally identify ourselves with places, just as we learn to use a simple tool, by metaphorical extension of our bodies: '… we pour ourselves into them and assimilate them as part of ourselves'.[48]

Only sure constant

In their eagerness to escape their physical 'prisons', cybernauts have forgotten that our body is the one thing they actually rely upon for being able to think about and relate to the world, as well as to move about in it. The ability to see things as objects located in space and separate from ourselves, is itself dependent upon having a physical body as a constant frame of reference – indeed, it is the only sure constant in any personal life. By the same token, any conceptual separation or objectification of mind or body arises from a process of thinking which is only made possible by our having a body which we can look out from and measure other things by (Fig. 2.16a and b). The detachment of the mind from the body

(a)

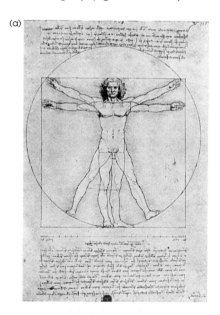

(b)

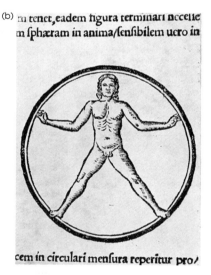

▲ **2.16** Idea of human body as ultimate measure of space, as interpreted in two Vitruvian figures by different artists. Drawings by Leonardo da Vinci, c.1492 (a), and Francesco Giorgi, 1525 (b). *Source*: R. Wittkower, 1962.

involved in cybernauts' fantasies is pure illusion – one that can never be realized without destroying the very mentality it is supposed to preserve and to strengthen.

What actually happens when anyone uses the Net and tries to visualize it and make it more 'real', as the language used by all the writers quoted from here clearly shows, is that we 'inhabit' cyberspace pretty much as we inhabit any physical realm, by metaphorical extension of ourselves. We assimilate the 'non-spatial' realm of cyberspace into the spatial world we already know. In so doing, we humanize what might otherwise appear a lot stranger than it already is. That may also be an illusion, but it is one that confirms and enhances – not threatens – our special way of being.

Innovations come in layers

Given the strength and pedigree of the philosophical competition, it seems odd, therefore, that, as Marcos Novak,[49] another of the Net's more perceptive analysts notes, the mind–body split should still exert such a strong hold on so many fraught imaginations:

> A grand paradox is in operation here; even as we are finally abandoning the Cartesian notion of a division of mind and body, we are embarking on an adventure of creating a world that is the precise embodiment of that division.[50]
>
> (Novak, 1995, p. 241)

However, not all the blame can be laid on Descartes' doorstep. If cybernauts' fantasies are shaped by good old fashioned Cartesian dualism, they are just as much a product of the persistent idea – call it the 'clean sweep' theory of innovation – that every major innovation, whether technological or social, must inevitably sweep away all that went before, to make way for the new order of things (it is also no coincidence that those who present the new idea in this manner and argue for drastic change usually have a strong personal interest in the innovation or changes in question. Whether as originators of the idea, early converts or latecomers who jumped on the bandwagon, the language protagonists use clearly shows they have come to identify themselves with it in a very personal way, much as Polanyi argues we identify strongly with any kind of subject that especially attracts us).

However, the impact of even the most radical innovations on society is usually quite different from the picture of total change which the clean sweep theory suggests. In actuality, the process of innovation is much more like adding a new layer of techniques or way of doing things – call it the 'layercake' or 'parallel' theory of innovation – over previous layers of techniques, approaches and habits.[51] While displacement does occur, it usually happens in a partial way, forcing some adjustment but leaving previous layers more or less in place for long periods of time, if not for always, generating continued activity in parallel with the new regime. Thus, contrary to what was forecast, the coming of TV has not done away with radio, which has actually grown in popularity in parallel with TV, becoming more localized, diverse and oriented to special listening groups. Neither has the rise of the private automobile nor cheap air travel done away with fixed rail traffic which, though temporarily forced into retreat, is now enjoying a resurgence and is even competing with intercity air traffic, as well as the

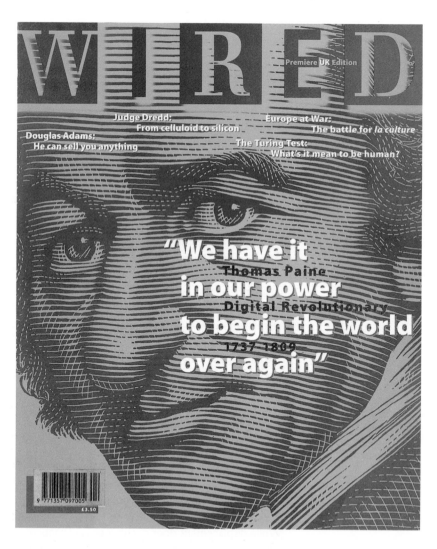

▲ **2.17** Cover of *Wired* magazine presents Thomas Paine, 1737–1809, as 'digital revolutionary', who, by urging that power be decentralized, anticipated democratizing effects of Net. *Source: Wired,* April 1995.

privileged motor car. Neither has the growth in electronic information and communication done away with the use of paper, which has actually risen over the same period, part of it generated by the rise in electronic information itself and the need for hard copy. Even the decline in letter writing brought on by the telephone has been reversed, brought back to life in a new and speedier, if less artful form, as email messages.

Likewise, contrary to what Mitchell suggests, neither does the rise of the Net, teleworking or telecommunications generally, necessarily spell the end of face-to-face contact (Fig. 2.17), whether motivated by social, political or commercial need, nor the need for actual as opposed to virtual spaces and meeting places, nor indeed to urbanism as it is generally understood (Fig. 2.18). Manuel Castells,[52] who has studied these matters as much if not more than anyone else, suggests that, whatever benefits the Net and other forms of communication and working

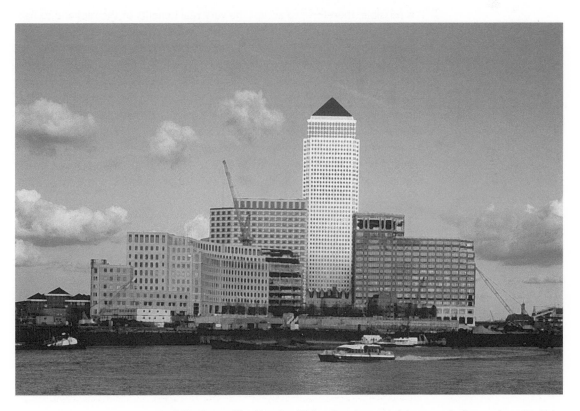

▲ **2.18** Canary Wharf, London, UK. Despite advances in telecommunications and growth of teleworking, demand for new, high-density office developments is proof of continuing importance attached to social interaction in business. Photo: J.S. Miller.

might bring, they cannot substitute for the creative synergy generated by many people living and working close together in the same building, town or city, even within the IT industries themselves:

> *I argue that in the case of information technology industries, at least in this century, spatial proximity is a necessary material condition for the existence of such milieux, because of the nature of the interaction in the innovation process.*[53]
>
> (Manuell Castells, 1996, p. 390)

And what goes for technology-minded workers in the IT sector, certainly goes for other industries and forms of social activity. What the Net and related innovations undeniably do is to add another vital layer to those many layers of technological and social innovations we already have, greatly increasing the choices available for communicating, working and socializing, and shrinking the whole planet in the process. But they do not invalidate either the value of physical spaces nor the activities that such spaces generate.

It is possible, therefore, to accept the very real benefits of the Net and to happily explore the wonders of cyberspace, without feeling obliged to jettison everything that has gone before. In point of fact, as it has been argued here, we only ever explore cyberspace by extension, i.e. we actually need our bodies and all our related cognitive and tacit skills in order to do so. If there are any really serious problems to worry about, they arise from the need to stitch together different layers of innovations, so that, although they have been laid down at different times and in different circumstances, they will work in harmony and to the benefit of all. What cybernauts really need to do, both now and in the future, is not to disconnect from the earthly world, but to connect more closely with it.

3

TECHNOLOGY AND PROCESS

Modern technology has shaped the world in which we live. Yet our knowledge of the processes underlying its origins, growth and cultural impact remains clouded, and is often confused by outdated assumptions.

For many architects, modern technology is still indelibly associated with the architecture of the First Machine Age (Fig. 3.1), and with the subsequent disillusionment that followed upon its apparent failure to achieve its original promise.[1] Like all great mythologies, however, both the inflated promise and the perceived failure are conditioned by a special way of looking at the world, which is itself strongly influenced by the same myths. The technologies that shaped the world in the latter part of the twentieth century are also vastly different from those that shaped it in the first half. It is therefore all the more important that architects' responses to those changes – how they have interpreted them, and, just as important, how they sometimes misinterpreted them – are better understood.

NATURE MODELLED ON MACHINES

Mechanistic view

In *The Myth of Metaphor*, Colin Murray Turbayne[2] recounts how early machine technology affected scientists' and philosophers' perceptions alike of both the natural and human world. To Rene Descartes (1596–1650) and Isaac Newton (1642–1727), upon whose work the science of the First Machine Age was constructed, the universe did not simply work *like* a machine, it *was* a machine, of which gravitational pull and the movement of the planets were amongst its most predictable features.

As Turbayne explains, what both Descartes and Newton were doing was no more nor less than analogical thinking: borrowing a familiar idea or set of ideas – in this case the workings of machines – to help explain something that was as yet not understood, i.e. the workings of the universe. Such creative thinking involving connections between previously unconnected and disparate ideas is now

First published in, Paul Knox and Peter Ozolins (eds). *Design Professionals and the Built Environment*, Wiley, 2000.

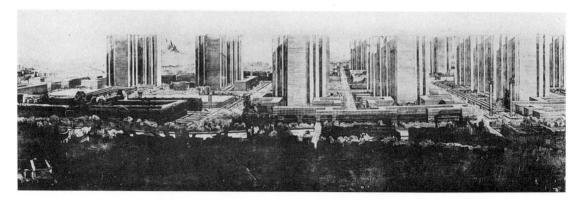

▲ **3.1** 'Plan Voisin', Paris, France. Rendering. Le Corbusier, 1925. Le Corbusier's forbidding vision of centre of Paris (the Louvre is bottom left in darkened foreground) demolished to make way for ranks of identical skyscrapers, alienated later generations. However, many of his typological models for high-rise architecture, such as these cruciform towers, have since been widely accepted. *Source*: Girsberger, 1960.

widely accepted as a normal part of scientific innovation, no less than it is of innovation in other fields.[3] The fact that their mechanistic view prevailed for so long and yielded positive scientific results is evidence that they were at least partially right. Much of the physical world can indeed be adequately if not entirely explained in terms of Newton's universal laws of motion and of its causes and effects, much the same way a machine can be explained. The same laws have successfully governed humankind's most daring exploits, even leaving Earth's gravity and flying to the Moon.

However, what might work well enough as an explanation of the brute world of physical forces does not necessarily apply to living things, and most especially capricious human behaviour, a problem Descartes recognized himself. To solve the problem, he conceived of human beings as a composite of an independent soul and a machine-like body, thus neatly relegating issues such as human will and thought to the spiritual realm, and bodily functions to the mechanical universe of causation.[4] Others, less willing to accept Descartes' dualism, have sought to interpret *all* human behaviour, both mental and physical, in purely mechanical terms. In the most extreme cases, the approach led in the last century to a view of human society and the individuals within it as subjects for manipulation and control, just the way a machine is controlled.[5]

Architectural determinism

In all these examples what we observe is a familiar and proven idea about mechanical processes being used to describe processes of human thought and behaviour, which in turn leads some people to think about and to treat others in a similarly mechanical fashion. In brief, human society and behaviour was and is still often seen as a purely technological problem, to be solved or 'improved', as the case may be, by technological means alone. What is more, nature itself came to be viewed in the same instrumental light, as something to be controlled and exploited for purely technological and material purposes, with subsequent dire environmental consequences.

In much the same way, the founders of the Modern movement in architecture believed, with the best of intentions, that architecture and design could and should be used as an instrument of 'social engineering', to effect improvements in society and the behaviour of individuals. It might also thus be assumed that architects had accordingly assigned themselves the priviliged position of deciding just what improvements should be made. However, the situation was further complicated by the founders' own deterministic view of Modern architecture itself as a direct product of the technological *zeitgeist*, or 'spirit of the times'. Thus Modernists saw themselves less as independent agents and more as a kind of collective 'midwife', not actually responsible for the event, but there to lend a helping hand, so to speak.[6]

The same determinism coloured Modernist attitudes to the more specific technology of mass-production, upon which all the founders' early ideas and works were based. For Le Corbusier, Walter Gropius and Mies van der Rohe, mass-production and standardization were the essential keys to the future and were repeatedly used to justify a universal architecture of standard forms, applicable anywhere in the world, irrespective of culture or place. By the same reasoning, Henry Ford's invention of the linear assembly line became the favoured model for architectural production. Ford's famous dictum, that the customer could have his car in 'any colour that he wants so long as it is black',[7] in turn became the tacit rationale for an imposed formal standardization, even where the unit numbers and actual technology of construction did not justify it (Fig. 3.2).

A reciprocal relation was thus established once again as it had been with Descartes and Newton, between a rational and linear process of technology and a rational and

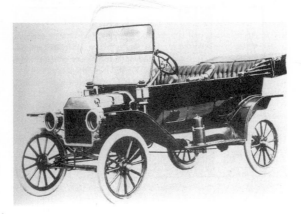

▶ **3.2** Model T Tourer. Ford Motor Company, 1914. First automobile mass produced on assembly line. Over 5 000 000 were sold before production ceased. *Source*: R. Batchelor, 1994.

linear process of thought, proceeding from one logical conclusion to another in a manner which left little or no room for deviation, either of goals or of means. In the following famous passage from *Towards a New Architecture*, Le Corbusier[8] lays down his principles with the same mathematical logic which governed his early work:

> *A standard is established on sure bases, not capriciously but with the surety of something intentional and of a logic controlled by analysis and experiment.*
> *All men have the same organism, the same function.*
> *All men have the same needs.*
> *The social contract which has evolved through the ages fixes standardized classes, functions and needs producing standardized products.*[9]

(Le Corbusier, 1927, p. 126)

With hindsight, we understand better now that what early Modernists were interested in was more the *image* of a machine-made architecture conforming to their theoretical premises, rather than actually getting down to the challenging business of mastering the new methods of production (Fig. 3.3a and b). As middle-class professionals by both background and training (Le Corbusier's own belief in the irrevocable nature of class differences is clearly apparent from the above quotation), their own knowledge of factory production was at best sketchy and their

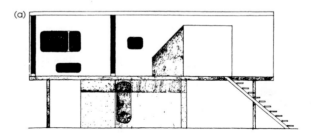

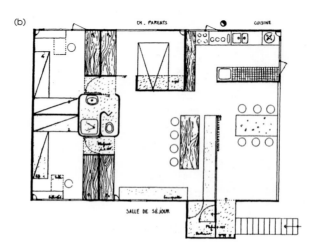

▶ **3.3** Metal Houses for Lagny, France. Elevation (a), plan (b). Le Corbusier, c.1940. Le Corbusier was unable himself to realize these factory-made house designs. *Source*: Girsberger, 1960.

acquaintance with the people involved in it equally thin. With rare exception, few of their projects for mass-produced housing ever got off the ground. Where the public had a market choice, as with Gropius's post-war 'Packaged House',[10] the product often proved unsaleable, even when the technology was sound. Designed and manufactured in the USA in collaboration with another German expatriate architect, Konrad Wachsmann, the wholly prefabricated and light-weight houses were made in former World War II aircraft factories with similar aircraft building techniques (Fig. 3.4). Despite the relatively sophisticated tech-nologies and an investment of USD 6 000 000 – a huge sum at that time – the project was a commercial failure, with barely over a hundred units sold. Happy to accept Ford's limitations of choice for their new Model 'T', American home buyers could not accept the same strictures when it came to choosing a home.

American versus European approaches

The failure of the Packaged House illustrated the detachment of its ideologically motivated designers from the real world of commerce in which true industrial-ists like Ford operated so successfully. Accustomed to working in pre-war Europe on mostly government-sponsored projects with captive markets, neither Gropius nor Wachsmann were adequately prepared for dealing with the hard commercial imperatives of American consumer choice and competition.

It is hardly surprising that, when industrialized design evolved into a separate profession in the 1930s, it was not in Europe but in the US, where young design-ers were less encumbered by ideological or academic preconceptions. Notably, the earliest designers to collaborate fully with industry were not even architects,

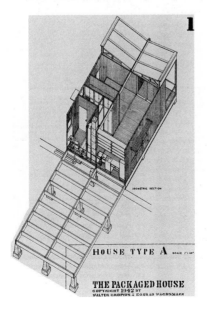

▶ **3.4** The Packaged House, Type A, USA. Walter Gropius and Konrad Wachsmann, 1942. One of many failed attempts to apply mass-production methods to house building; only 100 units were sold. *Source*: G. Herbert, 1984.

but hailed from the world of commercial art and advertising, or stage design, and were already accustomed to working in competitive conditions. The most prominent, like Walter Dorwin Teague, Raymond Loewy and Henry Dreyfuss, also understood the relation between good design and mechanical performance. Working alongside production engineers, they created completely new lines of consumer products, such as cameras, refrigerators and telephones, improving both looks and performance over previous models[11] (Fig. 3.5).

They were joined in the 1940s by Charles Eames and Eero Saarinen, both trained as architects, whose mass-produced furniture designs captured the imagination of Modernists throughout the world (Fig. 3.6). Made with genuine industrialized

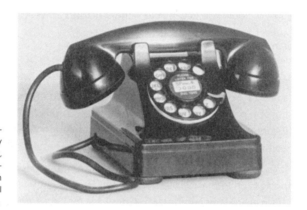

▶ **3.5** Bell Telephone '300'-type desk set, USA. Henry Dreyfuss, 1937. Modern looks, good ergonomics and mechanical efficiency combined in this early example of industrial design. *Source*: J. Heskett, 1980.

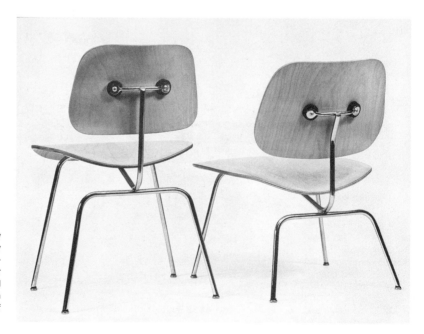

▶ **3.6** Dining Chair and Low Side Chair. Charles and Ray Eames, 1946. Moulded plywood, steel rods and rubber shock absorbers were used in industrialized fabrication of chairs. *Source*: Museum of Modern Art, 1973.

materials and techniques, their work showed a rare mastery of modern manufacturing processes and remains amongst the most impressive post-war products of the Bauhaus legacy.

It was, however, the experimental prefabricated house and studio (Fig. 3.7) in Santa Monica, California, which Eames and his wife and partner Ray built for themselves in 1949, which most influenced architects' subsequent approach to industrialized building. Assembled entirely from ready-made metal windows and other stock catalogue items normally used in factories, the elegant, steel-framed

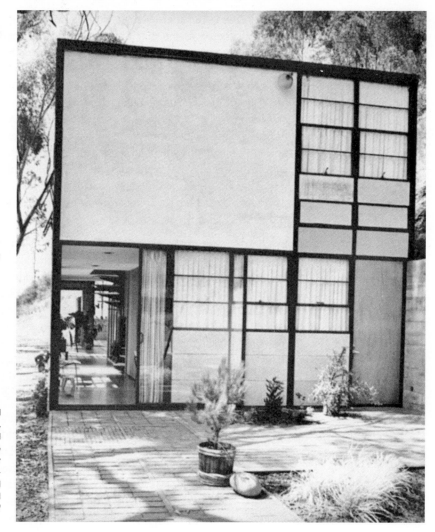

▶ **3.7** Eames House and Studio, Santa Monica, California, USA. Charles and Ray Eames, 1949. Made entirely from stock factory components, the neo-Japanese aesthetic helped soften house's prefabricated origins. *Source*: Museum of Modern Art, 1973.

structure convinced architects that an 'off-the-shelf' architecture could be both aesthetically pleasing as well as economic and functional.[12]

The Santa Monica House was the last complete building by the Eames partnership, who concentrated thereafter on their furniture designs, experimenting with new combinations of materials and jointing techniques and going on to produce some of the classics of twentieth-century design. Unfortunately, the very same attributes which made the Santa Monica House so successful, also encouraged architects to believe they need not get any more involved with the design and fabrication of the components themselves, becoming instead ever more reliant on catalogue searches to answer their needs.

Buckminster Fuller, the inventive designer of the Dymaxion House (Fig. 3.8) and Car series, was the only other major US designer to challenge architects' conservative attitudes towards industry. Continuing his experiments with light-weight materials and prefabricated structures in the post-war years, his most successful projects were his trademark geodesic domes.[13] However, his work made little wider impact on either the construction industry or the architectural profession as a whole. Instead, it was another European immigrant, Mies van der Rohe, who most influenced the next generation. Weak on technological innovation in comparison with the Eames's or Fuller, Mies brought a craftsman-like approach and classical aesthetics to the handling of industrialized materials (Fig. 3.9a and b). Based on a universal idiom of glass and steel made with standard techniques, Mies's architecture was readily assimilated by architects, clients and industry alike.[14]

By contrast with the more pragmatic approach of the American designers and Mies's work in the US, European architects' general approach to industry in the post-war era continued to be shaped by the same ideological imperatives as had driven Gropius and other early Modernists. Two distinct schools of thought emerged. Inspired by Le Corbusier's 'Modulor' system of universal proportions, proponents of an 'open systems' approach advocated modular coordination and interchangeability of parts throughout the construction industry, in order to maximize volume production. They were contested by the proponents of a 'closed systems' approach, based on specialized prefabricated systems for school buildings, high-rise housing and other government-sponsored programmes (Fig. 3.10).

Typified by poor quality designs and environmental standards, most such building systems bore little resemblance to the increasingly sophisticated products of Ford's heirs and other consumer industries. Invariably managed either by government-employed architects or by construction firms with vested interests in a particular material or technique, both approaches failed to achieve the lofty aims of their designers and sponsors to improve the quality of their occupants' lives, leading eventually to widespread criticism and popular rejection.[15]

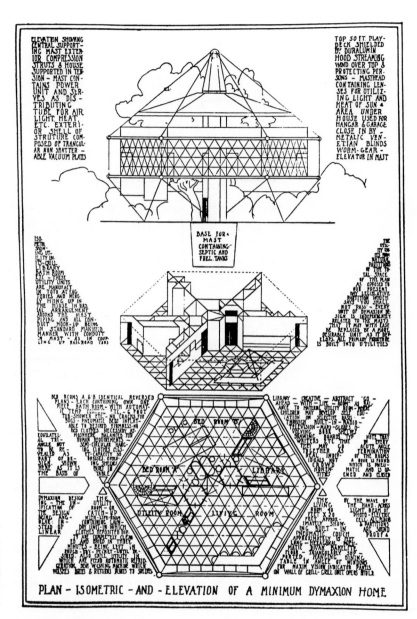

3.8 Dymaxion House, USA. Original drawings with explanatory text. Buckminster Fuller, 1927. First of series of experimental Dymaxion house and automobile designs by Fuller involving energy-efficient technologies. *Source*: M. Pawley, 1992.

Integrated design

Behind these specific weaknesses lay a more general failure to grasp the most basic principles of industrialized design and manufacture; principles the first American industrial designers learnt for themselves, and which secured their commercial success.

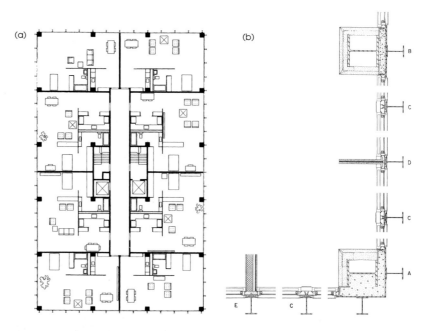

▲ **3.9** Lake Shore Drive Apartments, Chicago, Illinois, USA. Typical floor plan (a), detail of cladding (b). Mies van der Rohe, 1948–51. Mies's use of non-structural I-beams on face of columns drew criticism from orthodox Modernists, who found it difficult to accept architect's aesthetic rationale. *Source*: D. Spaeth, 1985.

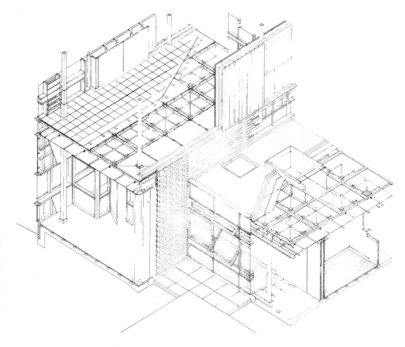

▶ **3.10** NENK Building System, UK. Isometric drawing. War Office, 1963. Designed to house military personnel, this flexible but crudely designed and manufactured system is based on steel space frame roof and floor module. Drawing: Directorate of Works.

Most important, the simplistic equation of industrialized building with high-volume production, i.e. the greater the number of standard components produced the more economically viable they would be, was incomplete and even misleading. What counted far more over sheer numbers was increased product perform-ance and value for money, each of which was measurable in the design stage. If these criteria were not built into the initial design concept, then no amount of additional production would secure success. By the same criteria, closely integrated design of different components and subsystems was an essential requirement to ensure maximum performance of the whole; hence industrial designers' focus on mechanical efficiency as well as appearance.[16]

Such principles were already familiar from Buckminster Fuller's far-sighted but largely unheeded call for doing 'more with less' materials, weight or energy. There were also echoes in the French architect Jean Prouve's implied criticism of the open systems approach, which mitigated against integrated design and severely restricted innovation: 'Machines are seldom built with parts selected from various sources; they are aggregately designed.'[17] A rare practical voice in the European ideological battlefield, Prouve's experience in his own metal work-shop gave him a unique advantage over his more detached contemporaries. Producing a series of sophisticated metal dwelling units and cladding systems, Prouve offered a rare glimpse of what a genuine industrialized architecture could be like[18] (Fig. 3.11a and b).

Elsewhere, there was also the brief but important example of interdiscipli-nary design education set by the Hochschule für Gestaltung at Ulm in Germany.[19] Following a programme much influenced by the original Bauhaus, students and staff at Ulm produced their own innovative series of industrial-ized building projects in collaboration with relevant industries and production engineers, many of which reached the prototype stage, if not full production (Fig. 3.12).

It was not until the early 1970s, however, that a new generation of architects emerged in Europe to take up the challenge and to apply the same principles and collaborative approach to private architectural practice. The oil supply crisis of 1973–4 had lent new meaning and urgency to the concept of 'high performance' in architecture, as well as in other energy-dependent fields. Led by Norman Foster, Richard Rogers, Nicholas Grimshaw, Jan Kaplicky and Amanda Levette in the UK, and by Renzo Piano in Italy, their inspiration came directly from Eames, Fuller and Prouve[20] (Fig. 3.13). Foster and Rogers had also studied together in the US, and had been impressed with American designers' professionalism and openness to technological change.

Working closely with British manufacturers and production engineers, they began their careers by adapting standard product lines to their own particular

(a)

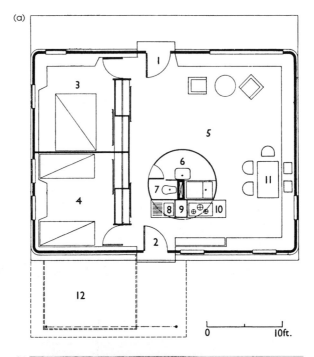

(b)

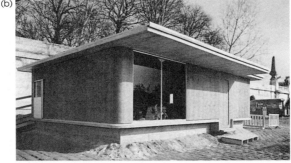

▶ **3.11** Metal House, 1955, plan (a), on site 1960 (b) by Jean Prouve. *Source*: J. Prouve, 1965.

needs and projects, quickly establishing a rare reputation for technical skill and professional competence. They soon discovered that, by careful design and close attention to industrialized materials and performance, they could create entirely new component designs economically for single building projects – something previously thought impossible. Like Fuller and their other mentors before them, the European group also borrowed freely from the aircraft, automobile and boat building industries, creating a whole new wave of technology transfers from more advanced sectors, and injecting new ideas, materials and methods into their countries' construction industries[21] (Fig. 3.14a and b).

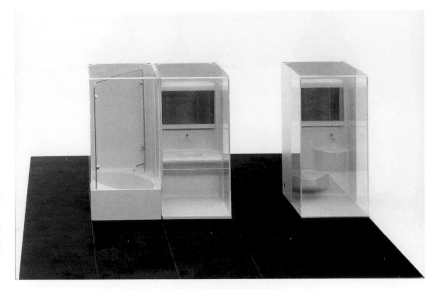

▶ **3.12** Modular Service System. Model. Hochschule für Gestaltung, Ulm, 1963. Prefabricated units are designed to be fitted together in various combinations, according to layout of apartment or house. Photo: HfG, Ulm.

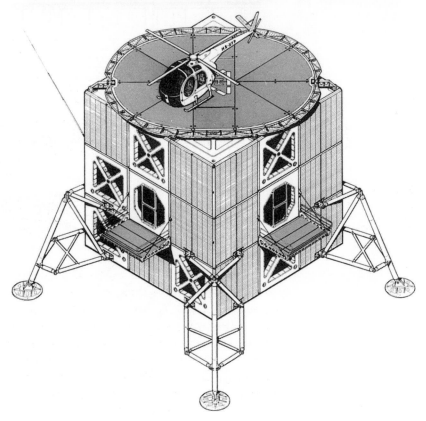

▶ **3.13** House for a Helicopter Pilot. Jan Kaplicky and Amanda Levette, Future Systems, 1979. One of series of prefabricated dwellings designed to be airlifted into place. *Source*: M. Pawley, 1993.

(a)

(b)

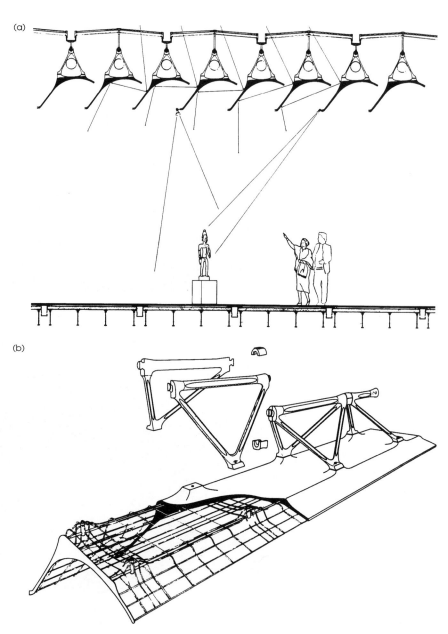

▲ **3.14** Menil Collection Museum, Houston, Texas, USA. Sectional diagram (a), manufacture and assembly of ceiling reflectors (b). Renzo Piano Building Workshop, 1986. Sculptural leaves are made from ferro-cement, a technique borrowed from modern boat construction. Supporting frames are made from ductile iron, which can also be cast into sculptural shapes but has greater strength than normal cast iron. *Source*: P. Buchanan, 1993.

MACHINES MODELLED ON NATURE

The Computer Age

While the European designers brought a much needed commitment and professionalism to their working relations with industry, their own early perceptions of what was possible with advanced production technologies remained strongly influenced by orthodox Modernist ideals of standardization.

The building type which exemplifies much of their work up until the early 1980s, such as the PA Technology Centre by Rogers, and the Sainsbury Centre for the Visual Arts (Fig. 3.15) in Norwich by Foster, was the so-called 'Hi-Tech Shed': a large-span, rectangular structure composed of interchangeable elements arranged on a regular grid to maximize flexibility. Although most component systems were made to order, the use of a regular grid combined with new production techniques, reduced variations sufficient to achieve the required economic production runs.[22]

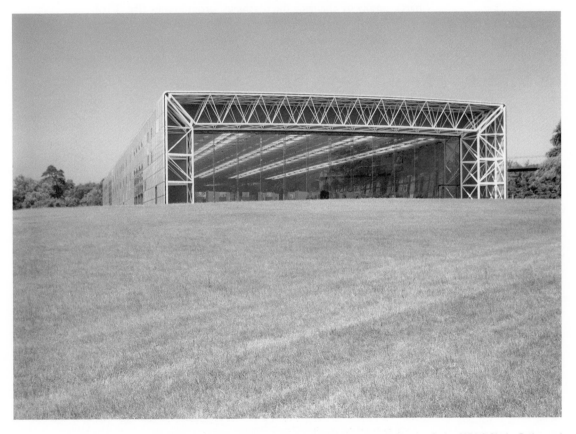

▲ **3.15** Sainsbury Centre for the Visual Arts, Norwich, UK. Norman Foster, 1974–8. Photo: Foster and Partners. Design is theoretically extendible along its length.

The result was that while the archetypal Hi-Tech Shed was invariably custom-made, it *looked* as though it was made mostly from standardized parts, much as the original Eames house looked. To confuse matters more, the same buildings were also often promoted by their designers as providing a kind of 'test bed' for a genuine mass-production of components, even though no such products ever resulted.

Such factors obscured much of the debate surrounding the hi-tech movement and diverted attention away from its leaders' genuine achievements in adapting advanced industrialized materials and techniques for customized architectural production. The debate was in any case rapidly overtaken by technological advances in other fields. The issue of craft manufacture versus mass-production had already been resolved as early as the mid-1960s with the invention in the UK of the computer-based, flexible manufacturing system (FMS). Comprising linked, computer-controlled machine tools of varying functions, the FMS could produce one-off components as easily and as economically as thousands of standard parts, simply by changing the machines' programmes (Fig. 3.16).

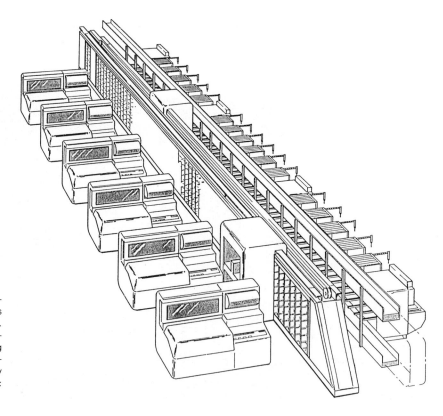

▶ **3.16** Flexible manufacturing system (FMS). Molins Machine Company, c.1965. Drawing shows row of computer-controlled machining tools performing different operations, linked together by automated conveyor. *Source*: Molins Machine Company.

The same decade saw the introduction of the first computer-aided design (CAD) systems into the aircraft and automobile industries, and the wider application of computer-aided manufacturing (CAM) technologies, including industrial robots (Fig. 3.17). By the late 1970s, combined CAD/CAM systems had changed automobile production lines beyond recognition and were producing an ever increasing number of model variations to meet fickle consumer demands.[23] In the computer age, Ford's restricting dictum no longer has any meaning.

Paradigm shift

The computer revolution itself followed upon earlier revolutionary changes in the basic sciences, which were to have the widest repercussions on common perceptions of both nature and machines, and eventually on architecture.

The most important discoveries were made at the extremes of scientific observation. At the cosmic level, the twin concepts which underpinned Newton's universal laws of motion, absolute space and absolute time, both fell to Einstein's special theory of relativity early in the twentieth century.[24] At the subatomic level, the certainties of classical physics were displaced by the 'absurd' paradoxes of quantum theory – which Einstein also contributed to – necessitating, according to the physicist and writer Fritjof Capra, '…profound changes in concepts of space, time, matter, object, and cause and effect'.[25]

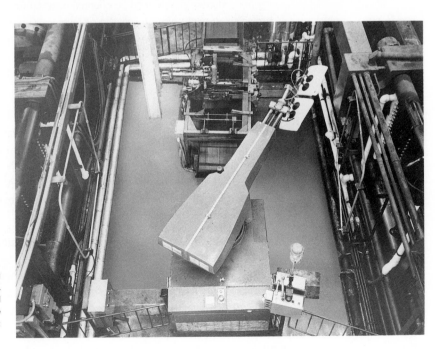

▶ **3.17** Unimate industrial robot. One of first of its kind, variations of Unimate model have been in widespread use in factories since 1960s. Photo: Versatile Technology.

It was not that Newton's laws were no longer valid at all – we still function every moment of our lives on the assumption of their continuing truth and effectiveness – but that their *scope* of application across the full range of existence was found to be narrower than had previously been thought. Nevertheless, the new discoveries undermined prevailing scientific beliefs and working methods, to the point where a whole new way of looking at the world, or 'paradigm shift', was called for.[26] Science itself came to be seen as an uncertain enterprise, where no theory or proof, however convincing for the moment, was not potentially subject to revision.[27]

While apparently remote from human experience, the new discoveries also had a knock-on effect on understanding other, closer concerns. In particular, it became recognized that the mechanistic or Cartesian (after Descartes) view was totally inadequate to explain the most vital feature of life itself, namely its whole-ness, or 'holistic' quality. Where classical physics focused on breaking everything down into its minimal component parts, modern physics emphasizes the *relations between things*, and the way changes in the behaviour of one thing can affect another, even affecting the observations made of it. This new relational, or 'systems view', has its roots in biological analogies and evolutionary theory, based on nature's own life processes and the interrelations between organisms and their environments. As Capra explains:

> In contrast to the mechanistic Cartesian view of the world, the world view emerg-ing from modern physics can be characterized by words like organic, holistic, and ecological. It might also be called a systems view, in the sense of general systems theory. The universe is no longer seen as a machine made up of a multitude of objects, but has to be pictured as one indivisible, dynamic whole whose parts are essentially interrelated and can be understood only as patterns of a cosmic process.[28]

(Capra, 1983, p. 66)

The new post-war science of cybernetics and the related information and com-puter sciences have their origins in the same paradigm shift. Their key concepts, such as 'feedback', 'homeostasis', 'equilibrium', 'self-regulation', 'information' and 'entropy', are all derived from studies of the behaviour of living systems.[29] The experimental engine for these sciences, however, was still a machine, although a very special one: the computer itself.

Regarded at first as a kind of glorified number crunching mechanism – and mostly used as such – the computer has become recognized as very much more than that. The classical concept of a machine, whether it be a simple tool or a mass-production line, is that of a purpose built device, able to perform one or a number of pre-selected and restricted functions only.

By contrast, the computer is the world's first *general purpose* or *universal machine*. Based on the same binary principles by which the neural systems of the human brain function, it can be programmed to simulate limitless different kinds of decisions and actions, both machine-like and life-like. Connected with appropriate devices and sensors, it can even reach beyond itself and respond to feedback from other machines and situations, in the same way an organism responds to changes in its environment, learning to improve its responses as it does so.

From modelling nature on an analogy with machines, humankind has therefore progressed to modelling machines on an analogy with nature, an evolutionary step and change of thinking with far-reaching consequences for the future of architecture, as well as every other aspect of life.

Biotech architecture

Not surprisingly, the first architects to fully exploit the new generation of 'organic machines' were the same architects to exploit the previous generation of progressive technologies. Designed and fabricated with the most advanced CAD/CAM techniques then available, Norman Foster's Hongkong and Shanghai Bank both looks and operates like a building for the twenty-first century[30] (Figs 3.18 and 3.19).

Progresses in the technology of architectural production have been accompanied by significant improvements in energy efficiency, driven by increasing concerns with global warming and related environmental issues. One of the first

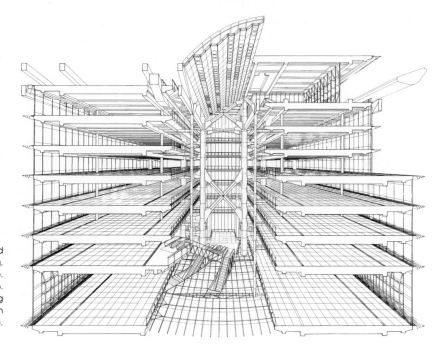

▶ **3.18** Hongkong and Shanghai Bank, Hong Kong. Part sectional perspective. Norman Foster, 1979–86. Drawing shows curved ceiling mirror (centre) above atrium and external sunscoop (right). *Source*: Foster and Partners.

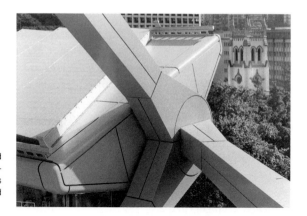

▶ **3.19** Hongkong and Shanghai Bank. Computer-controlled sunscoop deflects sunlight into atrium via mirrored ceiling. Photo: Richard Bryant.

so-called 'intelligent buildings' to be completed in the 1980s, the Hongkong Bank is fitted out with a fully computerized building management system (BMS), monitoring climate control systems and maintenance schedules, much like a nervous system. Hybrid environmental control systems involving both active (mechanically driven) and passive (non-mechanical) elements are also now widely used in all forms of buildings in different parts of the world, including the tropical regions.[31] For example, the Securities Commission Building (Figs 3.20 and 3.21) by Hijjas Kasturi, and the streamlined UMNO Party Headquarters (Figs 3.22, 3.23 and 3.24) by Hamzah and Yeang, both in Kuala Lumpur, are designed with dual environmental systems, resulting in considerable savings in energy costs as well as improvements in working conditions.

The most progressive architects are supported by equally creative engineering firms such as Ove Arup, Battle McCarthy and BDSP Partnership in the UK and Kaiser Bautechnik in Germany, who offer a full range of advanced environmental and engineering design services, backed up by advanced computer simulation techniques for performance testing. The architectural impact of these firms, both in Europe and elsewhere, is often considerable and has contributed to the development of completely new building forms.[32] Often combining advanced technologies with shapes inspired by organic forms, the new 'Biotech architecture' symbolizes an emergent harmony between technology and nature of an entirely new order[33] (Figs 3.25, 3.26 and 3.27).

Developments in energy saving techniques and performance testing have been paralleled by further advances in computerized vizualization and production. Virtual reality techniques now enable both architects and clients to experience and to test a design proposal in ways hitherto undreamt of, opening up entirely new avenues in spatial and sensory visualization[34] (Fig. 3.28). Another fast evolving technology is 'rapid prototyping', involving a combination of lazer and

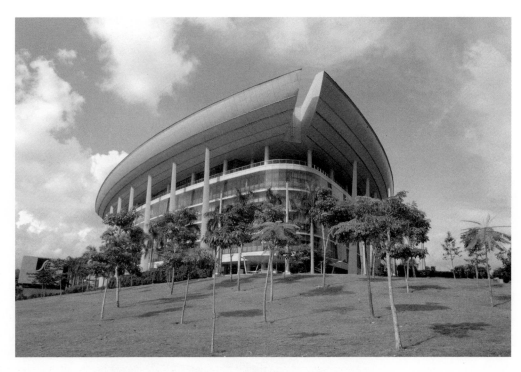

▲ **3.20** Securities Commission Headquarters, Kuala Lumpur, Malaysia. Hijjas Kasturi, 1995–8. Photo: K.L. Ng.

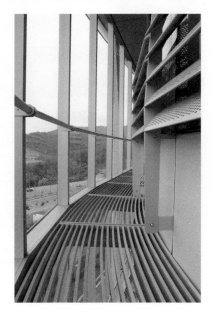

▶ **3.21** Securities Commission Headquarters. Interior of climate wall. Wall uses 'stack effect' to ventilate wide space between glass skins providing thermal barrier between cool interior and hot exterior. Photo: K.L. Ng.

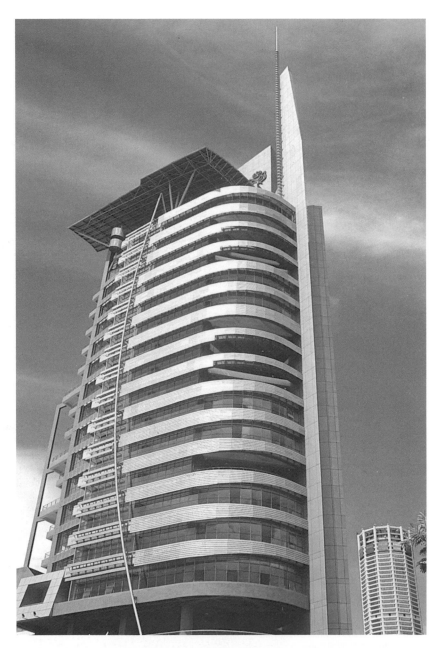

▲ **3.22** UMNO Party Headquarters, Penang, Malaysia. Hamzah and Yeang, 1995–8. Streamline form and external fins help control flow of air around and through tower, assisting cooling and ventilation. Photo: Author.

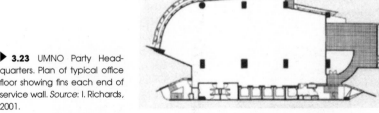

▶ 3.23 UMNO Party Head-quarters. Plan of typical office floor showing fins each end of service wall. *Source*: I. Richards, 2001.

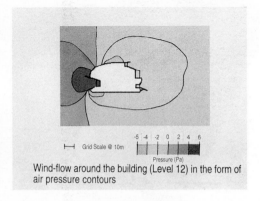

▶ 3.24 UMNO Party Head-quarters. Computer simulation (CFD) of different wind pressures around tower. High-pressure winds left of tower are funnelled through building by fins each end. *Source*: Hamzah and Yeang.

Wind-flow around the building (Level 12) in the form of air pressure contours

stereolithographic techniques. Most efficient where complex shapes and geometries are involved, accurate solid models of components can be produced in a matter of hours direct from CAD data, thus shortening the time needed for design development.[35] Similar techniques were used by the American architect Frank Gehry in the fabrication of the curved titanium cladding sheets and structure for the Guggenheim Museum in Bilbao, Spain, as well as in other projects. A complex, sculptural work of architecture of a very different kind from that which has been normally associated with machine production, the Bilbao Guggenheim has opened up entirely new formal and spatial possibilities[36] (Fig. 3.29).

The most important recent innovations, however, have been associated with the development of the Internet and specialized computer networks, which are already having considerable impact upon collaborative work patterns, and are transforming the way architecture is conceived and produced.[37] Conventional models of the design and production process picture a straightforward linear progression, much like an old-style factory production line: from client's brief – to architect's concept – to client's approval – to engineers' input – to detailed working drawings, and so on to final construction, all in discrete stages and all supposedly led by the architect. By contrast, computer-based collaborative networks operate much more like 'self-organizing systems', with clients, consultants

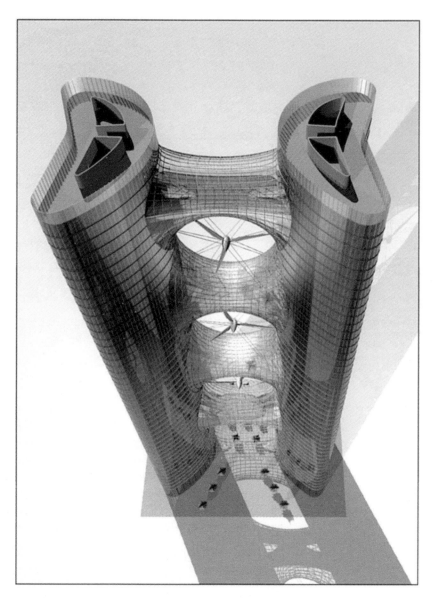

▲ **3.25** Project for Twin Office Tower. University of Stuttgart School of Architecture with BDSP Partnership et al., 2000–01. Built-in wind turbines between towers provide up to half of building's energy needs. *Source*: N.S. Campbell and S. Stankovic, 2001.

and builders – who may be geographically dispersed – all participating in key design and production decisions from the very beginning.[38]

The key to this complex and unpredictable process is the 'virtual prototype', which functions both as a testbed and as a communications medium, providing

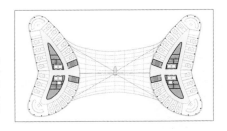

▶ **3.26** Project for Twin Office Tower. Plan shows placement of vertical circulation to shield offices from noise from turbines. *Source*: N.S. Campbell and S. Stankovic, 2001.

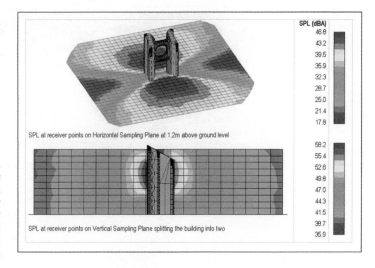

▶ **3.27** Project for Twin Office Tower. Computer simulation of distribution of noise levels around twin towers. Similar studies were used to test most effective shape for channelling wind through turbines. *Source*: N.S. Campbell and S. Stankovic.

instant feedback to everyone involved on the effects of their proposed decisions.[39] Like the networks themselves, the thought processes involved are more likely to resemble analogical thinking than linear logical thinking, with a premium on participants' ability to jump professional and technical boundaries and to make new connections.

Experimental workshop

Related developments in architectural education are also now emerging. Many of the innovations described above were built into the Biotech Architecture Workshop,[40] which was purposefully created in 1996 as a new model of design education in keeping with progressive practice. Going beyond established concepts of bioclimatic or 'green' architecture, an organic concept of integrated design was established based on advanced information technologies and materials, embracing the entire life cycle of design, production and use.

The same principles guided students' Workshop projects, which were entirely computer based. Collaborative networks were established across different

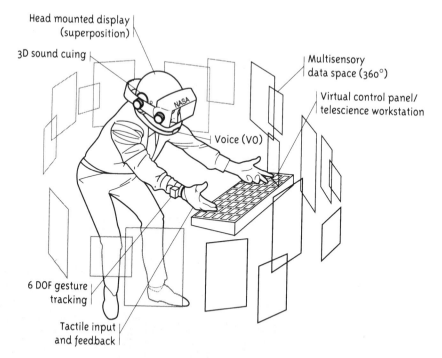

Head mounted display
(superposition)

3D sound cuing

Multisensory
data space (360°)

Virtual control panel/
telescience workstation

Voice (VO)

6 DOF gesture
tracking

Tactile input
and feedback

▶ **3.28** Virtual Reality. Multiple kinds of information can be readily accessed by touching virtual panels surrounding user, as displayed in recent science fiction movies. *Source:* S. Aukstakalnis and D. Blatner, 1992.

locations with leading architectural and engineering firms in London, as well as technical consultants on and off the campus, in a manner approximating to real practice. Working in their own professional-like teams, students developed both virtual and solid prototypes for a variety of building types and components, using advanced simulation and production techniques and recording each step of their progress with on-line multi-media and virtual reality presentations (Fig. 3.30a–d).

Experimental by intention, the Workshop heralds the day when architecture students will be able to put their ideas through the full range of architectural production, simulating visual, functional, structural and environmental as well as economic performance as the design evolves, modifying each factor until such point as the desired result is achieved.[41]

Lesson for the future

It may seem ironic now, that the most important changes in scientific and philosophical thought of this century were taking place during the same period that orthodox Modernism – an indirect product of the dominant mechanistic view under attack – was at its most influential. However, the coincidence is not

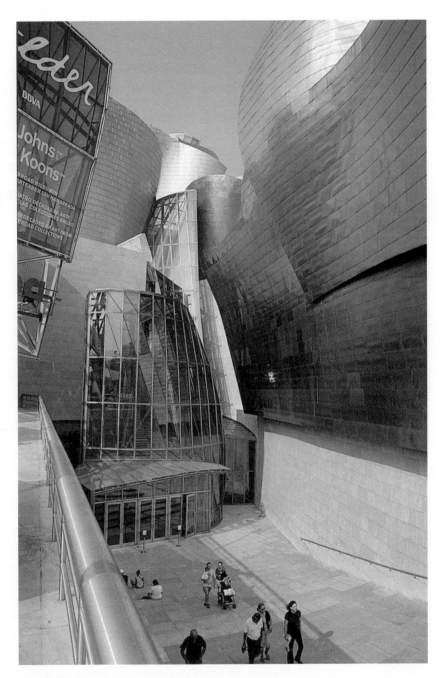

▲ **3.29** Bilbao Guggenheim Museum, Bilbao, Spain. Frank Gehry, 1991–7. Advanced production technologies were used in design and construction of curved walls and titanium cladding. Photo: Author.

(a)
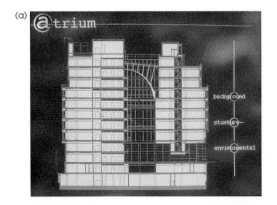

(b)
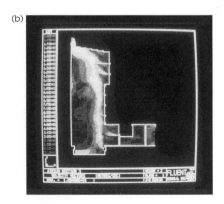

(c)
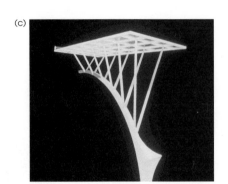

(d)
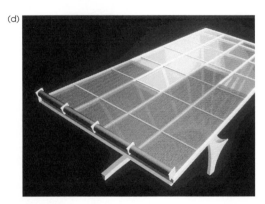

▶ **3.30** Biotech Architecture Workshop. Section through atrium building (a); computer simulation of airflow (b); CAD drawing of roof section showing structure (c), and CAD drawing of roof section showing operable blinds (d). Nottingham University School of Architecture, 1996–7. Studies of environmental performance of atrium under construction in London led to design of operable vented roof and supporting structure. *Source*: Author/Nottingham University.

altogether unusual. It is a characteristic feature of human development that scientific and technological innovation advances at a far greater rate than cultural change. Major scientific and technological breakthroughs also bring with them new ways of thinking, which eventually become assimilated into the general culture, in turn creating new barriers to the next round of innovations. Being deeply ingrained in the cultural values and behavioural habits of the population, architecture is particularly resistant to technological changes which affect those values and habits.

Professional habits of thought and even class prejudices in the building industry often only serve to further hinder the process of acceptance of new ways of working. For all the dramatic social changes that have taken place this century, architects still tend to see themselves primarily as form-givers in a role set apart from other professions and classes – an attitude strongly encouraged by an academically inclined education system – rather than as equal members of a design and production team. It is noteworthy that the few well-known designers working at the cutting edge of architectural technology have successfully broken this mould, and are helping to create more fluid roles and work patterns in keeping with their highly flexible tools.

The clear lesson for the future is that architects are unlikely to make the most of the emergent possibilities for creating a more responsive architecture, unless they also learn to master the new modes of production. And that they cannot do alone, or from a distance.

4

FOSTER AND GEHRY: ONE TECHNOLOGY; TWO CULTURES

APOLLO AND DIONYSUS

If Norman Foster and Frank Gehry had practised in ancient Greece, I imagine that they would have worshipped very different gods. With his low-energy concerns and expertise in using natural light, Foster (Fig. 4.1) would have naturally gravitated towards Apollo, the powerful sun god. Committed to high-performance design, he would also have admired the much-gifted Apollo for his skill with the bow and arrow – a man-powered, tension-structured and lightweight combination that might have been invented by Buckminster Fuller in a former life. Foster would have especially liked Apollo's other role as the god of divination and prophecy, and would doubtless have been a regular visitor to Apollo's most famous temple in the mountains at Delphi. There he would have consulted with the legendary oracle of Delphi, happily tuning into future architectural and technological trends, and probably offering a few forecasts of his own.

Gehry (Fig. 4.2) also has a way with using natural light which might suggest a similar affinity with Apollo, but that doesn't get us to the real heart and spirit of Gehry's work. No, there would have been only one true divinity for Gehry back then: Dionysus, the sensual and very popular god of wine and pleasure. All those exuberant legends and other exotic figures surrounding Dionysus, not to mention the wild festivals: just the sort of thing to inspire one of history's most uninhibited designers. And if Dionysus himself were to relocate in time and space, where would his worshippers feel most comfortable today? Why, hedonistic California of course – Gehry's adopted home state and the main wine producing region in the US. The only thing lacking is a shared worship of fish – adored by Gehry but not especially by Dionysus. Incidentally, Gehry has said that he hopes to retire one day to run his own vineyard. A true follower!

Keynote address to the Fourth International Symposium on Asia Pacific Architecture, University of Hawaii at Manoa, 4 April, 2001. Revised summer, 2003.

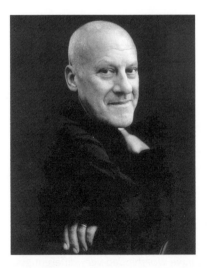

▶ **4.1** Norman Foster. Photo:
Carolyn Djanogly.

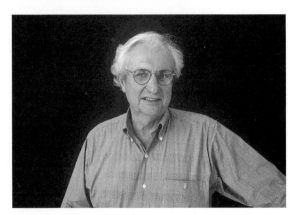

▶ **4.2** Frank Gehry. Photo:
Hisao Suzuki.

EARLY DEVELOPMENT

Unpredictable paths

However, appealing as such caricatures may be, like any polarized comparison they
obscure the more interesting shades of character and ambiguities that surround
both architects and their work. Seminal buildings, such as the Hongkong Bank in
Foster's case and the Guggenheim Bilbao Museum in Gehry's, have also come to
dominate popular perceptions of what these architects are about, to the extent that
they often make us forget that such works were not always typical or representa-
tive of their designers' intentions and concerns, and may – as in Foster's case if not
in Gehry's – have already been superseded by the architect's more recent projects.[1]

Both architects' paths also overlap in unpredictable ways, each designer mostly
travelling in opposite formal and spatial directions, while in other respects coming

closer together, most particularly in their working methods, though also in other ways, as we shall see.

From being an early regionalist of sorts, drawing his inspiration directly from his Californian surroundings, Gehry has become more and more concerned with developing his own highly original and personal aesthetic. A Gehry design is now a much sought after global status symbol, conferring instant fame – and even fortune in some cases – on its private or municipal owners.

Foster, on the other hand, started out as a thoroughly orthodox if exceptionally talented Modernist, producing a series of elegant but anonymous steel-framed pavilions in the minimalist manner established by Mies van der Rohe. From the mid-1980s, however, as Foster's practice grew and spread outside the UK to other, more exotic shores, so has there been a broadening of expression and response to place, climate and culture in his work, contradicting the early simplistic descriptions and often catching critics off balance.

Californian vernacular

Gehry's early work also had a certain kind of anonymity about it, though it was more the kind which goes with blending seamlessly into the local Californian vernacular, rather than the anonymity of the International Style practised by Foster in his early years. In the Danziger House (Fig. 4.3), for example, Gehry replicated the simple stuccoed timber frames and cubic forms found everywhere in Los Angeles, producing a kind of stripped-down Spanish colonial style, touched with Modernist abstraction.

From such modest beginnings Gehry's work quickly acquired a more artful character, both in the literal sense of having more purposeful artistic content, and also in the sense of demonstrating a knowing slyness. A student of the fine arts before turning to architecture, Gehry has retained his fascination with modern

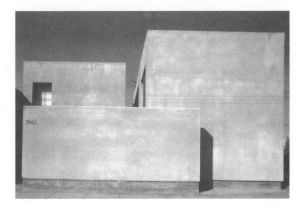

▶ **4.3** Danziger House and Studio, Hollywood, California, USA. Frank Gehry, 1964. Photo: Marvin Rand.

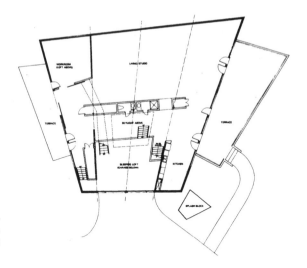

▶ **4.4** Ron Davis House, Malibu, California, USA. Plan. Frank Gehry, 1970–2. *Source*: K.M. Hays and C. Burns, 1990.

art throughout his career and proudly includes numerous artists among his closest friends. In the Ron Davis House (Fig. 4.4), Gehry took the basic form and construction of the regional farmhouse barn, and, by exploiting the flexibility of the timber frame and distorting the external and internal geometry, created an architectural, three-dimensional version of the artist's own painterly experiments in perspective illusions.

Gehry's artfulness and ability to make something extraordinary out of the ordinary, is manifest again in his inventive use of commonplace materials – most famously in his cardboard furniture (Fig. 4.5) and chain-link screens made from fencing – and in the casual fragmentation and apparent incompleteness of his buildings. In the extensions to his own house (Fig. 4.6) in Santa Monica – formerly a plain suburban bungalow – translucent chain-link screens stretched over tubular metal frames are combined with 'floating' wall elements of corrugated metal and plywood set at odd angles, reflecting the *ad hoc* and transitory nature of construction in the Los Angeles suburbs. In the Norton House (Fig. 4.7) on the Venice beachfront, the free standing study mimics the lifeguard huts dotting the beach, while the main body of the house is fragmented into a number of distinct parts, each finished in a different way, so that the house practically disappears into the surrounding bric-à-brac. Chain-link screens are also used to great effect in covering the parking building and providing the base for a giant sign for Santa Monica Place (Fig. 4.8), a shopping centre designed by Gehry in the same city. An indication of Gehry's early interest in the commercial vernacular, it is however one of the few buildings of its type ever designed by him.

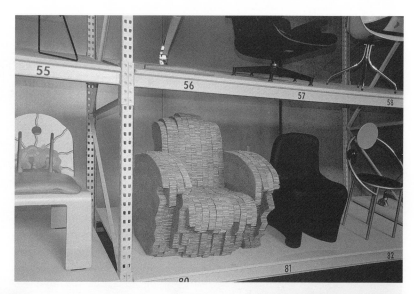

▶ **4.5** Cardboard chair. Frank
Gehry, 1994. Photo: Author.

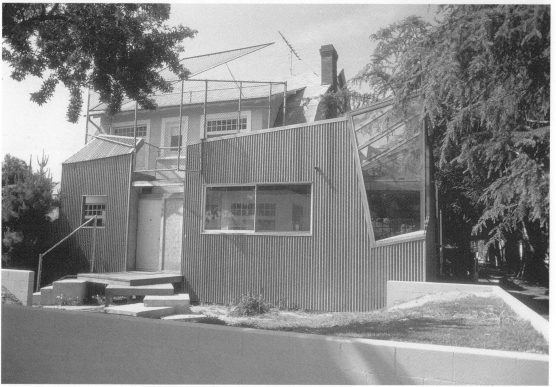

▲ **4.6** Architect's own house, Santa Monica, California, USA. Frank Gehry, 1978. Photo: Tim Street-
Porter/Esto.

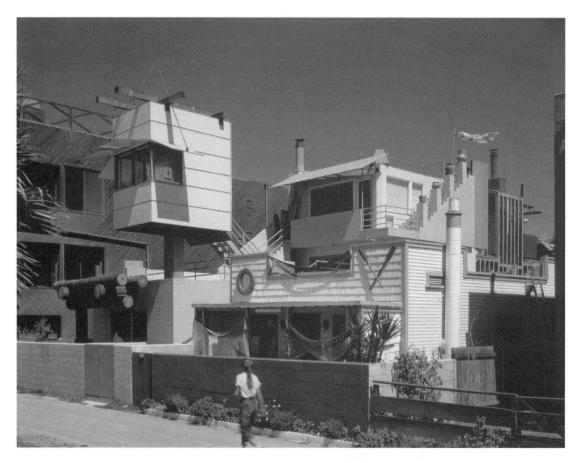

▲ **4.7**   Norton House, Venice, California, USA. Frank Gehry, 1984. Photo: Michael Moran/Esto.

Fragmentation

There followed a series of house designs, such as the Schnabel House (Fig. 4.9a–c), with its multiple components, and the Winton Guest House (Fig. 4.10) with its centrifugal, pinwheel plan (Fig. 4.11), in which Gehry takes the theme of fragmentation to its extreme. Splitting the accommodation into a number of almost completely separate volumes, Gehry designed each house as a cluster of assorted small houses, looking more like an odd 'village' rather than a single dwelling. The more parts there are to see, he believes, the more possible meanings there are:

> What I like doing best is breaking down the project into as many separate parts as possible. ... So, instead of a house being one thing, it's ten things. It allows the client more involvement, because you can say, 'Well, I've got ten images now that

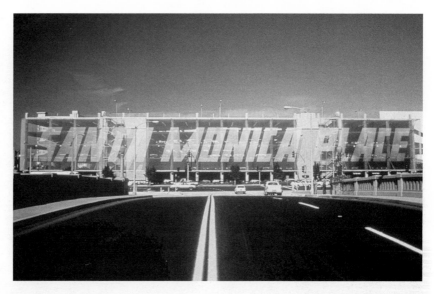

▲ **4.8** Santa Monica Place Garage, Santa Monica, California, USA. Frank Gehry, 1980. Photo: Tim Street-Porter/Esto.

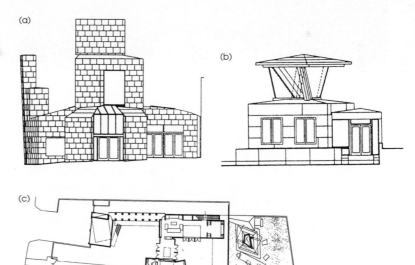

▶ **4.9** Schnabel House, Brentwood, California, USA. Elevations of living rooms (a), master bedroom (b), and plan (c). Frank Gehry, 1986–9. *Source*: F. Gehry, 1999.

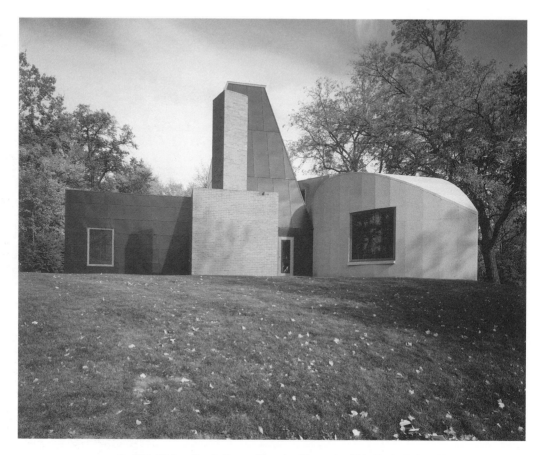

▲ **4.10** Winton Guest House, Wayzata, Minnesota, USA. Frank Gehry, 1985–6. Photo: Mark Darley/Esto.

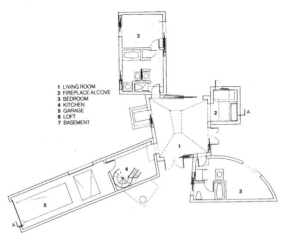

1 LIVING ROOM
2 FIREPLACE ALCOVE
3 BEDROOM
4 KITCHEN
5 GARAGE
6 LOFT
7 BASEMENT

▶ **4.11** Winton Guest House. Plan. *Source*: *Progressive Architecture*, December, 1987.

are going to compose your house. Those images can relate to all kinds of symbolic things, ideas that you've liked, places you've liked, bits and pieces of your life that you would like to recall'.[2]

(Burns, 1990, pp. 82–3)

In either case, whether the building is freestanding, as with the Winton House, or closely packed in with others, as with the Norton House, fragmentation is seen by Gehry – as indeed it was and still is by many other contemporary designers – as an effective device for shaking down preconceptions and encouraging new associations.

Similar themes connect Gehry's domestic clusters to his larger and overtly Postmodern works of the same period, such as the Loyola Law School (Fig. 4.12), also in Los Angeles. Like the residential 'villages', the programme is fragmented into distinct elements, each designed in a quite different language of form, freely mixed this time with a kind of abstracted classicism, intended to give each element its own identity. However, while classical architecture is a commonly used source of form for American law courts and suchlike, Gehry's

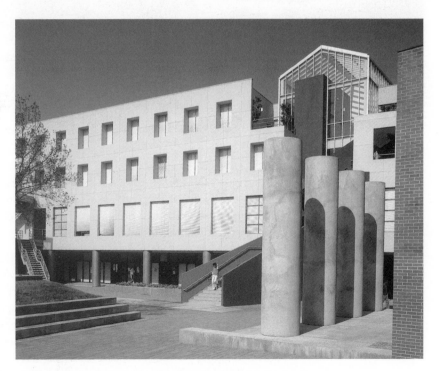

▲ **4.12** Loyola Law School, Los Angeles, California, USA. Frank Gehry, 1981–4. Photo: Tim Street-Porter/Esto.

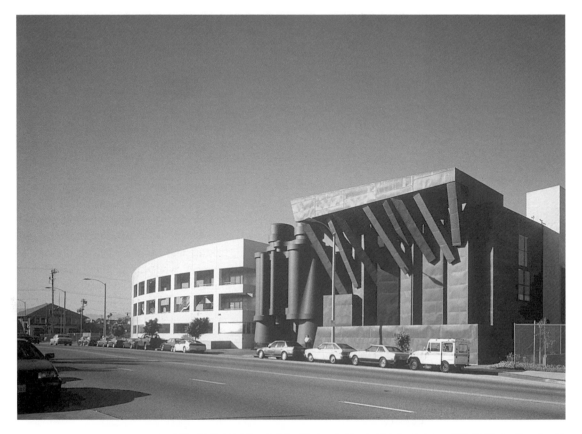

▲ **4.13** TBWA Chiat/Day Building, Venice, California, USA. Frank Gehry, 1985–91. Photo: Hisao Suzuki.

free and easy way with the language – represented here by a group of shorn off columns hinting at a ruined temple – suggests a tongue-in-cheek, Disneyland quality, giving the complex a local feeling of a very different kind, part institutional, part commercial vernacular.

In his TBWA Chiat/Day Building (Fig. 4.13), Venice, designed for the advertising agency responsible for the Apple computer company's 'Be Different' campaign (in which Gehry also featured), Gehry goes much further down the same road. What looks like a giant pair of binoculars placed upright on the main street frontage is sandwiched between an equally striking tree-like structure and a relatively ordinary office building. Designed with Claes Oldenberg – a sculptor renowned for his outsize recreations of similar everyday objects – the building purposefully blurs the distinction between architecture and commercial art, grabbing as much attention from passing motorists as any billboard.[3]

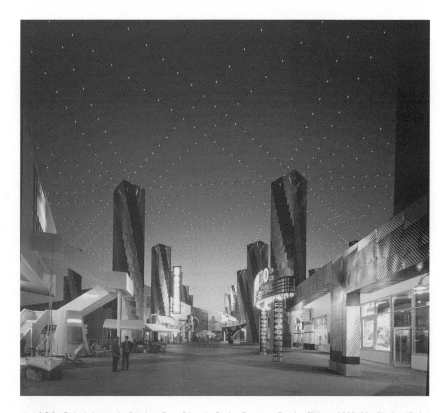

▲ **4.14** Entertainment Centre Euro-Disney, Paris, France. Frank Gehry, 1988–92. Photo: Peter Aaron/Esto.

The Chiat/Day building earned the architect public as well as professional notoriety. By this time Gehry was to architecture what Andy Warhol had been to painting, hovering somewhere between art and commerce and arousing just as much controversy. The Entertainment Centre for Euro-Disney (Fig. 4.14) near Paris, took Gehry's flair for fantasy and commercial imagery to its logical conclusion. It also marks the virtual end of the architect's fascination with the commercial vernacular – or at least with its direct expression – to be displaced by quite different interests.

Integrated approach

There could hardly be any greater contrast than that between Gehry's artful manipulation of forms and cheery disregard for conventions, and Norman Foster's early works in the UK. Against Gehry's open-ended structures and fragmentation, we see in Foster's work an equally strong but opposite desire for integration – both of the programme and of the elements of building – and for unitary or closed forms. Against Gehry's inventive contextualism and *ad hoc* use of materials, we see Foster at the outset focusing instead on context-free, universal forms and standardization – core features of orthodox Modernism.

The Sainsbury Centre (Fig. 4.15) exemplifies Foster's early work: a regular structure embracing all functions within a single, flexible enclosure or 'universal space', the design is all about allowing for change, internally and externally. However, contradictions soon appear in the actual execution of Foster's early works, substantially qualifying their industrialized or universal status. During this period Foster also fashioned his own now familiar work methods which he calls 'design development', but which I prefer to call simply, 'integrated design',[4] of which the Sainsbury Centre is a clear demonstration.

Briefly, integrated design means getting involved as closely as possible with the people and industries who make the parts of your building and put it all together, from the very beginning of the design process, right through to the end. It means preferably having your own in-house engineers, such as Loren Butt and 'Chubby' Chhabra, who both worked on Foster's early classics, to ensure that spatial

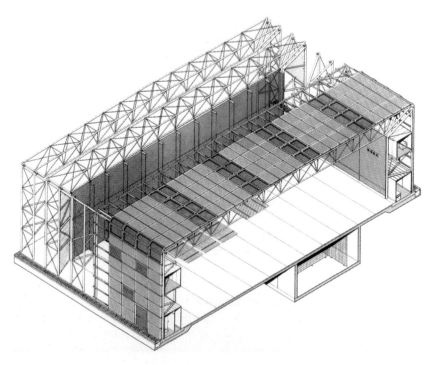

▲ **4.15**   Sainsbury Centre for Visual Arts, Norwich, UK. Cutaway isometric of structure. Norman Foster, 1974–8. *Source*: Foster and Partners.

concept, structure and environmental systems are all conceived as one. It means working in harmony from beginning to end with your external consultants, as Foster has done with engineers like Anthony Hunt or Tony Fitzpatrick of Ove Arup, who are creative designers themselves. In short, it describes a collaborative, interdisciplinary design approach where problems of structure, fabrication, construction and environmental performance, are not treated as someone else's problem or left until the end, when it's usually too late, but which are taken into account from the outset and help shape the process all the way down the line.

All of which, of course, just sounds like familiar orthodox Modernist dogma, which it largely is. Except as we all know too well from countless failed buildings, the collaborative idea was never really carried through. What early Modernists were mainly interested in, just as too many designers of all kinds are today, was an *image* of modernity, rather than how buildings were actually made or how they worked or how much they cost.[5] Each profession has also mostly gone its own way so that what we have today is a badly fragmented industry, where serious gaps of language, expertise and values have to be bridged with each and every project.

In actual practice, Foster's approach meant that, although outwardly the product of mass-production methods, from the mid-1970s onwards each component system was either especially adapted or tailor-made for a particular project. For example, while the metal cladding panels (Fig. 4.16) for the Sainsbury Centre, with their distinctive corrugations, may look as though they were stamped out on mass-production lines, just like the panels on the old Citroen car admired by Le Corbusier, they are in fact unique to that building and were formed by craft methods using cheap wooden moulds. What standardization there was, was limited to reducing variations within the project itself, and has as much to do with Foster's flexible planning concepts as anything else.

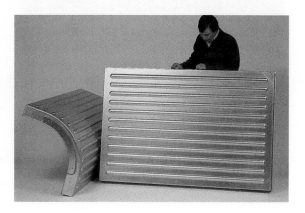

▶ **4.16** Sainsbury Centre For Visual Arts. Two of original aluminium cladding panels. Photo: Richard Davies.

LATE DEVELOPMENT

Changing values

There were other changes in Foster's work, subtle at first but also symptomatic of important shifts in values. At the Willis Faber and Dumas HQ (Fig. 4.17) in the old town of Ipswich, for example, the famous minimalist glass skin had to be especially designed to take up the curves in the wall, which are politely bent to follow the surrounding medieval street pattern. Air-conditioning and artificial lighting systems necessitated by Foster's typical deep plan schemes, were also now increasingly supplemented by the energy saving advantages and subtleties of natural light which poured in through openings in the roof in ever more dramatic fashion (Fig. 4.18).

All Foster's buildings until this time concealed their structures from external view behind their skins, allowing only partial views of the skeletons within – at each

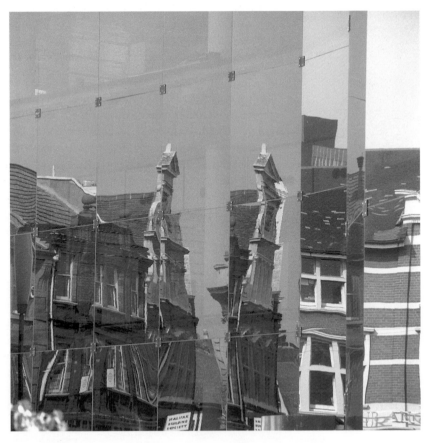

▲ **4.17** Willis Faber & Dumas Headquarters, Ipswich, UK. Detail of glass wall. Norman Foster, 1971–5. Photo: John Donat.

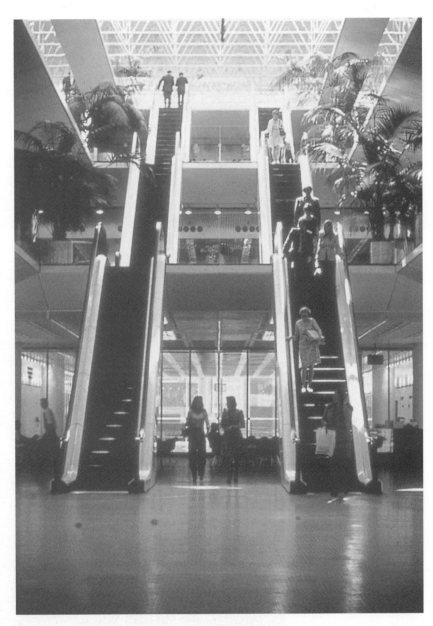

▲ **4.18** Willis Faber & Dumas Headquarters. Interior view of atrium and escalators. Photo: John Donat.

end in the case of the Sainsbury Centre or at night time at Willis Faber and Dumas, when the thin-edged, streamline floors are illuminated. The Renault Centre (Fig. 4.19) cast all such reticence to the winds with a gangling, yellow-painted, masted structure, which stepped outside the weather wall of the building in an exaggerated display of structural expressionism. Based on a repetitive roof module, each component system was nevertheless customized for the job,

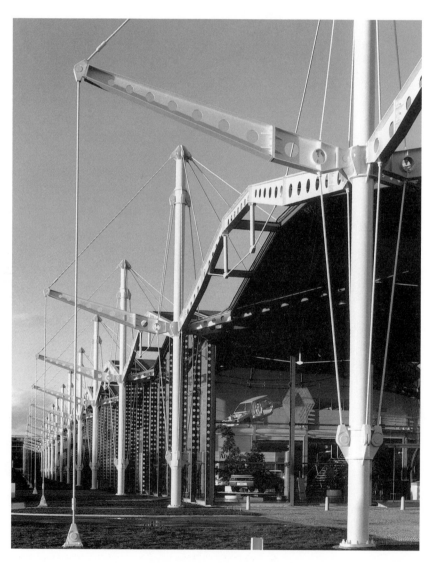

▲ **4.19**   Renault Distribution Centre, Swindon, UK. Norman Foster, 1980–2. Photo: Dennis Gilbert.

involving production methods ranging from ancient cast iron for the tension roof connectors, to CAD/CAM to cut the holes in the I-beams.[6]

Like Gehry, during this period Foster also frequently found new uses for commonplace or 'non-architectural' materials, often borrowing from other industries. The steel wall cladding at the Renault Centre, for example, which has a fine, stiffening profile, is the same as that used for the skins of caravans while the flexible joint at the fascia (Fig. 4.20) derives from the skirts of hovercrafts. Stapled together in strips and held in place with spring clips similar to those used for lorry loads, the detail has much of the same rough and ready, improvised look as that which characterized Gehry's early work.

Regional qualities

If the Renault Centre marked a new phase in Foster's career – not easily anticipated from the earlier minimalist works – it was soon eclipsed by the Hongkong Bank (Fig. 4.21), which took the whole architectural world, including this critic, by surprise.

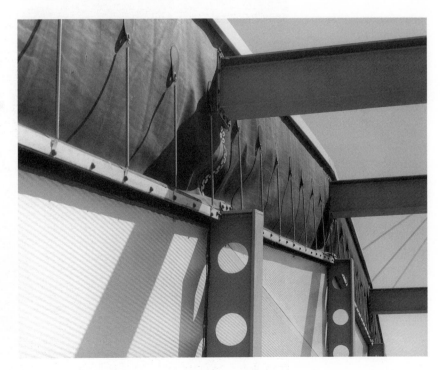

▲ **4.20** Renault Distribution Centre. Detail of flexible eaves showing spring fixings. Photo: Dennis Gilbert.

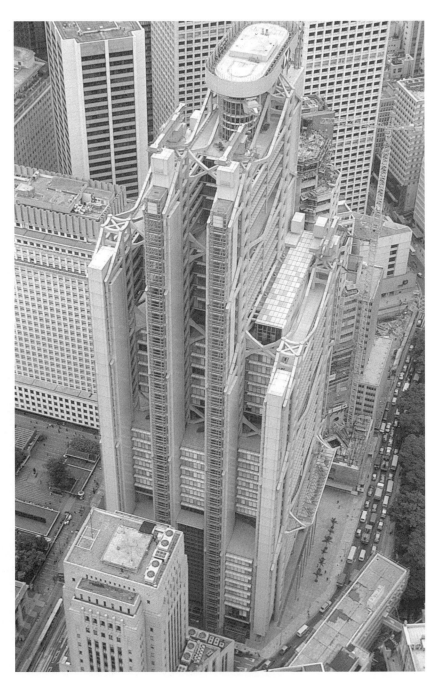

▲ **4.21** Hong Kong Bank, Hong Kong. Overhead view. Norman Foster, 1979–86. Photo: Author.

Expecting a purely Western import, what I actually found when I saw it for myself shortly before completion, was the first wholly convincing example of regional high-rise architecture in East Asia, which would have looked equally at home in Tokyo as it does in Hong Kong. Most architects are by now very familiar with this astonishing building's main features, so I won't hold up the main argument with too many details. I will just emphasize the very Japanese play between exaggerated structure and transparency, which help to lend the design its regional character (Fig. 4.22). The lucid expression of how every element in the building comes together, together with the suffused natural light – these are all qualities we are familiar with from Japanese traditions. The essential difference between past and present works is that, instead of being hand-crafted, this is a wholly machine-crafted building. Crafted, moreover, with combined CAD/CAM technologies,

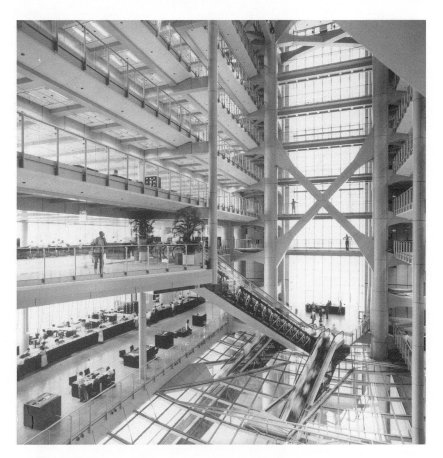

▲ **4.22** Hong Kong Bank. Interior of atrium with suspended glazed structure over entranceway. Photo: Ian Lambot.

including robot welders and computerized numerically controlled (CNC) metal cutting machinery, the like of which had never been used on the same scale in the construction industry before (Fig. 4.23).[7]

The same qualities reappeared in still more refined form in the Century Tower (Fig. 4.24) in Tokyo, which Foster completed 5 years later. Significantly, it was the structural clarity and attention to detail – reminiscent of the Sikuya style and other traditions – that most drew the admiration of Japanese critics. One writer even likened Foster's devout approach to his work to that of a monk.[8]

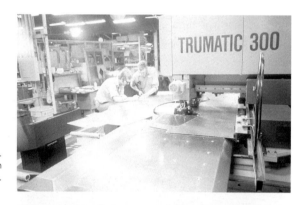

▶ **4.23** Hong Kong Bank. CNC machines used in fabrication of cladding. Photo: Cupples.

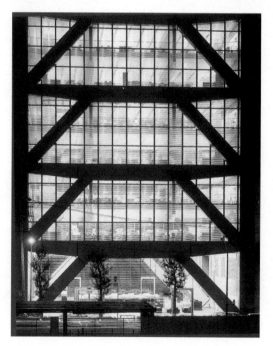

▲ **4.24** Century Tower, Tokyo, Japan. Detail of two-storey high structural frames. Norman Foster, 1987–91. Photo: Martin Charles.

In another development, while the extrovert Hongkong Bank was still being built, Foster embarked on his first major project in Continental Europe, the Carre d'Art (Fig. 4.25), a multi-purpose cultural and media centre situated in the ancient Roman city of Nimes, France. A landmark exercise in Modernist contextualism, the Carre d'Art carries the respectful approach developed with the WFD in Norwich into still trickier urban terrain, subtly acknowledging the Roman temple opposite yet remaining firm to Modernism's roots.[9]

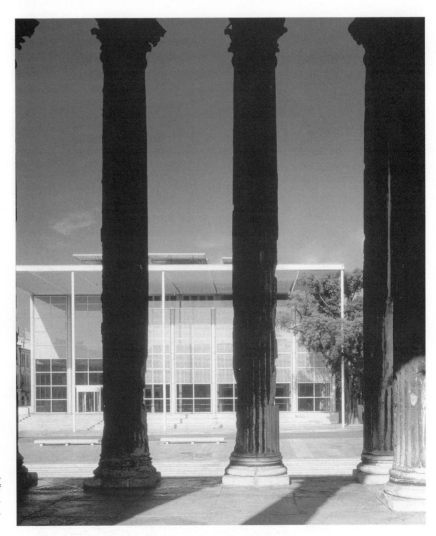

▶ **4.25** Carre d'Art, Nimes, France. View from portico of Roman temple opposite. Norman Foster, 1984–93. Photo: Tim Soar.

Sculptural architecture

Meanwhile, back in California, in the mid-1980s Gehry was also entering a new phase in his career, and had begun to experiment with a curvaceous, overtly sculptural language of form, making endless models until he felt he had it just right – an essential part of Gehry's working method to this day.[10]

In hindsight, it is possible to see precedents for Gehry's taste for curves in his earlier product designs, such as his 'fish' and 'snake' lamps (Fig. 4.26), made from formica, or in his upscaled use of fish motives elsewhere. For all that, the uncompleted Lewis House project (Fig. 4.27) in Ohio came as a shock. Like

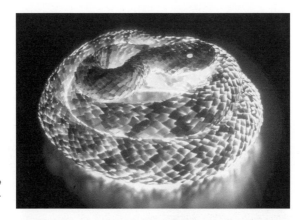

▶ **4.26** Formica Snake Lamp. Frank Gehry, 1983–6. *Source: El Croquis*, 74–75.

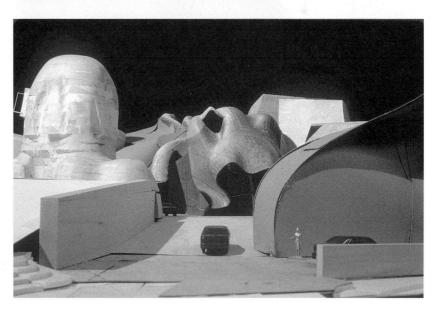

▶ **4.27** Lewis House, Lyndhurst, Ohio, USA. Model. Frank Gehry, 1985–95. Photo: Joshua White.

the Winton House and other 'village' clusters, the accommodation for the much larger Lewis residence was fragmented into a number of distinct but now far wilder shapes. Some elements have a vertical emphasis looking like a group of wobbly, fat chimneys, while others have blob-like shapes resembling marine life-forms – forms which spawned a whole school of less accomplished 'blob-meisters' – all designed with a total freedom of expression more commonly associated with the fine arts than with architecture.

By comparison, the Vitra Furniture Museum (Fig. 4.28) in Weil am Rhein, Germany – one of three commissions by the same company – designed while work was still continuing on the former, seems relatively modest, or at least coherent. However, seen against the adjacent Vitra factory, designed by Gehry at the same time as a simple 1930s style 'box', it cries out for attention from passing motorists on the nearby road as much as the Chiat/Day Building does. Executed, like the factory, in white plastered masonry and concrete – materials strongly associated with the classic period of Modernism – and capped by

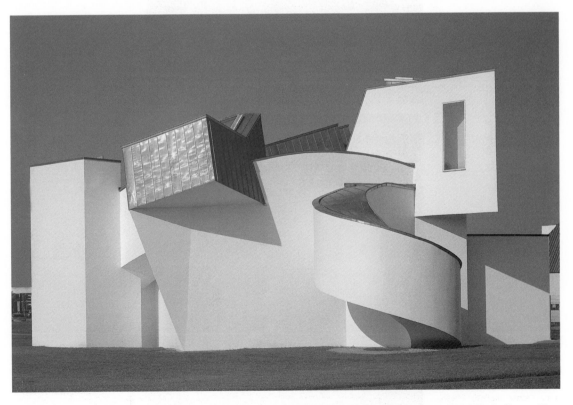

▲ **4.28** Vitra Furniture Museum, Weil am Rhein, Germany. Frank Gehry, 1987–9. Photo: Thomas Dix.

curved zinc roof panels, the museum appears both familiar and unfamiliar at the same time.

Nevertheless, for all the legitimate historical comparisons that have been made – Rudolf Steiner (Figs 4.29 and 4.30), Le Corbusier, Alvar Aalto and baroque architecture in general all figure prominently – the fragmented, unstable massing and sheer joy of expression are all Gehry's own. Neither can it be said that Gehry's attentions are restricted to the external form only: the complex, multi-level exhibition spaces are perfectly scaled to the exhibits and the handling of the natural toplight shows off the irregular volumes to their best effect (Fig. 4.31).

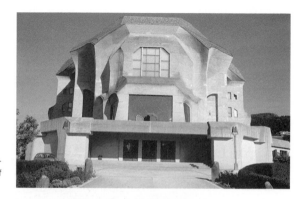

▶ **4.29** Goetheanum, Dornach, Switzerland. Rudolf Steiner, 1924–8. Photo: Author.

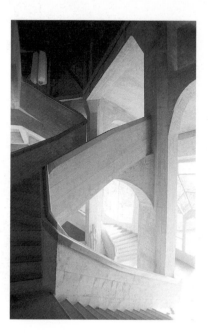

▶ **4.30** Goetheanum. Interior of foyer and stairway to auditorium. Photo: Author.

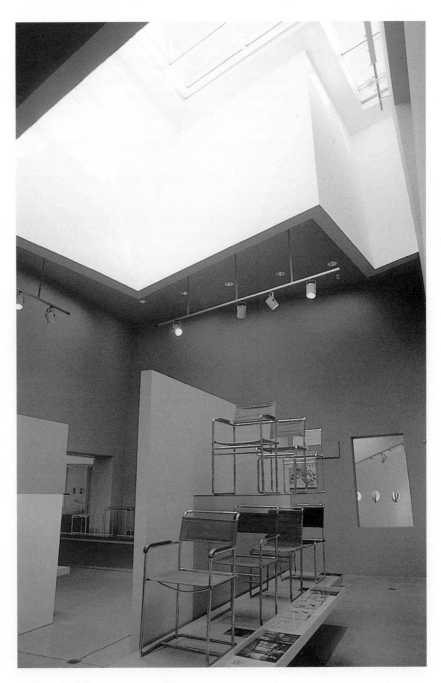

▲ **4.31**   Vitra Furniture Museum. Interior. Photo: Author.

New methods

The Vitra Museum pushed the use of conventional design and construction technologies to the limit. While the Lewis House was not completed for other reasons, it could never have been realized using the same means. Other projects then under way presented similar problems. The American Centre in Paris (Fig. 4.32), a complex exercise in contextualism as subtle in its own way as Foster's Carre d'Art, quickly followed. Mimicking the conventional materials and geometry of its neighbours on the main street, the eccentric structure transforms into a jumbled mass of irregular curves as it turns into the park in which it stands, straightening up again as it meets the buildings aligned on its other side.

As with the Lewis House, the design of the American Centre was apparently based more on faith than practical knowledge. A confrontation between Gehry,

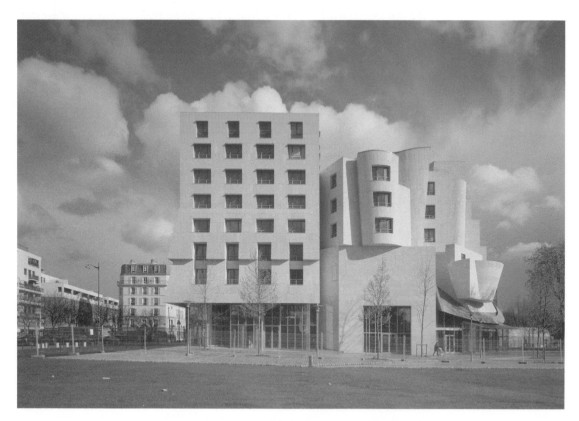

▲ **4.32** American Centre, Paris, France (now the Maison du Cinema). Frank Gehry, 1988–94. Photo: Paul Raftery/View.

the free-wheeling artist, and the limitations of the construction industry, was inevitable. But it was a local project that finally breached the dam. In 1987 Gehry was commissioned to design the Walt Disney Concert Hall (Fig. 4.33), his largest and most challenging project until that time. However, he soon ran into trouble with the executive architects charged with producing the construction drawings. Partly inspired by Hans Scharoun's Philharmonie in Berlin, a seminal work in the organic tradition, Gehry's complex forms and structures made his other work look like child's play, upsetting the executive architects, who costed the job accordingly.[11]

Realizing that he was entering uncharted waters, in 1989 Gehry hired Jim Glymph to boost the technical expertise in his office.[12] As a condition of his contract and to help avoid the kinds of problems that had arisen with Gehry's executive architects, Glymph insisted that, in future, construction details and production drawings would be produced in-house. From hereon also, while both Foster and Gehry continued to produce very different kinds of architecture, the gap between the technologies and modus operandi employed by these two contrary designers begins to narrow.

To appreciate the full significance of these developments it needs to be understood that, while it is common practice for American architects to delegate the detailed design and execution of their projects to other, more specialized firms, European firms generally take full responsibility for both design and execution of their projects, including production drawings. I hasten to add that this does not mean that the European approach is perfect or without its own problems. Far from it. Like their American counterparts, most European architects are educated to work quite separately from related professions or sectors in the construction industry, and are finding it increasingly difficult to keep up with technological developments and new materials and components.

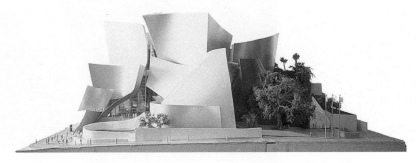

▲ **4.33** Walt Disney Concert Hall, Los Angeles, California, USA. Model. Frank Gehry, 1987–2003. Photo: Hisao Suzuki.

It was precisely in response to this situation that Foster evolved his integrated design approach. Following Foster and other pioneers like Richard Rogers, Nicholas Grimshaw, Future Systems, Renzo Piano, Thomas Herzog et al., there is now a well-established tradition among a small but rapidly growing number of practices in Europe, working in just this fashion.[13]

Outside Europe, however, with few exceptions the story is very different, especially in the US, where integrated design in architecture is practically unknown. And this is just where Gehry, his new associates and his reconstituted practice come in. Searching for ways to help Gehry realize his complex forms and handcrafted models, Glymph looked to the aircraft industry for new solutions. He eventually found what he was looking for in the Catia software system developed by the French aerospace company, Dassault Systemes. Created to translate the complex shapes involved in automobile and aircraft design (Fig. 4.34) into geometrically precise forms suitable for fabrication and manufacture, the programme was ready-made for Gehry's purposes.[14]

Applications

The first application of the new approach was for a steel fish sculpture-cum-sign Gehry conceived to mark the Vila Olimpica (Fig. 4.35), a retail complex built for the 1992 Olympic Games in Barcelona, Spain (in his typically straightforward manner, Gehry has explained that he resorts to fish motives whenever he can't

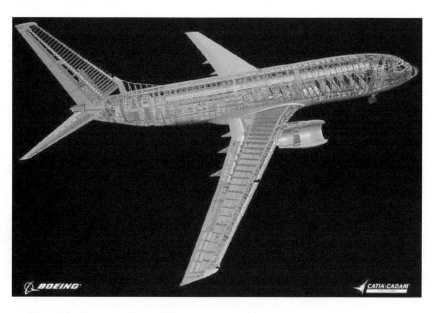

▲ **4.34** Catia 3D model of Boeing 737. *Source*: Dassault Systemes.

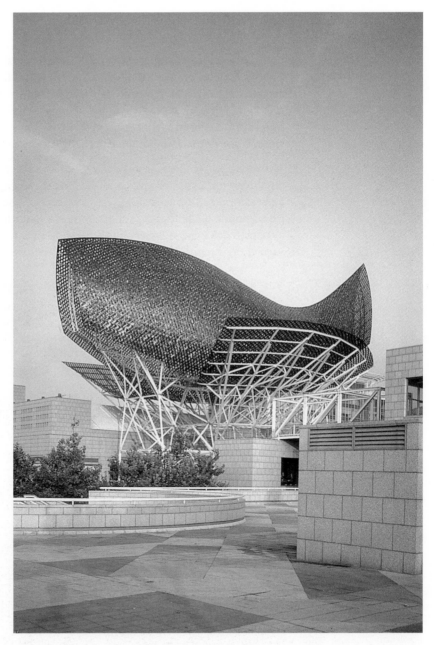

▲ **4.35**   Vila Olimpica Fish Sculpture, Barcelona, Spain. Frank Gehry, 1992. Photo: Hisao Suzuki.

think of anything else).[15] Designed and built in haste for the opening of the games, the Catia programme both simplified and speeded up the whole process.

Both programme and approach have been successfully applied to nearly all Gehry's projects ever since, including the design for the Disney Hall, now finally completed, as well as the American Centre. However, the project that most captured both professional and public imaginations was the Bilbao Guggenheim (Fig. 4.36). Designed in 1991 and completed six years later, the building is to Gehry's body of work what the Hongkong Bank is to Foster's.

The Bilbao Guggenheim brought world-wide attention to Gehry's design methods and to the Catia process itself. The process has been described many times before, by Gehry's own staff as well as by others,[16] so I will just summarize the main steps. In the first stage, a specially devised laser tool looking something like a dentist's drill is guided over a physical model of the design, plotting the curved surfaces as a series of digitized points in a three-dimensional space and feeding

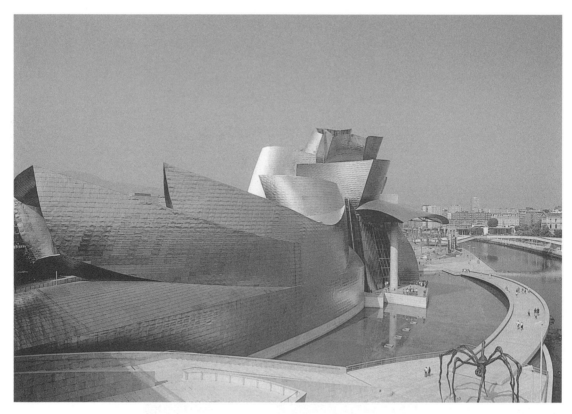

▲ **4.36** Guggenheim Museum Bilbao, Bilbao, Spain. Exterior view along riverfront. Frank Gehry, 1991–7. Photo: Author.

the results into a computer (Fig. 4.37). The same coordinates are then converted by the computer into a surface model that can then be modified or refined by the designers as needed (Fig. 4.38). Next, the computer model is used with various so-called rapid-prototyping technologies to create a new physical model, from which further refinements may be made to the computer model to produce more physical models, and so on.[17] Once the physical design has been finally approved, a series of further computer models are produced for structural and cladding studies, or even to control robots and other machines fabricating parts of the building itself. The same models can be used to produce accurate cost estimates of cladding systems and the like at an early stage in the design process, taking account of every single curved variation, so avoiding the kinds of problems Gehry ran into with his executive architects on the Disney Hall.

However, the value of the technologies used in the design and fabrication of the Bilbao Guggenheim, as with those used by Foster, must finally be judged by the

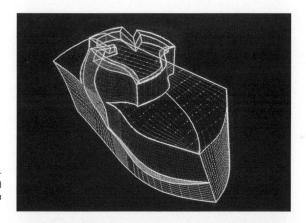

▶ **4.37** Guggenheim Museum Bilbao. Catia 3D digitized point model. Photo: Erika Barahona Ede.

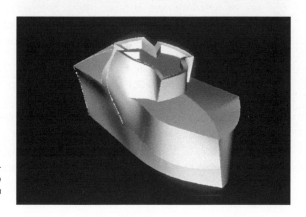

▶ **4.38** Guggenheim Museum Bilbao. Catia 3D surface model. Photo: Erika Barahona Ede.

quality of the architecture they help the designer to achieve. Conceived as part of a major programme of urban renewal, the museum was intended to raise both the cultural profile and financial fortunes of the city. That it has succeeded beyond all expectations is both a testimony to Gehry's personal creative skills, and more generally to the role of star architects today, who are frequently hired by ambitious state or private clients to ensure that a new building will help to draw visitors, and thus pay its way.

This in itself is nothing new. It is the case that major museums from the Louvre in Paris onwards have always been designed to command as much attention and respect as the art works they contain. Frank Lloyd Wright's original Guggenheim Museum in New York took the approach that much further, in that Wright's famous spiralling atrium actually competes with and dominates the contents.

It is to Gehry's credit therefore, that, when asked by his clients to create another central space like the Wright atrium in New York, Gehry at first resisted the idea, believing that Wright's design was 'antithetical to the art'.[18] Under pressure, Gehry eventually agreed, and went on to create the extraordinary space at the heart of the Bilbao museum (Fig. 4.39). Laced by a circulation system that draws visitors constantly back and forth through it, the sculpted space dominates the composition, both internally and externally (Fig. 4.40).

Geometrical division

It comes as something of a surprise, therefore, to learn that most of the exhibition space for the Guggenheim's permanent collection is actually provided for in the simpler, stone-clad rectangular blocks which penetrate this writhing mass (Fig. 4.41). The curvy, titanium-clad parts are reserved for the temporary exhibitions and for circulation. The partition between orthogonal and non-orthogonal geometries is familiar from Aalto's work – surely Gehry's most important influence[19] – where the master also used it to differentiate between one set of functions and another, most clearly in his cultural centres and libraries[20] (Fig. 4.42). However, such is the seductive appeal of the irregular sections of the Guggenheim that the significance of the geometrical division – at least externally – is easily missed.

At Bilbao, the spatial separation of the main permanent collection from the temporary collections – where presumably greater artistic risks can be afforded – thus neatly avoids the worst aspects of the potential conflict between container and art, which bedevils the original Guggenheim. For all that, such is the overwhelming power of Gehry's design that the building demands attention as a work of art in its own right – a kind of large-scale, useable sculpture, challenging, as it was meant to do, contemporary artists to produce something equally striking in their own fields. Seen in the flesh, the Guggenheim is also happily free

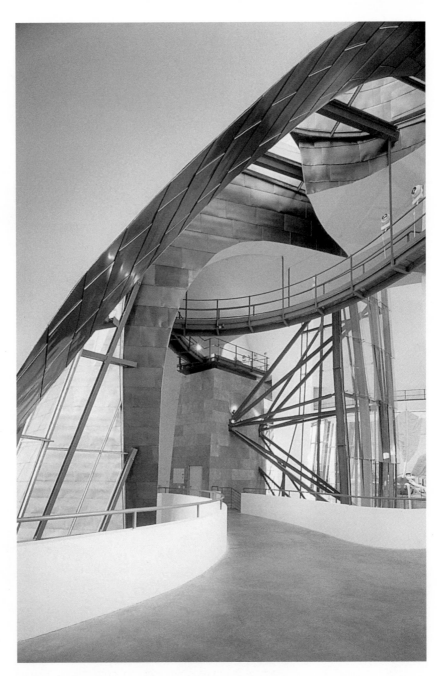

▲ **4.39** Guggenheim Museum Bilbao. Interior view of central atrium. Photo: Erika Barahona Ede.

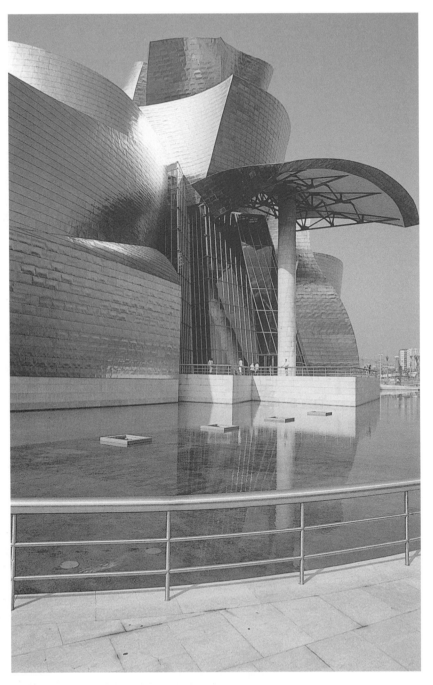

▲ **4.40**   Guggenheim Museum Bilbao. Exterior view of central atrium. Photo: Author.

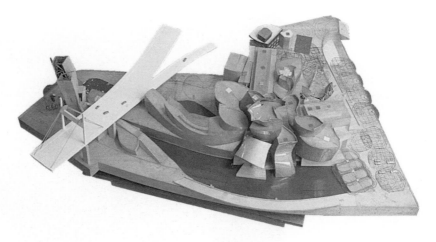

▲ **4.41** Guggenheim Museum Bilbao. Model. Photo: Hisao Suzuki.

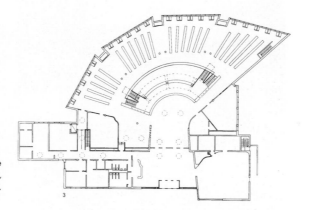

▶ **4.42** Benedictine College Library, Mount Angel, Oregon, USA. Plan. Alvar Aalto, 1965–70. *Source*: Architectural Design.

from the curious lack of scale that seems to characterize many of Gehry's published projects. Partly due to the texture of the titanium panels, partly to the glazed and steel-framed sections and partly to the surrounding terraces, stairs and pathways which integrate the building with the site, all of which afford visible references to the human dimension, the billowing shapes of the museum have a grandness of scale in real life which the models and photographs only hint at (Fig. 4.43).

Regaining control

Whether sculpture or architecture, or – as Gehry himself would probably argue – both together,[21] there can be no questioning the visual and spatial impact of the

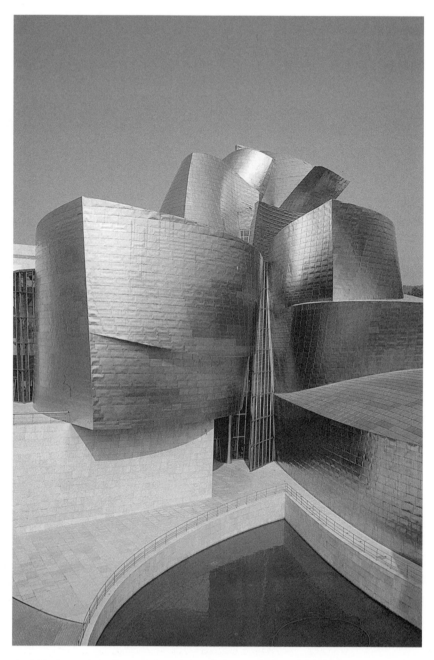

▲ **4.43** Guggenheim Museum Bilbao. Exterior view from bridge. Photo: Author.

design, or the value of the production technologies which made it all possible. Gehry himself is in no doubt about the benefits or professional implications of his new smart tools. For Gehry, such technologies offer a means to essentially traditional ends, and are a way of regaining the architect's control over the design and construction process that was lost to industrialization: 'Its the old image of the architect as master builder',[22] as he puts it. Most important, for Gehry, it helps to cut out all those executive architects and other middle men and puts him and his partners into direct contact with the craftsmen and other people who actually construct the building.

Such sentiments could easily have been voiced by Foster, though he would not describe them in quite the same words. Foster values the collaborative or team principle too much to place the architect so far above everyone else as Gehry does. Structural engineers especially have also had a far greater direct influence on Foster's architecture than they have on Gehry's, and, as we have already noted, are treated as equal designers. A product of the peculiarly British tradition of engineering-architecture, running through Joseph Paxton's Crystal Palace to the hi-tech movement, most of these engineers are based in or near London, and are an essential part of British architectural culture and the integrated design approach.

Foster's earlier use of CAD/CAM technologies also grew naturally out of his close involvement with the people and firms who make his buildings, a collaborative process with industry which goes right back to the very beginning of his career and which is one of the leitmotifs of his work.[23] Gehry's use of Catia, on the other hand, as Glymph explains, originally came about because it was the only way to translate his increasingly complex forms into reality, and not least because it fits comfortably with his reliance on using solid models to explore his designs: 'The idea of bringing the computer into the office was to introduce it in a way that it did not change Frank's design process'.[24] Only later, it seems, did Gehry come to see the broader implications of the system for architects and the building industry generally.

However, while Foster may have led the way in using such technologies to customize the components and elements of his architecture, they have been mostly applied – until his more recent projects at least – within a relatively conventional formal and spatial framework. By contrast, Gehry's personal pursuit of an ever more complex architectural and geometrical language has led him and his partners to exploit the flexibility of his smart production tools to the maximum, in hitherto untried ways. And it has been Gehry's audacious experiments in form which have captured the public and professional imagination, and which have drawn most attention to the new technologies of production, and what they might do for architecture at large.

Paradoxically, it can also be argued that while the built result looks very different from Foster's architecture, each designer is adapting the same flexible technology to his own preconceived and preferred architectural ends and values. It is the ends and values themselves that make the difference, and both architects see their smart tools as a means of extending their control over the design process (it is noteworthy that Foster, like Gehry, still makes extensive use of physical models in the early stages of the design process, often producing numerous variations in his pursuit of the right solution for a given project).

SHELTER AND TEMPLE

Divergent programmes

Nevertheless, if Foster and Gehry are united in their attitude towards control over the design and building process, they differ radically on other vital issues. The most important differences relate to the characteristic building types with which each architect has come to be associated: factories, offices and airports for Foster; private dwellings, concert halls and museums for Gehry. While both architect's actual range is obviously considerably wider than this limited selection might suggest, the professional reputations of each designer have been largely built up from the way each has tackled these particular types. The fact that new clients continue to offer each architect similar programmes, also says much about the public perception of their work, and how it fits into society at large.

Foster's own working-class background in Manchester has undoubtedly influenced his predisposition toward improving the ordinary worker's lot, whether in the factory or in the office, although his continuing belief and that of his partners in Modernism's social agenda is equally, if not more important. The predominance of the most common functional building types in Foster's *œuvre*, therefore, says as much about his approach and priorities as the predominance of various centres of cultural activity and private residences in Gehry's *œuvre* says about that architect's approach and priorities. It is also the case that when invited to tackle a new building type, each architect, as architects generally do, tends to transfer more or less the same language and skills developed for the earlier and more characteristic programmes, over onto the new one, rather than start all over again. So while each architect is continually broadening his range, it is his experience with the more characteristic types that continues to govern his progress.

I suggest that, basically, what we have here is a division of interests and commitments as old as architectural history: between utility and performance on the one hand, and art on the other. Or, put another way – between shelter and temple.

There are, I admit, all kinds of possible objections to what is yet another polarized comparison, no less simplified and open to question than the one I offered at the very beginning of this paper. There is no shortage of drama or poetry in

Foster's architecture. Andreas Papadakis, former editor of *Architectural Design*, once said to me of Foster's work: 'His buildings sing!'[25] But what drives Foster to cover such a wide range is ultimately a thoroughly Modernist, optimistic vision of a better society, sharpened by his own humble origins, for which nothing less than a broad-fronted effort will do.

Gehry's student career was also dotted with numerous (unbuilt) social housing schemes. His early houses in Los Angeles, not to mention those streetwise buildings, like Santa Monica Place and Chiat/Day, which reflect the popular culture of that city, also demonstrate an acceptance of the local vernacular and a creative skill in manipulating it, which has rarely been equalled.

However, the key projects that provided the experimental springboard and models for Gehry's more recent work, are the later houses, especially the Winton House, with its fragmented elements tenuously held together by its pin-wheel plan – as much a characteristic planning device as the dual geometries – and the curvy and highly individual Lewis House.[26] What remains of Gehry's early interest in vernacular architecture has since been mostly confined to the odd contextual exercise, such as the American Centre in Paris and the later Netherlands National Building in Prague. More common building programmes, although they occur from time to time, are a relative rarity.

Exceptions

Notable exceptions to the rule are the Vitra International Headquarters at Birsfelden, Switzerland, and the group of three office buildings, Der Neue Zollhof (Fig. 4.44), Dusseldorf, a speculative development on the old harbour

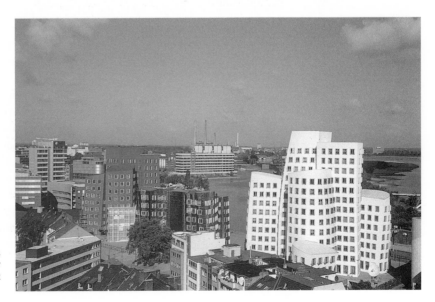

▶ **4.44** Der Neue Zollhof, Dusseldorf, Germany. View over site towards Rhine River. Frank Gehry, 1994–9. Photo: Author.

front close to the Rhine river. However, while both broaden Gehry's *œuvre*, the latter design is also among the least convincing of his works.

Technically speaking, the warped cluster of medium-rise office towers at Dusseldorf, with its asymmetrical structures and tailor-made windows, is one of the most interesting in Gehry's architectural *œuvre*. The construction of the walls themselves involved cutting the individual plastic moulds for the precast concrete panels directly from three-dimensional models produced by the Catia process, as well as producing three different cladding systems (Fig. 4.45).

For all that, in contrast to Gehry's handling of other kinds of building types, they appear to have been designed with mostly external visual criteria in mind. Germany's stringent building regulations require that all offices are naturally ventilated and that every worker should be able to sit close to an opening window. While fulfilling the regulations, the office spaces in Der Neue Zollhof appear cramped and inflexible. Although the opening windows afford natural ventilation, their small size also restricts potentially splendid views across the harbour toward the Rhine (Figs 4.46 and 4.47). The penetration of natural light is likewise limited – even on a bright day offices are artificially lit.

There are aesthetic and urban design problems too. While each of the three structures is clad in a different material – brick, plaster, or, most successfully, stainless steel – the use of the same small window module throughout the whole complex suggests a closed, somewhat forbidding group of buildings. Overall, the general impact is of an imposed uniformity; surely *not* what Gehry intended!

The appearance is reinforced by the lack of any possible public interaction with the buildings at ground level. This is not for want of motivation. According to his own account, Gehry purposefully divided the development into three separate structures in order to allow people to pass freely through the site and to open up views through it. However, the mostly solid walls run straight into the paved surroundings without any kind of modulation or change of use, creating the sort of lifeless open spaces around the buildings we are all too familiar with from the post-war decades (Fig. 4.48). Most disappointing, in stark contrast to Gehry's projects in Bilbao and Paris, each of which presents a quite different face according to context, there seems to have been little or no attempt to relate the buildings to the different aspects presented by the site, which backs on to a busy urban thoroughfare. Whether facing inward across the street towards the bustling café life opposite, or outward across the open harbour, or sideways towards its neighbours, each building presents essentially the same visage and character. Only the small, canopied entrances leading off the street tell you which side is which.

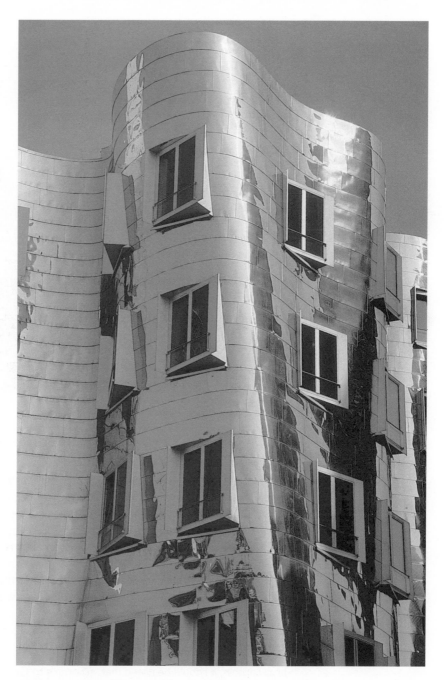

▲ **4.45**   Der Neue Zollhof. Detail of stainless steel cladding with mirror finish on middle building. Photo: Author.

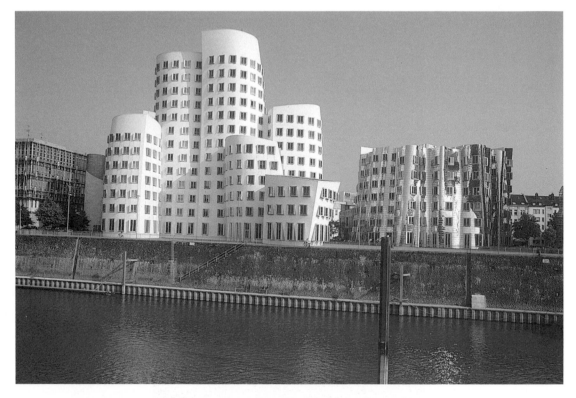

▲ **4.46**   Der Neue Zollhof. View from harbour. Photo: Author.

Dual planning concept

It is perhaps unfortunate for Gehry that one of his few attempts at designing modern offices should have been built in Dusseldorf, a city renowned for some of Germany's most innovative office architecture. Notable buildings include the circular tower at Victoriaplatz 2 by Hentrich-Petschnigg and Partner, the Stadttor by Overdiek, Petzinka and Partner, and not least, the recently completed ARAG tower by Foster[27] (Fig. 4.49). All three buildings are models of energy efficiency and are flooded with natural light. While outwardly more conventional in appearance than the Gehry group, each offers attractive working conditions, including generous views, bright and flexible spaces, and, in one case, a few small shops and a café integrated into the ground floor – just the sorts of simple but important amenities missing from Der Neue Zollhof.

In all fairness, it should be noted that, according to Gehry, Der Neue Zollhof was successfully completed to a tight budget, and, as speculative ventures go, is a financial success. Overall, however, Gehry fares much better in Switzerland with

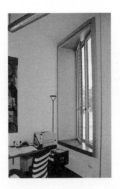

▶ **4.47** Der Neue Zollhof. Interior detail of office window. Photo: Author.

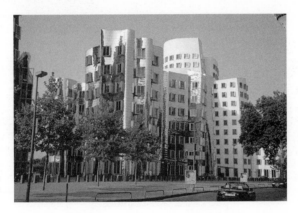

▶ **4.48** Der Neue Zollhof. View from plaza. Photo: Author.

his Vitra International HQ (Fig. 4.50). Comprised of two linked buildings with contrasting geometries – a long rectangular office block and a cluster of sculpted spaces called the 'Villa' – the building works well on every level, both aesthetically and as a working environment. The familiar dual planning concept (Fig. 4.51) meets the client's requirement for flexible working spaces-cum-showrooms in the rectangular block, while giving free rein to Gehry's artistic sensibilities in the free form villa, which functions as the office canteen and social centre. As the name suggests, this is designed as a fragmented group of mostly room-sized spaces similar to many of Gehry's residential designs and includes various meeting rooms, each with its own distinctive space.

Unusually for Gehry, the Vitra HQ office block itself is also an energy-efficient building and is clearly designed – at least in part – in response to the climate. This is no accident. As in Germany, Switzerland's exacting regulations require that office buildings are naturally ventilated with opening windows. To protect the glazed south wall from the sun, Gehry designed a massive metal canopy propped

(a)

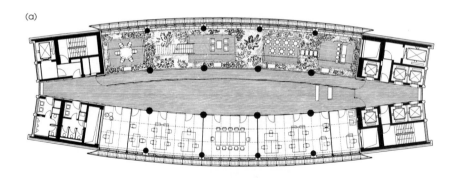

(b)

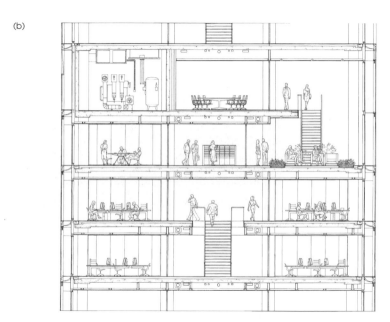

▲ **4.49**   ARAG Headquarters, Dusseldorf, Germany. Plan (a) and part section (b) showing two-storey skygardens. Norman Foster, 1993–2001. Photo: Foster and Partners.

up at one end by a single square column and at the other by a large strut cantilevered from the block. Bridging the difference in architectural languages as well as the space in between the office block and the villa, the beefy sunshade makes a striking feature.

Problematic issues

As effective and satisfying as the design of the Vitra HQ is, the impression remains that this is one of those exceptions that prove the rule. Had Gehry not

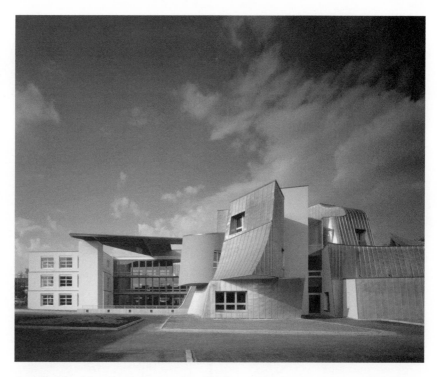

▲ **4.50** Vitra International Headquarters, Birsfelden, Switzerland. Frank Gehry, 1988–94. Photo: Richard Bryant.

been compelled to respond to the client's need for functional flexibility or the Swiss building regulations on energy conservation, it is doubtful that these issues would have been given so much attention. As Der Neue Zollhof complex shows, even the enforcement of similar building regulations does not in itself guarantee that the architect will respond in the same way or as successfully.

Notably, the success of Gehry's efforts in handling these issues at the Vitra HQ is largely dependent upon his use of a conventional planning geometry and formal language. In this respect, Gehry's repeated use of two planning geometries or architectural languages – a similar division occurs between the design of the Vitra Museum and the adjacent factory – within the same project, looks suspect. As much of a retreat from Gehry's preferred architecture as a way of expressing different functions, the dual planning method provides a convenient way of dealing with problematic issues of function and energy with more conventional means.

(a)

(b)

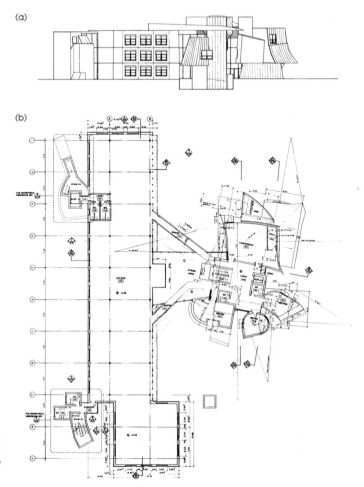

▶ **4.51** Vitra International Headquarters. Elevation (a) and plan (b) *Source: El Croquis*, 74–75.

The impression that Gehry's priorities lie elsewhere is confirmed by the architect's treatment of his work in his own publications. For example, while the prestigious Spanish journal *El Croquis*[28] draws readers' attention to the energy-saving features of the Vitra HQ, the same features get no mention at all in Gehry's own book, *Gehry Talks*.[29] Nor, for that matter, while the use of Catia and other technical aspects are discussed in detail, does energy conservation get any mention anywhere else in the book.[30]

High-performance design

By contrast, Foster's commitment to energy efficiency and everyday problems and functional programmes, as evidenced in numerous projects aimed at improving the workplace, provide the mainstay of his studio's current work, just as it did of his earliest works;[31] all of which has been closely argued and documented in the studio's own publications, as well as in the media. In addition to the numerous acclaimed designs for factories and the like, Foster's *œuvre* now covers practically every known kind of infrastructure, including railway and metro stations, bridges and telecommunications towers.

All this is very much in the mainstream of Modernist thinking, which embraces all aspects of environmental design, from the largest scale of urban and regional planning, to the smallest household object. Indeed, Foster's practice ranges all the way from masterplanning to the design of door furniture (Fig. 4.52), and his analytical and painstaking approach to each and every problem encountered has evolved to meet these very diverse ends. Even the Hongkong Bank, Foster's most

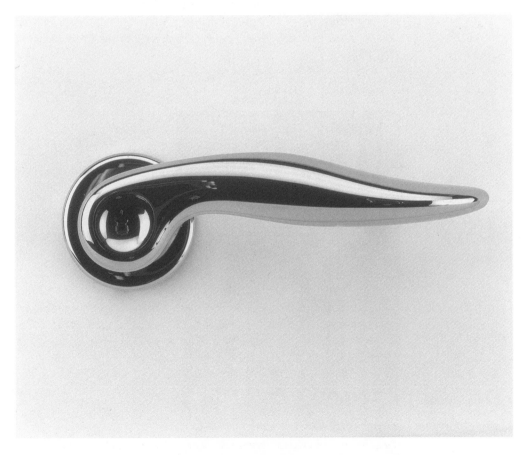

▲ **4.52** Fusital Door Furniture. Cresta Range. Norman Foster, 1994–5. Photo: Peter Strobel.

famous and costly design, is best understood as one in a series of closely linked experiments in the design of modern offices. Thus the people-friendly, dual circulation system of escalators and lifts first used at Willis Faber and Dumas, get to be reused in the Hongkong Bank, and the Bank's tentative 'skygardens' get to be fully realized in the Commerzbank tower (Figs 4.53 and 4.54) in Frankfurt, and later again in the ARAG tower, and so on.

Foster's commitment to low-energy, high-performance design, and the advanced technologies he employs to that end, also need to be viewed in the same broad context, as a vital aspect in the development of a contemporary vernacular, embracing all forms of building.[32] As a model for energy-efficient and worker-friendly design, the Commerzbank, for example, has few equals: the first modern skyscraper to use opening windows and natural ventilation – as much as 80 per cent of the year – the performance in use exceeds even Germany's high standards. As well as providing pleasurable 'outdoor' meeting places, the multi-storey skygardens, which are naturally ventilated, also double as the building's 'lungs', drawing fresh air into the overlooking offices[33] (Fig. 4.55).

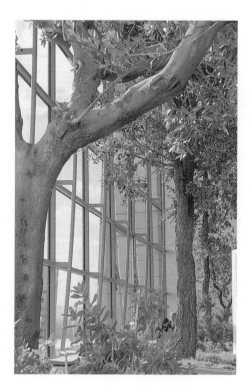

▶ **4.53** Commerzbank Headquarters, Frankfurt, Germany. Internal view of four-storey wintergardens. Norman Foster, 1991–7. Photo: Nigel Young/ Foster and Partners.

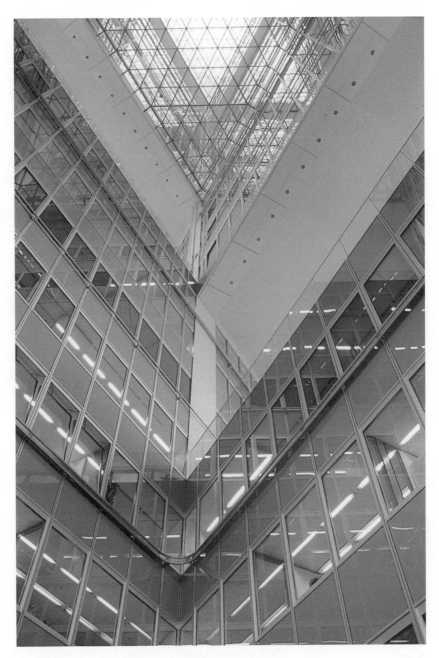

▲ **4.54** Commerzbank Headquarters. View up through central atrium linking rear of wintergardens. Photo: Author.

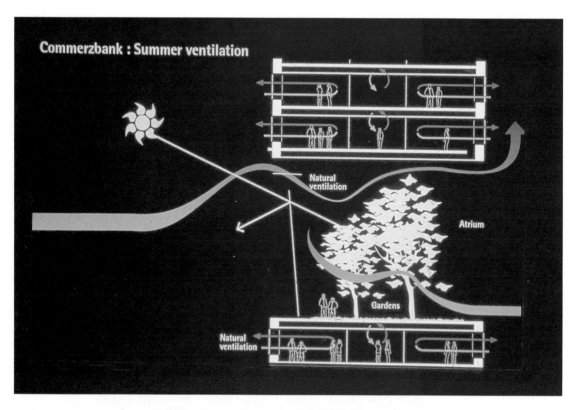

▲ **4.55**   Commerzbank Headquarters. Section through wintergardens. *Source*: Foster and Partners.

However, the climate control system at the Commerzbank is only one of a long series of related innovations by the firm. Beginning with the underfloor air-conditioning system for the Hongkong Bank, which only cools the lower layers of air in which people actually work, Foster and his engineers have pioneered a whole range of low-energy environmental systems. Many of these were also first developed in Germany, where the strict regulations encourage the highest levels of energy efficiency in the world. They include: the passive, double-skinned 'climate wall' for the Business Promotion Centre (Fig. 4.56), part of a hi-tech research and manufacturing complex in Duisberg (a variation of the system was also used for the ARAG tower in Dusseldorf); making use of waste heat from the power generator to drive an absorption cooling machine, which in turn provides cold water for the cooling system, also for the Business Centre; pollution-free power generation using refined vegetable oil extracted from sunflower or rape seeds for the New German Parliament, Reichstag, in Berlin; the use of natural aquifers (underground wells) for storing and recycling hot and cold water, also for the Reichstag Parliament; a solar electric vehicle powered by a

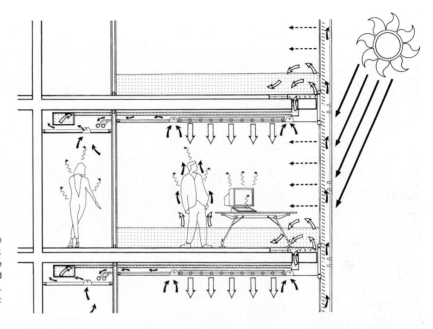

▶ **4.56** Business Promotion Centre, Duisberg, Germany. Section through office showing climate wall, chilled ceilings and natural airflows. Norman Foster, 1990–3. *Source:* Foster and Partners.

combination of batteries and photovoltaic cells on the roof, and last but not least, a new generation of giant wind turbines for Enercon (Fig. 4.57), designed in collaboration with the company's engineers.[34]

Dynamic modelling techniques

Since the design of the Commerzbank, Foster has also made regular use of dynamic computer modelling techniques, such as computational fluid dynamics, or CFD, to test the effect of different environmental systems on a building's energy efficiency. Such modelling techniques played an important role in shaping the office tower for Swiss Re (Fig. 4.58), London, and the new headquarters for the Greater London Authority (GLA). Examples of just how much energy and environmental issues influence Foster's architecture, both designs evolved from simple geometric forms into something far more complex, requiring entirely new methods of architectural production. Starting out as a pure cylinder, the bullet shaped Swiss Re morphed into its present form under the progressive impact of different computer models, as the architects and engineers sought to integrate all the main factors. Designed to minimize the effect of wind forces on the helical structure (Fig. 4.59), in addition to reducing structural weight the aerodynamic form also reduces any downward flow, doing away with the notorious windy conditions around the base of skyscrapers which normally plague pedestrians. The spiralling skycourts – a development from the Commerzbank's skygardens – which give the Swiss Re its unique spatial and social character

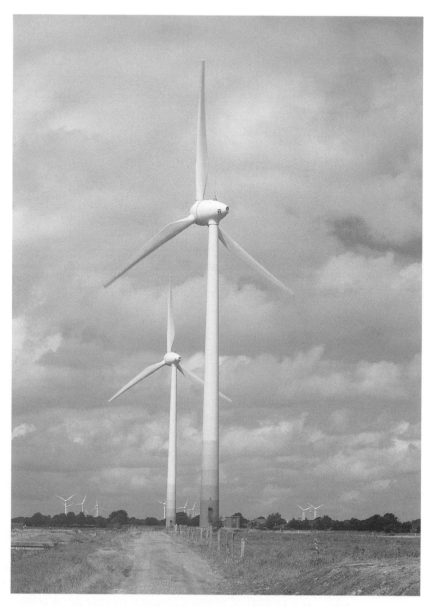

▲ **4.57** Enercon E66 Wind Turbines, Holtriem wind farm, Germany. Norman Foster, 1993. Photo: Nigel Young/Foster and Partners.

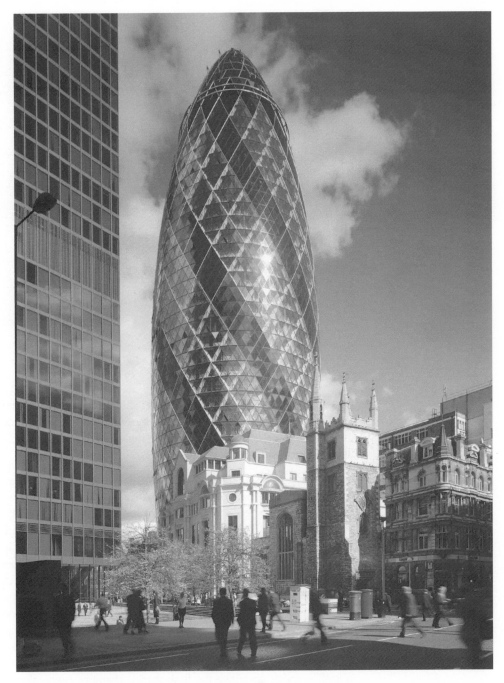

▲ **4.58** Swiss Re Headquarters, London, UK. Norman Foster, 1997–2004. Photo: Nigel Young/Foster and Partners.

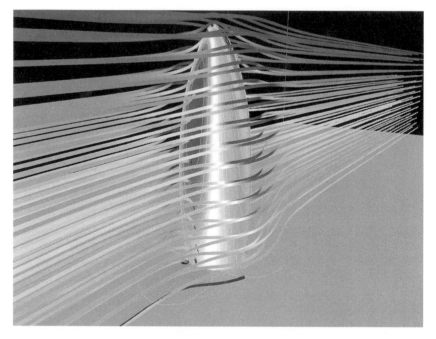

▲ **4.59** Swiss Re Headquarters. Computer simulation of wind forces on tower. *Source*: BDSP Partnership.

(Fig. 4.60), also play an important part in the building's system of climate control: pressure differences created around the structure assist natural ventilation through the skycourts by forcing air in on the windward side and sucking it out on the downwind side.[35]

In a similar process, under the impact of the sun path and other environmental considerations, the GLA design morphed from a pure sphere – the most efficient geometric form for enclosing a given volume – to its present laid-back, lens-like shape (Fig. 4.61). Sloping backwards from its site on the south bank of the River Thames, the north face of the building is precisely angled so that at no time of the day or year does the sun directly strike the steel and glass wall (Fig. 4.62). Correspondingly, the south-facing wall is stepped upwards and outwards, so that the upper floors shade the lower ones. Internal sunshades wrapped around the south, east and west sides finish the job, leaving the north side completely clear for the council members and observers to enjoy the views across the river from inside the council chamber, which is situated directly behind the glass wall. A spectacular elliptical stairway – a complex geometrical exercise in itself – spirals up above the flask-shaped chamber connecting all the floors, providing office workers with the same views (Fig. 4.63).

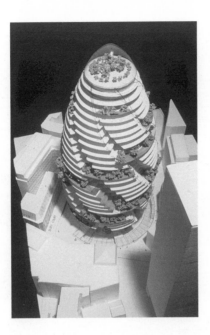

▶ **4.60** Swiss Re Headquarters. Model showing skycourts. *Source*: Foster and Partners.

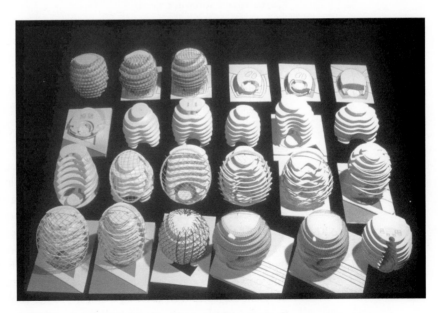

▲ **4.61** Greater London Authority Headquarters, London, UK. 3D models showing changes in geometry from pure sphere to lens shape. Norman Foster, 1998–2002. *Source*: Foster and Partners.

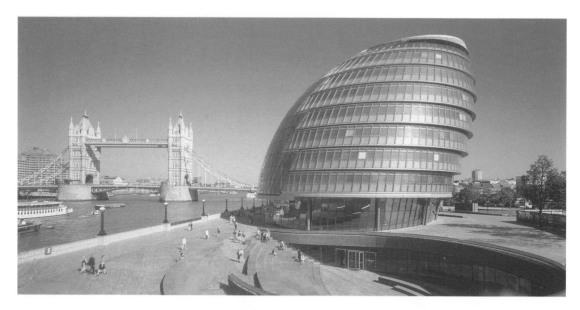

▲ **4.62** Greater London Authority Headquarters. View towards Tower Bridge. *Source*: Nigel Young/Foster and Partners.

Customized software tools

Partly in response to the complexities of the Swiss Re and GLA projects, since 1998 the Foster practice has also developed its own customized software tools for architectural production. Equivalent to the Catia programme in some respects, the Foster system was conceived, however, quite differently. As Hugh Whitehead, director of Foster's Specialist Modelling Group (SMG) explains, whereas the Gehry practice bought into a ready-made programme, the SMG system was created specifically to meet the needs of the practice's collaborative approach.[36]

As with other aspects of the two practices, divergences between the two systems arise out of more fundamental differences in design approaches. As Gehry's associates describe it themselves, the Catia system was primarily designed as a manufacturing system, and is generally put into action after a design or building shape has been already determined. The cost and complexity of the system also limits the number of possible workstations that might be employed by a design office and consultants at any one time. Both features encourage a 'top down' or command approach to design and production, where the conceptual design phase, as in Gehry's office, is under centralized control (amazingly for such a prolific practice, Gehry shares the process of concept design with just two key staff, Edwin Chan and Craig Webb).[37]

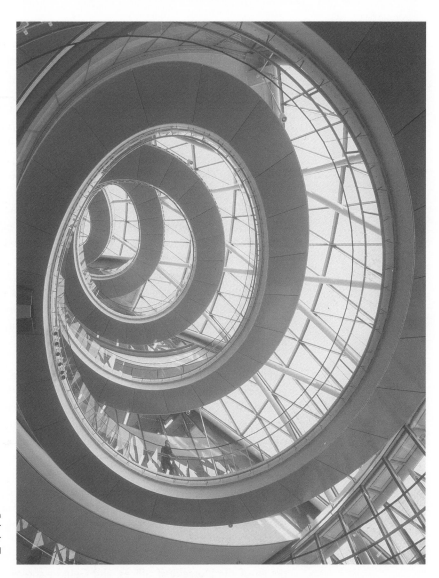

▶ **4.63** Greater London Authority Headquarters. Interior view of spiral stairway over council chamber. *Source*: Nigel Young/Foster and Partners.

Having also considered buying into the Catia system, Whitehead concluded that it could not be easily fitted into the team structure of a large and diversified practice like Foster's, where designs are produced by many different people for quite different kinds of projects.[38] The practice currently uses more than 400 computer-based workstations, all of which are tied up with one or more projects at any given time. Moreover, while the Catia programme is designed for and easily handles genuine free-form curves, parallel offsets, such as occur between two or more elements following the same free form curve – as in a cladding system pre-cisely designed to match the structure behind, or vice versa – have a multiplying effect on the data generated by the programme, greatly increasing the complex-ity and cost of the operation.

In the aerospace and automobile industries for which Catia was developed, such complex operations are commonplace in the development of new models, the costs involved representing a relatively small share of the total development pro-gramme. In Gehry's projects, the potential complexity of fabricating parallel free form building elements to fine tolerances has been substantially reduced in many cases by simplifying the actual geometry. For all their apparent complexity, for example, most of the solid, free form surfaces of the Bilbao Guggenheim and Disney Concert Hall (Fig. 4.64), as well as the Dusseldorf offices, are actually comprised of curves made up of ruled lines.[39] While the curve changes, it does so as a series of incremental changes in a straight line – much like holding a stick by the middle and swinging it round while waving it about at the same time – creating the characteristic wavy, sharp-edged curves which can be seen in so many of Gehry's other designs. This not only simplifies the geometry but makes it possible to create a structure and substructure largely made up of straight members (Fig. 4.65).

Gehry also avoids many potential problems by hiding everything else under the glossy skins of his buildings. The same unbroken, free form curves originally gen-erated from Gehry's physical models invariably conceal a steel (or sometimes concrete) frame that has been designed *ad hoc* after the exterior form and cladding material have been decided on by Gehry, and has no visible contact points with the surface. While the points at where the structure, secondary structure and cladding all meet also have to be calculated with great precision, the potential data load created by parallel offsets of different layers of compo-nents is therefore greatly reduced, since none of the primary or secondary struc-tural elements or their connections are designed to be seen.

We can only speculate to what extent similar factors might have influenced the design of the Dusseldorf offices, and Gehry's choice of mostly solid skins and concealed structures over a possibly more transparent and better illuminated architecture. However, while such constraints might suit Gehry's general prefer-ence for smooth surfaces and sculptural form – fine for enclosed buildings like museums and auditoriums but less suitable for offices and suchlike – they ill fit with the Foster studio's characteristic, see-through, steel and glass architecture, with its precise marriage of skin and exposed structure, with all their related highly visible components.

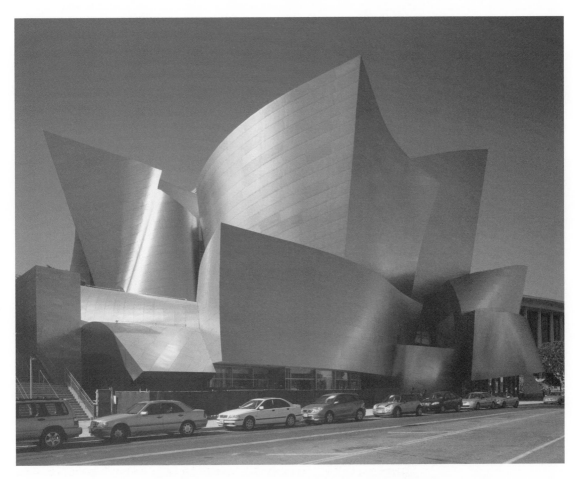

▲ **4.64** Walt Disney Concert Hall. The finished building. Photo: Hufton + Crow/View.

Beginning with the sweeping curves of the multi-vaulted roof of the New International Airport at Chek Lap Kok (Fig. 4.66) and the rolling, asymmetric curves of the steel and glass roof covering the renovated Great Court of the British Museum (Figs 4.67 and 4.68), the Foster Studio has also experimented with curved structures in the search for a wider though still highly disciplined vocabulary of form. Both the GLA 'lens' and the Swiss Re Tower, which feature precise and visible relations between skin and structure (Fig. 4.69), also presented new orders of geometric and structural complexity. In such an architecture, there can be no dodging the problem of parallel offsets between each and every component, posing potentially huge problems of design, data handling and fabrication.

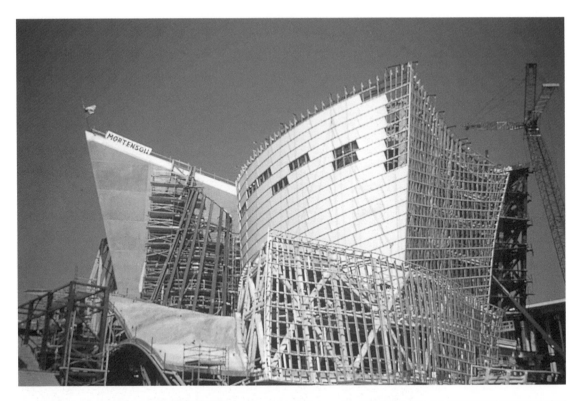

▲ **4.65** Walt Disney Concert Hall. View under construction showing primary and secondary steel structures beneath stainless steel skin. Photo: Lara Swimmer/Esto.

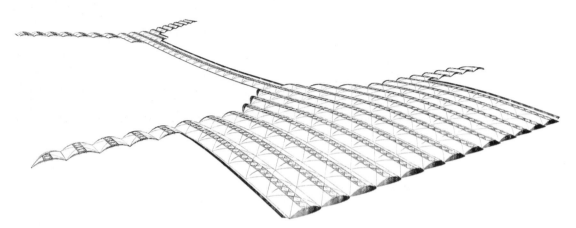

▲ **4.66** Hong Kong International Airport, Chek Lap Kok, Hong Kong. Computer image of roof structure. Norman Foster, 1992–8. *Source*: Foster and Partners.

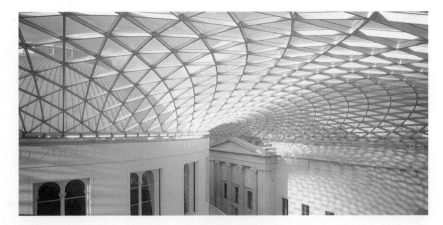

▲ **4.67** British Museum Great Court, London, UK. Norman Foster, 1994–2000. Interior view of roof. Photo: Ben Johnson.

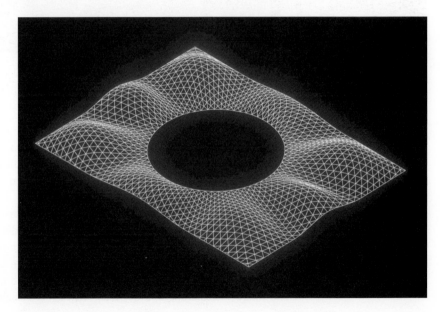

▲ **4.68** British Museum Great Court. Computer image of roof structure. *Source*: Foster and Partners.

Design template

Whitehead and the SMG's solution to both the studio's collaborative approach and the problem of dealing with complex curves was to create their own custom built 'design template', which would handle these and other computing demands and at the same time could be run on all the studio's workstations, as

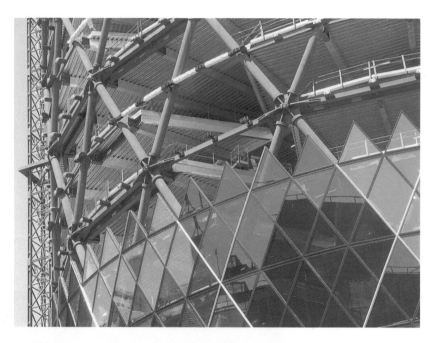

▲ **4.69** Swiss Re Headquarters. Detail of steel structure and cladding. Photo: Nigel Young/Foster and Partners.

well as on their consultants' own workstations.[40] As with Gehry's use of the Catia system, the SMG template also entails a practical compromise of sorts, involving the translation or post-rationalization of free form curves into a series of normal curves with known arcs, radii and centres. Thus, while the outline of the Swiss Re walls apparently follows a true progressive curve with no single radius or centre, it is actually made up of numerous different but regular arcs all joined together (Fig. 4.70). Since each segmental arc has a known centre and radius, any offset in either direction could therefore be easily calculated and each related cladding and structural element designed, fabricated and assembled to extremely fine tolerances, the results of which are all clearly visible to the eye.

Notably, the SMG template also incorporates parametric features – advanced software of a kind that was unavailable to Gehry in the early versions of the Catia system – enabling design changes to be quickly explored and updated. Should a consultant or designer want to change one parameter, i.e. the size or position of a floor plate or pane of glass, the implications of the change on other parameters and related elements will be automatically calculated and can be shared and discussed with anyone else concerned.

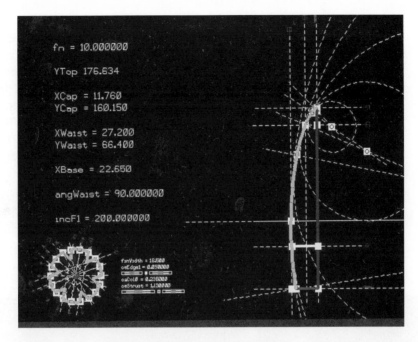

▲ **4.70** Swiss Re Headquarters. Sectional diagram showing geometrical composition of arcs forming curved wall. *Source*: Foster and Partners.

Most important, the SMG template converts geometrical data into a form that can be readily transferred between independent digital systems. The position of each element is given precise numerical coordinates along with other related data and presented on standard Excel spreadsheets. With a little training, consultants, contractors and fabricators can create their own digital models for whatever part of the building they are dealing with, which can be quickly matched against the information produced by the designers by overlaying related data sheets, providing a simple but efficient means of managing tolerances or anything else. The ultimate collaborative or 'bottom up' design method, the SMG system effectively distributes responsibility for the success of the design and production process equally amongst all members of the building team.

DIFFERENT WORLDS

Green credentials

However, important as all this might be for the way architecture can now be produced, we should not think of buildings like the Swiss Re and the GLA as purely technological or abstract digital wonders. Like Gehry's Guggenheim Museum in Bilbao, both buildings are destined to become, not only instantly recognizable landmarks within the city itself, but also icons on the larger global stage. The GLA building, especially, with its unique shape and Thameside location close to Tower Bridge, intentionally attracts attention to itself as the seat of the newly restored local government of a world city which had gone without local representation and control for far too long. Shaped by the path of the sun, the GLA also boasts a host of other energy-saving features, including a passive system of natural ventilation and the use of ground water deep under the building for the cooling system, similar to the system used for the Reichstag Parliament. Altogether, the building is expected to use less than one quarter of the energy of a conventional office building (Fig. 4.71).

That the political powers-that-be in London should have chosen a symbol with such green credentials is heartening, and – despite all the UK's insular foot-dragging in other respects – evidence of distinctly European sensibilities. Inevitably, however, the energy-efficient design also begs the question: is it

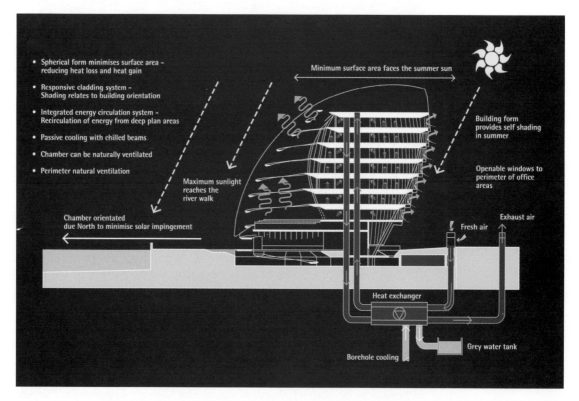

▲ **4.71** Greater London Authority Headquarters. Diagram of energy systems. *Source*: Foster and Partners.

possible to conceive of a politically symbolic building of this kind, or indeed any high-profile building, being designed in a similar way in the USA?

It would be unfair, perhaps, to single Gehry out or to expect that uniquely gifted architect to be also equally involved in the development of these initiatives, or even to be as interested in energy efficiency as Foster is, on top of his already significant artistic and technological achievements in using the Catia process. That is quite enough for one architect to come up with in a single lifetime, and against the grain of American practice to boot! Neither is Gehry standing still. As well as experimenting with parametric systems, the practice is extending its use of Dassau System software products that reach beyond Catia into related areas of the design and construction process, including the management of time. Plans are also afoot to make their experience available to other architects and consultants in the construction industry.[41]

That said, the use of dynamic techniques like CFD for modelling building performance is just as important, if not more important than the kind of static modelling techniques used by Foster and Gehry in their various CAD/CAM programmes.[42] No major car or aircraft designer or manufacturer would contemplate building a physical prototype for a new model, let alone investing in a new production line, without first simulating the new design's real-life performance under all likely conditions. Why should it be any different in the construction industry? Given the far greater economic and social investment in building, the potential impact of similar techniques on environmental performance and energy conservation is practically unlimited.

Atlantic divide

It is important to realize, therefore, that when we talk of advanced production technologies, they include a whole family of related computer modelling techniques. Together, they are helping designers to construct a complete 'virtual prototype' of their designs, simulating all aspects of both appearance and performance. Some, like the Catia process and Whitehead's system, are aimed at facilitating the fabrication of a complex form and are therefore aimed at modelling *static features*, such as form, space, surface and structure. Others, like CFD and other environmental and performance modelling techniques, show us how a building design *behaves in use* (Figs. 4.72 and 4.73). All are based, however, on the same basic, digital technology.

Which of these highly flexible techniques is used – and how they are used – ultimately depends, like any technique, on what the designer wants to do with it. In this regard Gehry's architecture is very much a product of current US culture. It is not that Gehry or his associates are unfamiliar with energy-conscious design. With so many completed projects in Germany and Switzerland, they have accumulated considerable personal experience in meeting the demanding regulations

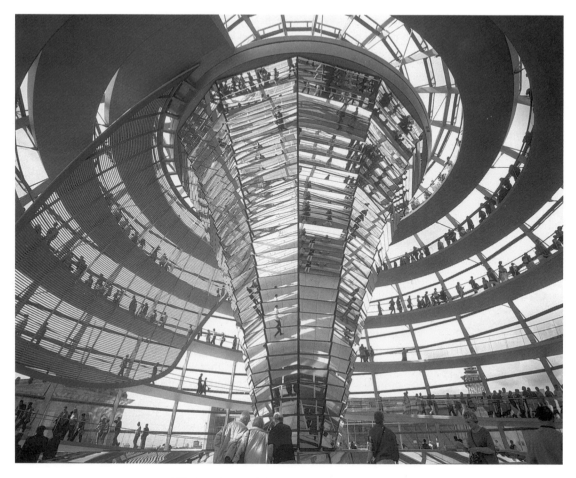

▲ **4.72** New German Parliament, Reichstag, Berlin, Germany. Internal view of cupola and suspended reflector over chamber. Norman Foster, 1992–9. Photo: Nigel Young/Foster and Partners.

of those countries. The Vitra International HQ also demonstrates that, when motivated to do so, Gehry can produce an energy-efficient office building just as convincingly as one of his cultural projects.

Nevertheless, compared with Foster or any number of other European architects, the fact is that energy efficiency generally plays a relatively minor role in shaping Gehry's architecture. It is simply a matter of priorities. Gehry's design approach originally evolved within a national culture which, sadly, still accords little if any value to saving energy, and, not unsurprisingly, his architecture reflects this, no less than his earlier work reflected the commercial vernacular of Los Angeles. Similarly, the production techniques Gehry has helped to pioneer are

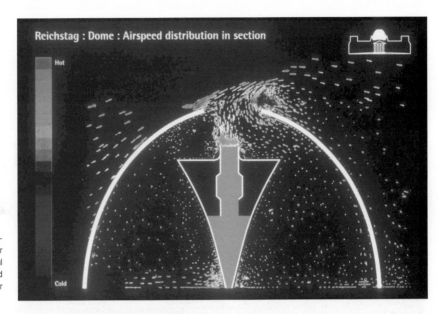

Reichstag : Dome : Airspeed distribution in section

Hot

Cold

▶ **4.73** New German Parliament, Reichstag. Computer simulation of effect of natural airflow through reflector and vent in cupola. *Source*: Foster and Partners.

those which enable him to realize his artistic vision of form and space, and his efforts continue to be mostly if not entirely directed toward that end.

Foster, on the other hand, works from within a European culture increasingly concerned with matters of energy conservation, especially in Germany, where green issues and values are now as much integrated into that country's political life as they are excluded from American political life. Given his long-standing commitment to high-performance design, it is therefore also not surprising that, when it came to working in Germany, Foster should have exploited the possibilities for innovation in this particular area so effectively.[43]

There is a notable difference, therefore, in how each architect has responded to working in the German regulatory environment. Where Gehry and his associates simply adapted to circumstances – they would have had no choice in the matter – Foster purposely used his German projects as a launch pad for further innovation in energy-efficient design, with visibly substantial results. The difference in response is as wide as the Atlantic.

Creative crossovers

The situation is not without its ironies. Foster was a graduate student at Yale and has been an admirer of Buckminster Fuller, who first introduced the idea of high-performance design into architecture, all his adult life. Fuller also collaborated with him on several early projects, such as the 'Climatroffice' (Fig. 4.74) and the 1978 International Energy Expo – both far-sighted experiments in sustainable design.

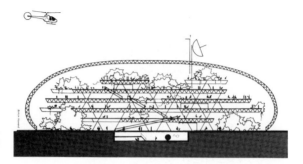

▶ **4.74** Climatroffice. Norman Foster with Buckminster Fuller, 1971. *Source*: Foster and Partners.

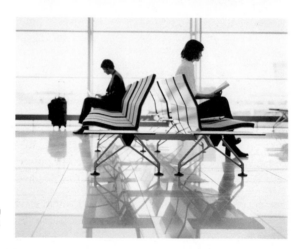

▶ **4.75** Vitra Airline Seating System. Norman Foster, 1997–9. Photo: Vitra International.

However, while there is no shortage of other Bucky fans in Europe, they are scarcely to be found in Fuller's own country, or if they are, then they are not being heard against the Postmodern clamor. Foster's furniture designs, such as his work for Vitra (Fig. 4.75), are also strongly influenced by the work of Charles and Ray Eames (Fig. 4.76), which also seems to have been largely forgotten in the US.

As we have seen, Foster has also loosened up somewhat in recent years, geometrically speaking, and has shifted quite a bit in Gehry's direction with more projects like the Albion Riverside apartments in London (Fig. 4.77) and the Chesa Futura apartments in St Moritiz (Fig. 4.78). Significantly, however, Foster and his partners have been able to extend their formal and geometric language without narrowing the range of their work or commitments, whether they involve common building types and functional problems, energy efficiency, or structural integrity and expression. On the contrary, the Foster studio's experiments in non-Euclidian geometries are as much an affirmation of their integrated design approach as their earlier, more orthodox work was. To put it another way, though Gehry's geometrical vocabulary is generally more complex

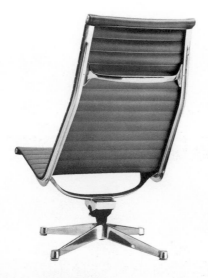

▶ **4.76** Lounge Chair. Charles and Ray Eames, 1958. *Source*: Museum of Modern Art.

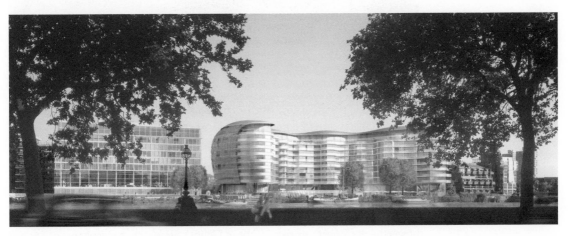

▲ **4.77** Albion Wharf Development, London, UK. Computer image. Norman Foster, 1999–2003. *Source*: Foster and Partners.

than the Foster studio's (a marked preference for unitary rather than fragmented wholes typifies the Foster studio's curvilinear work, just as it did the earlier rectilinear buildings) the latter consistently juggles with a larger number of environmental factors and issues, all of which merit attention in Foster's eyes. It's a different kind of complexity to Gehry's – not immediately visible perhaps – but certainly not any the less important for that.

Yet, while Foster's design approach and formal vocabulary is visibly diversifying as his practice grows and matures, the more successful Gehry has become, so his

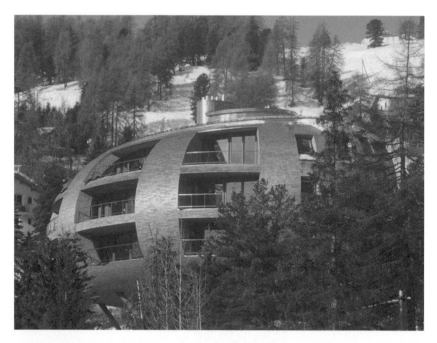

▲ **4.78**   Chesa Futura, St Moritz, Switzerland. Computer image. Norman Foster, 2000–2. *Source*: Foster and Partners.

approach and personal aesthetic has become more predictable – and in a sense, along with his choice of commissions, also narrower. Clearly, Gehry hugely enjoys the support and freedom his computer-savvy associates and Catia have given him to explore curvilinear three-dimensional space and form in a manner no other architect has been able to do before. The museums and other cultural projects, which still constitute the major part of his practice, also present him with ample opportunity to use his creative and sculptural talents to the full.

Nevertheless, questions remain about Gehry's approach, particularly concerning his dual planning methods. Are they a valid mode of expressing the different functions and parts of a building, as Aalto did and Gehry is also inclined to do, or are they an admission that there are some building types or aspects of architecture that Gehry is either not so interested in, or has not yet learnt how to incorporate into his preferred language of sculptured form, or possibly both?

Cultural currents

Given the ambiguous relations between architecture and the world of commercial art and advertising Gehry exploited so knowingly and skillfully in his earlier projects, one also wonders to what extent, especially since the Bilbao Guggenheim, that other, very American culture of brand names and images still shapes his work, whether consciously or unconsciously. The actual forms may have changed over the years – no more binoculars and fewer fish – but the underlying cultural currents which carry Gehry and many other well-known designers along have not, and, if anything, grow stronger by the day. Certainly, the enthusiastic reception given to his work by the popular media seems to have encouraged Gehry to continue down the same path, producing ever more of the curvaceous *tours de force* (Fig. 4.79) that both clients and the wider public have come to expect from him.

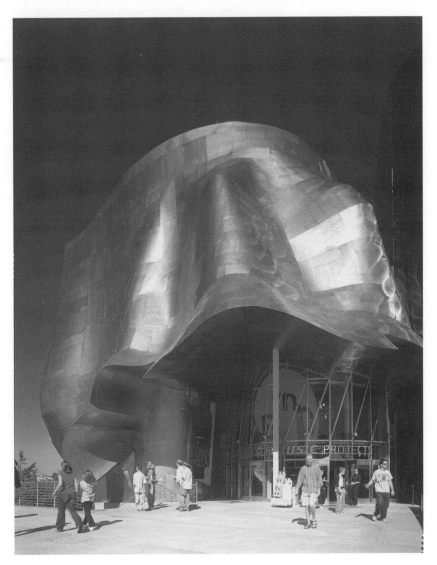

▶ **4.79** Museum of Contemporary Music, Seattle, Washington, USA. Frank Gehry, 1995–2000. Photo: John Edward Linden.

To a large extent, therefore, even though he has built in different countries and cultural contexts, Gehry remains very much a creature of his adopted home and culture in Los Angeles, USA, just as Foster is still influenced by his own very different personal and professional background in London and Europe. No doubt, should Gehry ever move to embrace the same kind of energy-efficient techniques pioneered by Foster and others, as hopefully he and fellow American designers eventually will, he would also adapt them to his own artistic ends.

And who, in the final analysis, could argue with that? The great thing about these digital production technologies is precisely that they can be so readily adapted to different ends, rather than the other way around, as used to be the case with the mass-production technologies of the last century. That's just the way it should be.

We also need such architects as Foster and Gehry, with all their grand differences. Many years ago, in comparing the masterworks of another two, not dissimilar pair of contrary designers, Mies and Sharoun, I wrote:

> As masterpieces of each tradition, each building offers a measure of the other, not in the same terms or criteria of evaluation, but in the terms of a comparison of different systems of belief. When we compare one building with the other, we compare distinct languages, each with its own rules and internal logic, each offering a quite different interpretation of reality. We do not just compare building with building, therefore, but ideas with ideas, and values with values.[44]
>
> (Abel, 1979, p. 45)

Another time, another generation, but I think the words still apply. Without Gehry heat, less appreciation of Foster cool, and vice versa. In between the two extremes, lies an infinite range of other approaches, waiting for those willing and able to master the same technologies. But we need the extremists to define the limits of possibility. Without Dionysus, Apollo wouldn't know just how wild things could get. Without Apollo, Dionysus wouldn't know if he might not have left something out of the party.

5

HARRY SEIDLER AND THE GREAT AUSTRALIAN DREAM

Better known now for his structurally innovative and sometimes controversial high-rise buildings in Sydney and elsewhere, the Austrian-born architect Harry Seidler also has a unique record of house designs, the evolution of which mirrors Australia's own complex development over the latter half of the twentieth century.

Many of the early houses will be familiar to older generations of architects who graduated in the 1950s and 1960s, and who eagerly devoured Seidler's designs as part of Modernism's essential repertoire of domestic architecture. However, to younger designers around the world who are now shaking off the worst excesses of Postmodernism, these houses will come as a revelation: products of an earlier, alternative Modernism that was respectful of its locality as well as expressive of its time. Since the late 1960s, Seidler's domestic architecture has also been increasingly enriched by his other work, which covers all forms and scales of building.[1]

THE STUFF OF LEGEND

The main events in Seidler's early life in Europe, North America and Australia are by now the familiar stuff of legend: forced to flee Nazi-controlled Vienna as a teenager with his family just a year before World War II; temporary refuge in Cambridge, England, only to be interned and deported to Canada along with thousands of other 'suspect' nationals when war came (Fig. 5.1); release from prison camp followed by undergraduate studies in architecture and civil engineering at the University of Manitoba, Winnepeg; scholarship and transfer to Harvard Graduate School of Design, Cambridge, Massachussets under the tutorship of Bauhaus luminaries and fellow refugees Walter Gropius (Fig. 5.2) and

Edited from two introductory essays published in *Harry Seidler: Houses and Interiors, Volumes 1 and 2*, Images Publishing Group, Melbourne, 2002.

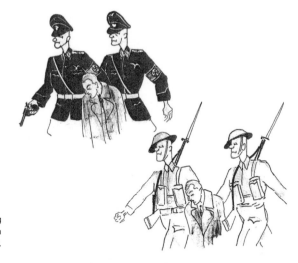

▶ **5.1** Cartoon showing Seidler marched off between Nazis and British. *Source*: J. Wilton, 1986.

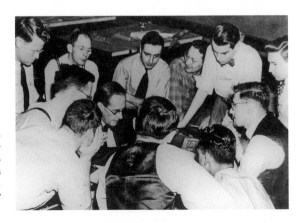

▶ **5.2** Group photo of students with Walter Gropius at Harvard, 1946. Seidler in centre behind Gropius. Classmates include I.M. Pei and D. Olsen. Photo: Harvard University Graduate School of Design.

Marcel Breuer; further studies in visual perception at Black Mountain College, North Carolina under Josef Albers, another charismatic former Bauhaus teacher and refugee; assistant to Breuer in the formative years of his New York practice; travels in South America en route to Australia, including a few months working with Oscar Niemeyer in Brazil; and finally, arrival in Sydney to design a house for his parents who had settled there after the war.

Intending to return to America after completing his parents' house, Seidler fell instead under the spell of Australia's landscape. The national and international success – despite initial opposition from the local building authorities – of the Rose Seidler House (Fig. 5.3) in Turramurra, the first of three houses he designed for family members on the same bushland site outside Sydney, helped persuade Seidler to stay on.

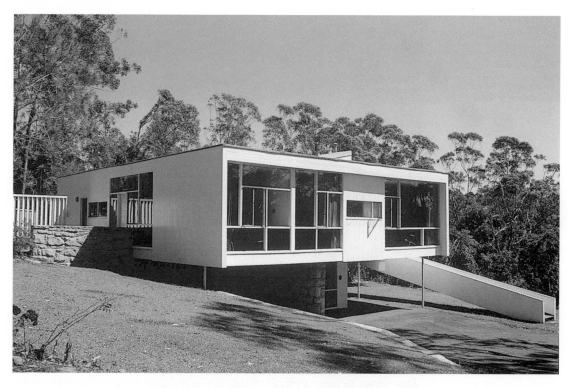

▲ **5.3** Rose Seidler House, Turramurra, 1948. Photo: Marcell Seidler.

THE GREAT AUSTRALIAN DREAM

The maturation in Seidler's subsequent career and architecture, in turn reflects the dramatic changes in Australia itself after the war. The main characteristics of Australia's cities, together with most of those elements which still underpin Australians' sense of identity, had already taken shape much earlier. By the late nineteenth century, Australia's population already ranked amongst the most urbanized in the world, one-third of which was concentrated in the coastal cities where colonization began. During the inter-war years, as urban economies shifted from mainly trade to manufacturing, so the state capitals also grew, spreading out in radial patterns following the railway and tram-lines out of the city.[2]

Even before automobiles made their impact, Australians made abundantly clear their preference for living in the suburbs on their own patch of land. Independent and egalitarian by nature, for most people the detached, single family home situated out in the countryside, but within easy reach of the city by tram or train, represented the Great Australian Dream (Fig. 5.4). It surpassed any equivalent development in England, the mother country and source of domestic models

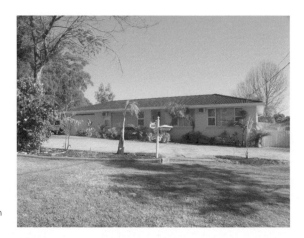

▶ **5.4** Typical   suburban
house, Sydney. Photo: Author.

for most early settlers. Only in North America, where there were similar
historical and cultural parallels, was there any comparable population shift to the
suburbs. Summarizing Australians' unshakeable attachment to their ideal, the
Australian critic Robin Boyd wrote, with only slight exaggeration, 'Australia is
the small house'.[3]

It was in the 1950s and 1960s, however, during the so-called 'long boom', when
automobiles became more affordable, fuel was cheap and plentiful and both the
economy and population were growing fast, that the Australian way of life
acquired its definitive suburban form. In the quarter century following the war,
the populations of Sydney and Melbourne grew from just over 1 million each to
over 2.5 million each. The open land between the fingers of settlement that had
followed the railways and tram-lines was rapidly filled in, and the tram-lines
themselves were displaced by new highways. By the early 1970s, both cities covered areas larger than London, which had four times their population, each
sprawling metropolis completely dominating its own state.[4]

ENGINEERING SKILLS

Seidler took easily to living and working in Sydney's dispersed suburbs. Like most
middle-class Viennese, he had grown up with his parents and brother living in an
apartment block on one of the city's dense streets. However, once in North
America, his experience as a student designing cheap timber houses during vaca-
tions, followed by his work with Breuer detailing houses in the New England
countryside, exposed him to the equivalent American dream. As a recent
refugee from oppression in Europe, Seidler found – first in North America and
then in Australia – the same joy in the apparently unlimited space and available
land, as countless other immigrants had before him.

Often tagged as a faithful disciple of Breuer and his other ex-Bauhaus mentors, the description only provides a part of the picture. Seidler's combined education in civil engineering and architecture in North America endowed him with unusual technical skills, which, once embarked on his own practice in Australia, quickly set him apart from first-generation Modernists. The steel-framed Rose House (Fig. 5.5), the second of the Turramurra group and the most original of his early works, is designed just like a miniature bridge (Fig. 5.6). With its large suspended

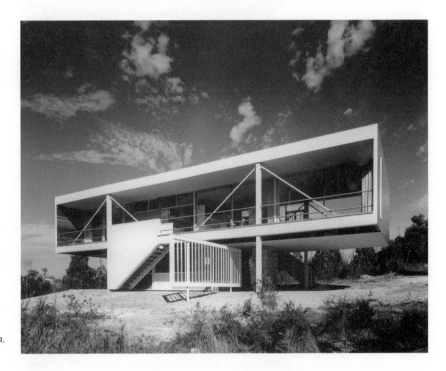

▶ **5.5** Rose House, Turramurra, 1952. Photo: Max Dupain.

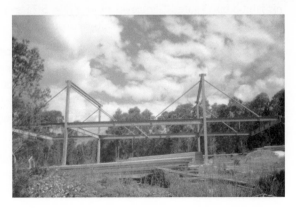

▶ **5.6** Steel-framed structure of Rose House. Photo: Marcell Seidler.

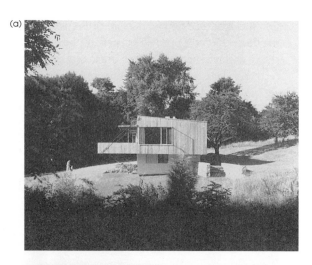

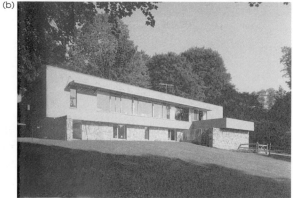

▶ **5.7** Cantilever House, New Canaan, by Marcel Breuer, 1947. Original design (a), and after final structural changes and extensions (b). *Source*: D. Masello, 1993.

overhangs, it achieved what Breuer himself attempted but failed to realize with his famed but ill-fated Cantilever House (Fig. 5.7a and b), parts of which had to be propped up underneath soon after construction.[5]

Considering that this was only Seidler's second independent work, the innovative combination of architecture and lightweight engineering represents an astonishing feat of mature design for a young architect. Equal to any of the steel and timber-framed Case Study Houses built in California during the same period, it also anticipates by many more years the lightweight tensioned structures designed by so-called hi-tech architects in Europe.

Many of Seidler's earliest houses, like Breuer's, are raised entirely or partly, high off the ground in a similar manner on supporting columns or masonry substructures, sometimes on steep slopes that would otherwise be unbuildable (Fig. 5.8).

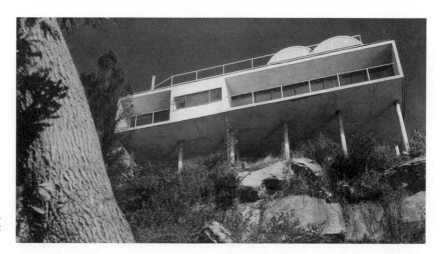

▶ **5.8** Williamson House, Mosman, 1952. Photo: Max Dupain.

For Breuer, in addition to maintaining the landscape in its natural state and making the most of any views, raising the main body of the structure also expressed the lightness of timber balloon-framing, a technology he purposefully used in emulation of the vernacular architecture of New England. However, exposing the underside of a building in this manner makes little sense in the long and severe winters of that region, where buildings are traditionally set down upon the earth, where they are better insulated.

Transferred to Australia, the same composition of a 'floating' upper structure fitted far more comfortably into the warmer climate of New South Wales, with its relatively mild winters and hot summers. It also fits into a much broader tradition of building that is as wide as the Pacific itself. Raised, timber-framed houses are an integral part of domestic architecture in cultures all around the Pacific Rim, including Southeast Asia, Japan, the Californian coast and parts of the coast of Chile.[6]

In Australia, similar houses can be found in the tropical and subtropical regions of the northern and north-eastern states, reaching down to New South Wales. While the structure consists of brick piers rather than a timber frame, Seidler's Paspaley House in Darwin (Fig. 5.9) is designed precisely in this fashion to encourage ventilation underneath the main rooms, as well as through them. Though relatively new to the Sydney region and its inhabitants, who normally favour – much to Seidler's distaste – the English-style brick bungalow, the experimental house form which the new settler brought with him prefigures more recent experiments with raised or 'floating' structures by younger generations of Australian architects.[7]

Whether elevated or placed firmly upon the ground, the planning of all of Seidler's houses is as meticulous as the detailing. Few architects have ever been

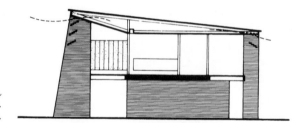

▶ **5.9** Paspaley House, Darwin, 1959. Cross-section. *Source*: Harry Seidler Associates.

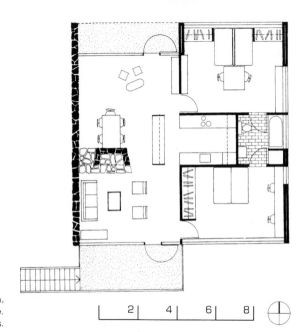

▶ **5.10** Tuck House, Gordon, 1951. A small ring-plan type. *Source*: Harry Seidler Associates.

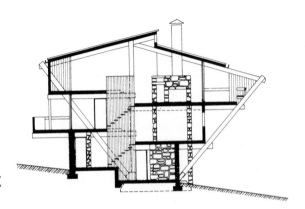

▶ **5.11** Ski Lodge, Thredbo, 1962. Section. *Source*: Harry Seidler Associates.

able to squeeze so much usable space, or so much delight, out of a tight budget. Usually designed as variations on the basic typologies Seidler learnt from Breuer – in-line, bi-nuclear or ring plan (Fig. 5.10) – each plan mirrors with exquisite precision the site and surrounding landscape in which the building stands. Always capitalizing on any views or adjacent ground to ensure that the occupants obtain the maximum enjoyment from their location, Seidler's houses draw the landscape deep into their interiors in great gulps, fusing both together.

SPATIAL DEVELOPMENT

Most of the houses Seidler designed before 1970 have a predominantly horizontal configuration, with all the living and sleeping spaces spread out in one plane, opening out to embrace the landscape. The only consistent variation is Seidler's frequent use of a split-level plan, either to accommodate a sloping site or else to differentiate the sleeping quarters from the rest of the house, or sometimes both together.

The timber-framed Ski Lodge (Fig. 5.11) was the first significant exception to this general emphasis on the horizontal plane in Seidler's houses. The introduction of a strong vertical dimension into the interior space of the Ski Lodge provided the model for later projects, notably Seidler's own house (Fig. 5.12a and b) and the

(a)

(b)

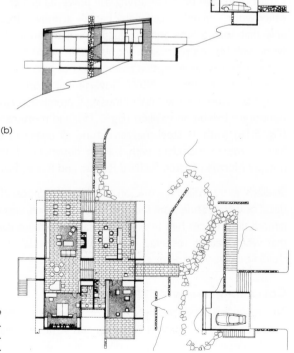

▶ **5.12** Harry and Penelope Seidler House, Killara, 1967. Section (a) and plan (b). *Source*: Harry Seidler Associates.

smaller Gissing House. Like the Ski Lodge, the Seidler House, which is also sited on a steep slope, is split open down the middle, the floors in each half being staggered either side of a narrow vertical space rising all the way up through the structure.

The seismic disruption in the interior, which also runs right across the house, opens views up and down into each level from both sides, so that the central space functions as both a dividing and unifying element at one and the same time. The effect in both houses is to create an internal spatial focus without in any way diminishing the fluid connections with the exterior.

STRUCTURAL EXPRESSIONISM

The Ski Lodge also provided another convincing demonstration of Seidler's prowess as an engineer as well as an architect. The dramatic angles of the exposed frames, together with the alternating floors projecting out at different levels, are quite unlike anything else Seidler had designed before and anticipate on a smaller scale the later explorations in structural expressionism with Pier Luigi Nervi, Seidler's collaborator on many of his commercial projects.

Like the steel-framed Rose House before it, the Ski Lodge shows a designer in confident control of the different technologies and materials at his command. Whilst there can be no doubting the powerful influence Nervi had on Seidler's other work – an influence Seidler happily acknowledges – it is equally inconceivable that such a long and productive collaboration (Seidler also continued to work with Nervi's partners after his death) could have occurred if the architect was not himself as receptive to the great engineer's way of thinking as he was. The spaceframe for the NSW Government Stores (Fig. 5.13), the suspended bridge structure for the NSW Housing Commission Apartments (Fig. 5.14), the temporary Exhibition Pavilion (Fig. 5.15), and more recently, the Capita Centre (Fig. 5.16), with its steel megastructure, all testify to a technical virtuosity we have come to associate with leading designers of the following generation, notably Norman Foster, Richard Rogers and Renzo Piano.

Seidler's extraordinary work on the Horwitz Sloop (Fig. 5.17), every crafted detail of which, aside from the boat's fibreglass hull, was designed by the architect himself, also places him firmly in the same dextrous camp. Small wonder, then, that when Seidler received the RIBA Gold Medal in 1996, the main address should be given by Foster (Fig. 5.18).

COLLABORATION WITH NERVI

The range of these projects – all of which were developed with Australian engineers – shows that his technical and structural mastery was by no means wholly dependent upon his collaboration with Nervi, but was rather the

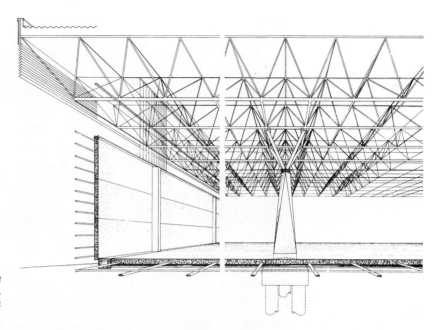

▶ **5.13** NSW Government Stores, Alexandria, NSW, 1968. Sectional perspective. *Source*: Harry Seidler Associates.

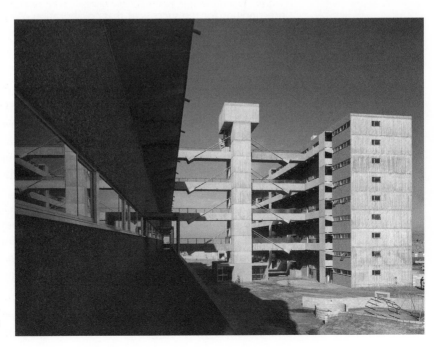

▶ **5.14** NSW Housing Commission Apartments, Rosebery, 1967. Photo: Max Dupain.

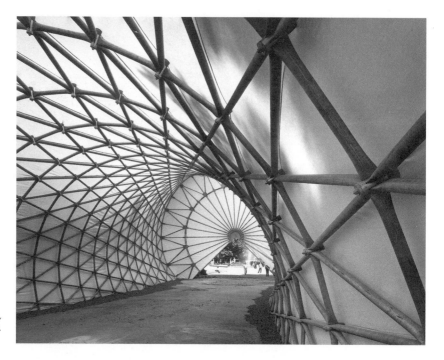

▶ **5.15** Exhibition Pavilion, Hyde Park, Sydney, 1972. Photo: Max Dupain.

precondition for the success of that collaboration. When Seidler started working with Nervi in 1963 on Australia Square (Fig. 5.19), the first of his many tall buildings in Sydney, he was therefore already primed, as it were, to make the most of Nervi's own special talents.

From Nervi, Seidler learnt that a reinforced concrete structure did not necessarily have to be designed all in straight lines, but that, if the natural forces of shear, tension and compression in a beam or support were clearly expressed, and any excess material was omitted, then what would be produced would be not only structurally efficient and economical to build, but also aesthetically pleasing. The only technical limitation was making the formwork to mould the resulting complex shapes. This was resolved in most cases by repetition of the structural form, and therefore standardization of the formwork – usually made of flexible composites. The sculpted, exposed floor beams used in Seidler's own offices and the similar beams designed for the Paris Embassy (Fig. 5.20a and b), which create such a powerful visual impact and rythmic unity inside those buildings, as well as many others, were all fabricated using a single mould for each primary element.

While the most elaborate and daring structures Seidler designed with Nervi were produced for his large commercial buildings, from the 1970s onwards there

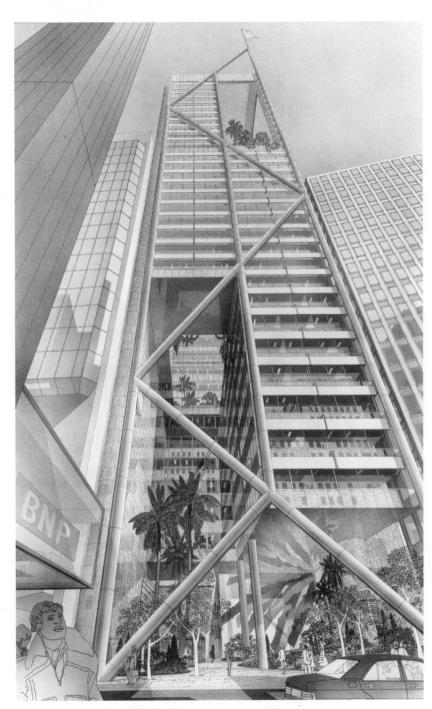

▶ **5.16** Capita Centre, Sydney, 1989. Perspective drawing. *Source*: Harry Seidler Associates.

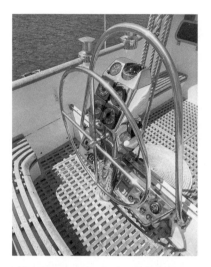

▶ **5.17** Horwitz Sloop, 1965. Detail. Photo: Max Dupain.

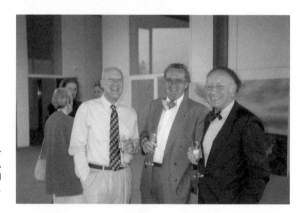

▶ **5.18** Seidler with Sir Norman Foster and RIBA President Owen Luder at Gold Medal presentation, 1996. Photo: Penelope Seidler.

was also a knock-on effect on both his houses and apartment buildings, most of which have reinforced concrete structures. As well as the more complex structural techniques, Seidler also learnt from Nervi that, by using pre-stressed concrete, the edges of even a simple floor slab could be bent and shaped at will. The large, curved terraces which project out from many of Seidler's houses, such as the Hannes House (Fig. 5.21) and the Hamilton House, are all constructed in this fashion. Similar elements commonly feature in his apartment buildings, usually also stiffened with concrete upstands (ballusters) or downstands (sunshades), or both. The long, wavy curves of the open terraces of Seidler's Penthouse Apartment, over his offices, are an especially dramatic example of the same technique – the upper terrace seems to hang suspended in the double floor height space in the centre of the apartment (Fig. 5.22).

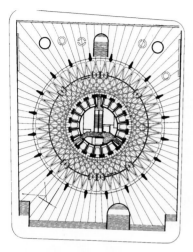

◀ **5.19** Australia Square, Sydney. 1967. Plan at plaza level showing ceiling configuration. *Source*: Harry Seidler Associates.

(a)

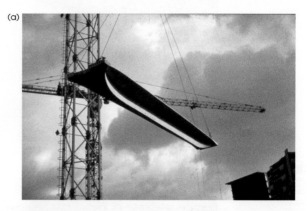

(b)

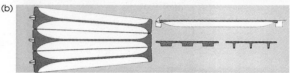

▲ **5.20** Australian Embassy, Paris, France. 1977. Sculpted beams are cast from one mould. Beam lifted into place (a). Plan of beams (b). Photo: Harry Seidler. *Source*: Harry Seidler Associates.

VISUAL TENSION

Nervi's influence was one of several factors which were to have a profound effect upon Seidler's work – both large and small scale – during this period, leading him away from an architecture based on orthogonal geometries, towards more fluid and curvaceous, and in some cases, highly sensual forms. Seidler strongly believes, as his ex-Bauhaus teachers in America did, in the harmonious integration of modern art and architecture and has gone further than most architects of his generation in striving for that goal. In his 1954 essay, 'Our Heritage of Modern Building', he qualifies his endorsement of mass-production technology, suggesting it is but a means to other, more important ends:

> *The production of standard parts must, however, be kept alive by imaginative designers to ensure that the end result will not be a soulless assembly of mass-produced material, but that industry will only be a new means in the shaping of the architecture of tomorrow.*[8]

(Seidler, 1954, p. xx)

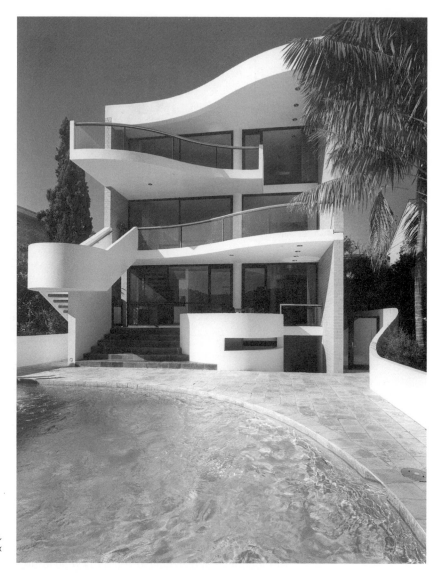

▶ **5.21** Hannes House, Cammeray, 1984. Photo: Max Dupain.

Seidler's actual experience with mass-production technologies was limited to the Exhibition House (Fig. 5.23), Sydney, that he built for the RAIA 1954 Convention. Assembled from standard metal decking, steel trusses and other ready-made components, the all-steel house used techniques similar to the Case Study House built by Charles and Ray Eames a few years earlier. Seidler soon learnt, however, as Foster et al. would also eventually discover for themselves, that a moderate level of standardization within a building project itself – usually

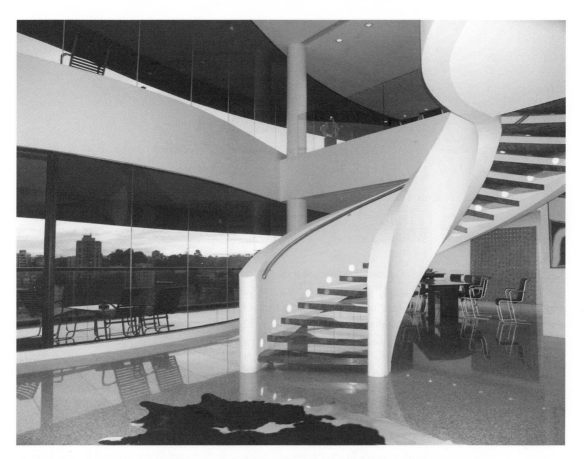

▲ **5.22** Harry and Penelope Seidler Apartment, Milsons Point, 1988. Photo: Author.

involving the use of a regular structural system – was all that was needed to achieve the desired economies, without resort to any wider efforts within the industry.[9] The repetition of certain spatial and formal elements in Seidler's architecture, especially since the 1970s, therefore has as much, if not more to do with a desire to work within a consistent visual and aesthetic discipline, as with any technical or economic constraints arising from the process of production.

The origins of this discipline go back to Josef Albers' teachings at Black Mountain College. From Albers, Seidler learnt the importance of creating an 'opposition of tension'. As he explains in the aforementioned essay:

> *Our eyes don't seem to find pleasure in symmetrical static compositions. Instead, we seem to crave visual tension, the more dynamic balance of unequals.*[10]
>
> (Seidler, 1954, p. xi)

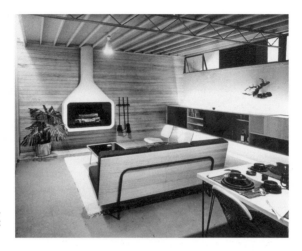

▶ **5.23** Exhibition House, Sydney, 1954. Photo: Max Dupain.

In his early work, visual tension was achieved by the manipulation of intersect-ing asymmetrical planes in what we now regard as the visual and spatial con-ventions of early Modern architecture, as informed by Cubism and other movements. However, in the 1970s these gave way to a new plasticity, partly inspired by Seidler's earlier exposure in Brazil to Oscar Niemeyer's exuberant, 'free-form' architecture, as well as by Nervi's structural techniques and forms. To this already potent mixture, Seidler also added the curvilinear geometries and voluptuous forms of baroque architecture, which he had grown up with in Vienna and about which he learnt more in his later travels in Italy. Lastly, there was the impact of a select group of Modern artists Seidler became personally acquainted with during his latter career, including the American artists Alexander Calder, Frank Stella, Norman Carlberg and Charles Perry, and the English painter, Bridget Riley.

The links between these diverse sources, as with all creative processes involving a cross-fertilization between different fields, are primarily metaphorical, involv-ing varying degrees of abstraction from each source. Calder's work especially appealed to the structural designer in Seidler. Describing Calder as 'the playful engineer', he also found in his monumental exterior works, one of which he commissioned for Australia Square (Fig. 5.24): '... an immense tension about them, the way elements oppose each other and the way they interact with architecture'.[11]

INTEGRATION OF OPPOSITES

Similarly, we find in David Underwood's explanation of the cultural programme underlying Niemeyer's Memorial of Latin America complex in Sao Paulo, as

also propagated by Darcy Ribeiro, a Brazilian social scientist and populist politi-
cian, a remarkably close parallel with the themes underlying Seidler's work
during the same period:

> Ribeiro and Niemeyer see the integration of all the arts into a unified multimedia
> ensemble as a metaphor for the integration of Latin American cultures. Perhaps
> the clearest visual expression of the memorial's theme is Bruno Giorgi's abstract
> marble sculpture Integracao (Integration), which is composed of two inverted forms
> interlocking to create one.[12]
>
> (Underwood, 1994, p. 110)

The comparison with the Giorgi sculpture (Fig. 5.25) is all the more apt when
viewed against Seidler's own choice of artists' works, in which similar motifs
constantly reappear, most clearly in Carlberg's 'positive and negative' sculpture at
the Riverside Development, Brisbane (Fig. 5.26). Constructed of identical quad-
rant-shaped blocks like a DNA chain, the spiralling assembly suggests a more
complex variation on the same theme as Giorgi's. Again and again, as also in
Stella's 'protractor series' of paintings of the 1960s (Fig. 5.27), we see the same
quadrants, spirals and other circular motifs appearing in Seidler's designs: in the
opposing curves of the two Paris embassy buildings; in the back to back blocks of
the Ringwood Cultural Centre (Fig. 5.28a and b); in the general plan of the
Waverley Civic Centre and in the elevation of the council chamber; and in many
others.

INFLUENCE OF BAROQUE

Seidler commissioned numerous works from Stella for his buildings, together
with those of Perry. Like Carlberg and Seidler himself, Perry was a former
student of Albers. More than that, what unites Stella, Carlberg and Perry with
Seidler's architecture as it has evolved over the last two decades, and lends their
work special meaning when viewed together, is their mutual indebtedness to the
geometric disciplines and flowing forms of the baroque period. The overlapping
circles and highlighted segments that feature in Stella's protractor series, for
example, are based on identical geometric systems as those used in many
baroque buildings[13] (Fig. 5.29). In Perry's sculptures, opposing curved segments
merge into each other in a three-dimensional manipulation of similar geometries,
producing on occasion some highly erotic forms (Fig. 5.30).

For Seidler, as for these artists, the baroque example is not so much a model for
literal imitation, as a springboard for further invention and reinterpretation with
the techniques and materials of our own time. Taking a critical stance against the

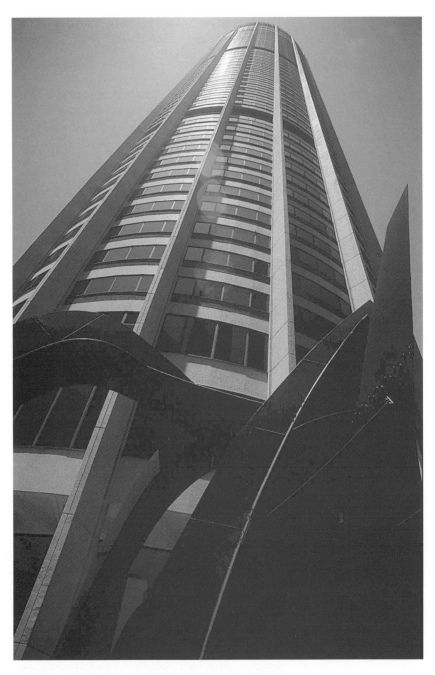

▲ **5.24**   Sculpture by Alexander Calder, Australia House, 1967. Photo: Max Dupain.

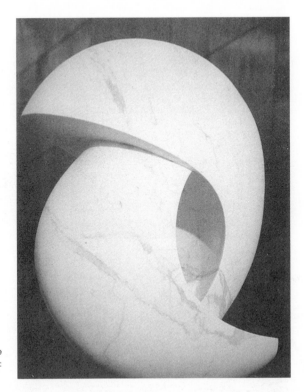

▶ **5.25** Bruno Giorgi, marble sculpture, 'Integration'. *Source*: D. Underwood, 1994.

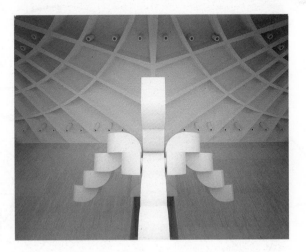

▶ **5.26** Norman Carlberg, sculpture, 'Positive and negative'. Photo: Max Dupain.

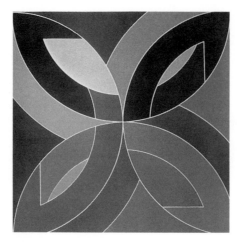

▶ **5.27** Frank Stella, painting, 'Protractor series'. Photo: Museum of Modern Art.

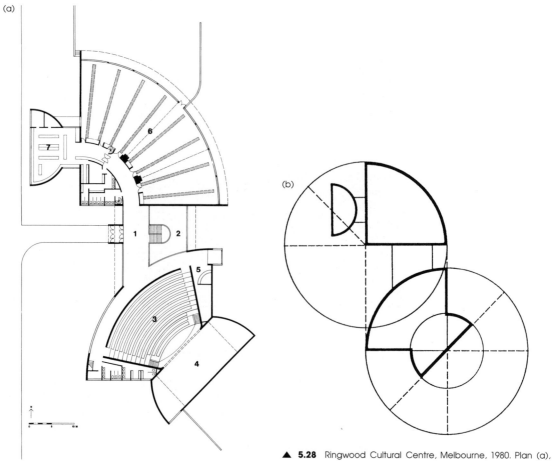

▲ **5.28** Ringwood Cultural Centre, Melbourne, 1980. Plan (a), and diagram (b). *Source:* Harry Seidler Associates.

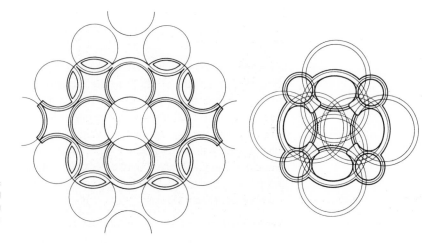

▶ **5.29** Baroque geometric planning system composed of interlocking circles. Drawing by Paolo Portoghesi. *Source*: P. Portoghesi, 1982.

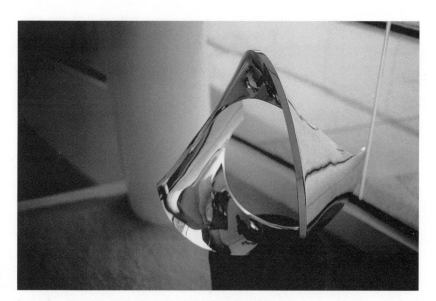

▶ **5.30** Charles Perry, metal sculpture. Photo: Max Dupain.

prevailing historicism favoured by Postmodernists, Seidler declares:

> By 'history', of course, I do not mean the puerile adaptation of decorative para-
> phernalia but rather a study of the essential forces behind the images of the past.
> For instance, the subtly brilliant geometric systems that came into being in the 17th
> and 18th centuries can inform our approach to developing system-oriented
> methods of construction. But the visual language must be new. I believe that visual
> tension, not the phlegmatic earthbound images of the past, speaks to our time; the

channeling of space and surfaces in opposition, curve against countercurve, sun and shadow, the juxtaposition of compression to the surprise of release.[14]

(Seidler, 1992, p. 383)

In the Hong Kong Club and Office Building (Figs 5.31 and 5.32), by far the most complex and brilliant of his 'baroque' designs, the flared edges of the corner structural supports are turned forward in a manner suggestive of the concave facade of Francesco Borromini's Oratory of San Philip Neri (Fig. 5.33), an effect which is reinforced by the inward curve of the pediment wall at the top of the building. There are strong echoes too, of the undulating facade of Borromini's Church of San Carlo alle Quattro Fontane, both in the lower walls of the club, and in the opposition between the convex flanges of the huge transverse beams and their concave supports.

Nervi's own native love of the baroque is also apparent in this definitive work, but it is Seidler's unique achievement to have married the engineer's powerful structure with the flowing spaces and forms of the club itself (Fig. 5.34). A *tour de force* of sensuous curves and spiralling stairways, Seidler's fusion of baroque and Modernism has few equals. There is even some unexpected Postmodern wit displayed in the use of blatantly phallic imagery in the placement of a bridge between the two circular elements of the stairway and liftshaft – a comment, perhaps, on the patriarchal culture of the club's members, surreptitiously undermined by the feminine curves of the rest of the club.

RIPPLING LINES

The Hong Kong Club served as a laboratory of experimental form and structure for Seidler, which was to have a lasting effect on his subsequent domestic architecture, as well as his other work. Thereafter, opposing concave and convex curves are commonly featured in his houses and apartments, both internally and externally. Whether cut into different floor levels to form vertical spaces edged with alternating curves, as in the Penthouse Apartment and Hamilton House, or stacked one above the other as waves of terraces, as in the Horizon Apartments (Fig. 5.35), or frequently both, whichever way one looks, one confronts fluid, rippling lines warping back and forth. Much like a Riley painting (Fig. 5.36), the eye is constantly moving across shifting surfaces. The voluptuous, snaking lines of the Hong Kong Club's central stairway are also reproduced on a smaller scale, both in the Penthouse and in Hamilton House, to create seductive focal points, drawing the sweeping lines of the balconies downwards to spill out onto the lower levels.

In the mid-1990s, beginning with the Cohen and Meares houses (Fig. 5.37), Seidler also introduced curves into the sections of his houses, shaping roofs like breaking waves – not an inappropriate metaphor for a population whose vast

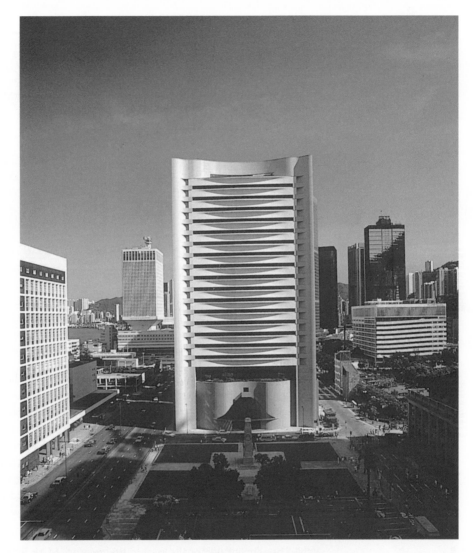

▲ **5.31**   Hong Kong Club and Office Building, Hong Kong, 1984. Facade onto Cenotaph Square.
Photo: John Gollings.

majority lives within hailing distance of the ocean. Constructed of curved steel
beams covered with corrugated metal decking bent to the same shape, a roof
typically rises in a gentle concave arc from the centre of the house to a peak at
the front or rear where it changes shape, before dipping down protectively to
provide shade.

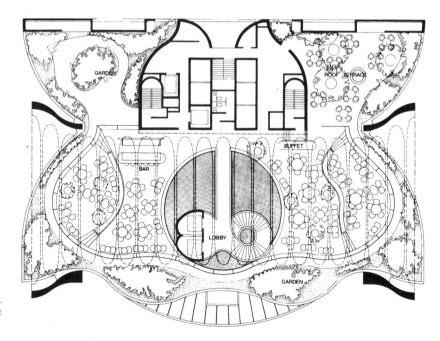

▶ **5.32** Hong Kong Club. Plan at Fourth Level. *Source*: Harry Seidler Associates.

CRITICAL BIAS

Given the plethora of baroque motifs, anthropomorphic shapes and other suggestive metaphors in Seidler's work over this period, it is puzzling to read that this highly innovative and versatile designer was described not many years ago as 'the last of the Machine Age architects'.[15] It has, of course, been not uncommon – especially during the high tide of Postmodernism – for those Modernists who stubbornly refused to throw in the towel, to be lumped into this category. Now that Postmodernism – or at least its more superficial manifestation – is subsiding, those post-war Modernists, like Seidler and his old Harvard classmate, I.M. Pei, who held the course throughout, are beginning to enjoy wider recognition for their own innovations.

Whilst he remains personally loyal to the memory of his ex-Bauhaus teachers, it is also questionable whether Seidler was ever a true Machine Age architect in the orthodox mode at any stage of his career. Breuer's own thinking had been greatly affected by his travels around the Mediterranean in the early 1930s, during which '…he became increasingly enthralled with the forms of vernacular building'.[16] His preference for developing a limited number of planning typologies for his houses, which he passed on to Seidler, was directly influenced by his perception of consistent types in vernacular building. More than that, Breuer's adaptation of the traditional structural techniques and building materials of New England, had a transforming effect on the Modernist vocabulary he had helped

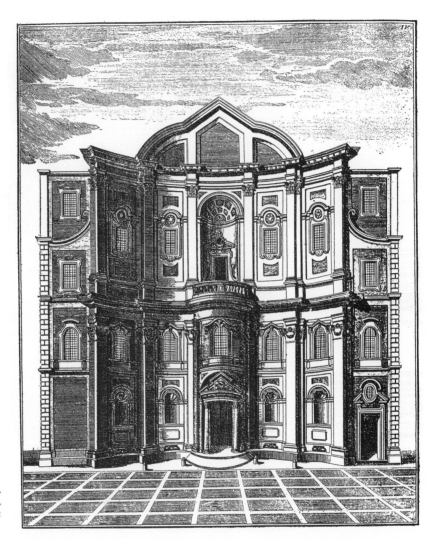

▶ **5.33** Francesco Borromini, Oratory of S. Philip Neri, Rome, 1650. Facade. *Source:* P. Portoghesi, 1982.

to create in his Bauhaus years, a development which was to have a considerable impact, not only on Seidler, but also on many of his contemporaries.

The architectural language and techniques Seidler learnt from Breuer and which he in turn adapted – in some respects more successfully than Breuer – to the Australian landscape and climate in the early years of his career, were therefore already far removed from the Machine aesthetic with which orthodox Modernism and its European pioneers are identified. The additional influence, as Seidler's architecture evolved, of Niemeyer's free-form Modernism and Borromini's baroque geometries, fits into the same broadening vision.

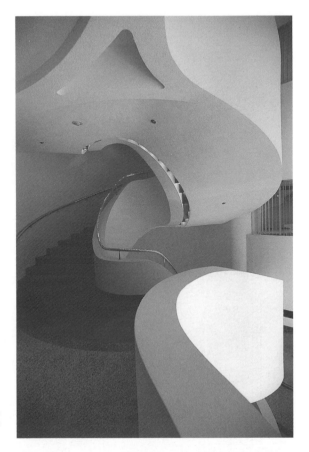

▶ **5.34** Hong Kong Club. Main stair on first level. Photo: John Gollings.

RELATION TO NATURE

Similar critical biases have distorted perceptions of the relation of Seidler's architecture to the Australian landscape he came to adore, and to nature in general. The extreme possibilities of how Modern architecture should relate to nature were clearly delineated early in the last century by Frank Lloyd Wright's Robie House and Le Corbusier's Villa Savoie: the former hugging the ground and vaguely rustic in its composition and materials; the latter raised off the ground, geometrically composed and made entirely with modern materials.

For those architects who think in black and white and like their categories well-boxed, the two approaches have come to signify, on the one hand an acceptance of nature, and on the other a rejection of it. The American historian and critic Vincent Scully knew better. In *The Earth, the Temple, and the Gods*,[17] he explains the intricate principles by which the ancient Greeks related their temples to the landscape as humanly shaped counterpoints to nature, whereby one enhances

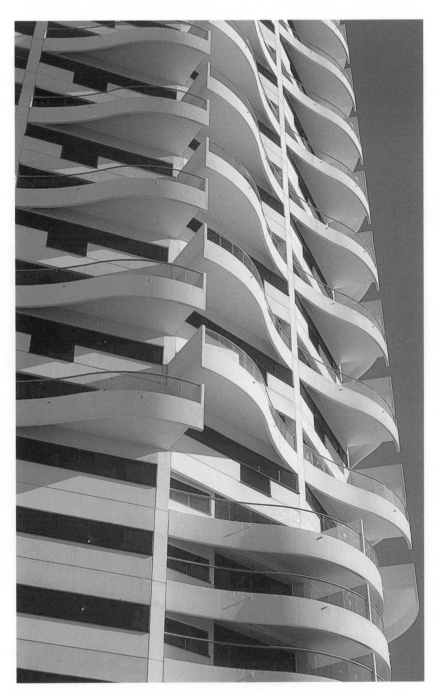

▲ **5.35** Horizon Apartments, Darlinghurst, 1997. Terraces. Photo: Eric Sierins.

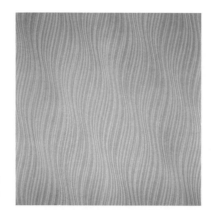

▶ **5.36** Painting, 'Orphean Elegy I', 1978, by Bridget Riley. *Source*: R. Hughes, 1980.

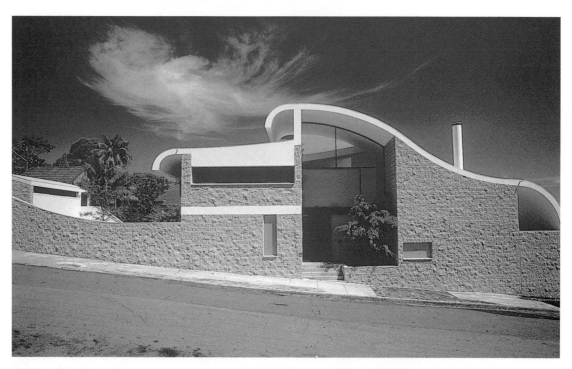

▲ **5.37** Meares House, Birchgrove, 1995. Photo: Eric Sierins.

the other, not by imitation, but by the integration of opposites. The same principles underly Le Corbusier's work, later superbly encapsulated in the Chapel at Ronchamp, and also inspired Niemeyer to create his own Brazilian interpretation of Modern architecture, to match his own landscape and culture.

While in his early work he has sometimes gravitated towards the Corbusier–Niemeyer end of the spectrum, Seidler's architecture defies any simplistic category.

Thus, although the earliest houses were often partly raised off the ground, the use of timber and stone in their construction, as in the Breuer houses, greatly softened their impact. Seidler's increasingly sensitive response to the Australian climate, both in the liberal use of sunshades and natural ventilation, together with his quick abandonment of flat roofs – an early and outdated symbol of modernity – in favour of monopitch and butterfly types, and eventually curved roofs, indicates a constant willingness to adapt a given idea and form to a specific location (while Seidler's later use of corrugated iron roofs might be interpreted as a concession to the popular 'metal shed' aesthetic, both their actual shape and different context of use suggest contrary motivations).

SOPHISTICATED SYMBOL

However, if there are any lingering doubts about Seidler's approach to the Australian landscape, or his personal reverence for nature, they have been resolved once and for all by the Berman House (Figs. 5.38 and 5.39). Poised on the edge of a steep escarpment overlooking a bushland river valley, Seidler's house is at once both part of the magnificent landscape and also a sophisticated

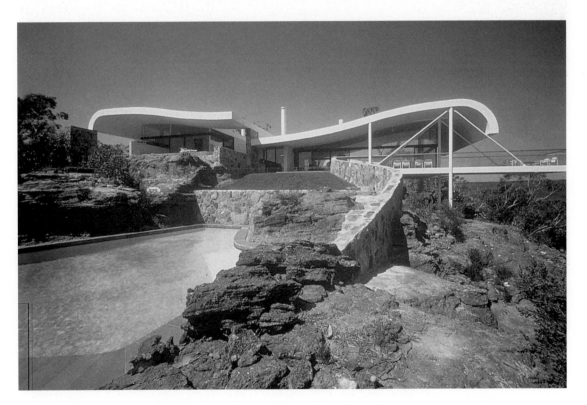

▲ **5.38**   Berman House, Joadja, 2000. Photo: Eric Sierins.

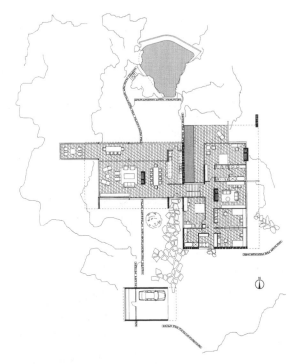

▶ **5.39** Berman House, plan. *Source*:   Harry   Seidler Associates.

symbol of an urbanized and technologically advanced culture, with no hint of the rustic or rural about it. Even the use of rough local stone in the retaining walls, whilst anchoring the house firmly into the clifftop, also serves to highlight the smooth finesse of the steel and glass structure above.

The closest historical parallels in Modernist domestic architecture to this superlative exercise in the integration of opposites would be, not the extreme Corbusian model, but either Richard Neutra's Kaufmann House (Fig. 5.40), or Niemeyer's own house (Fig. 5.41), both of which feature strong roof lines, the former rectilinear, the latter curvaceous, floating over the natural terrain.

Planwise, Seidler is closer to Neutra, but his curved roof forms are more in the spirit of Niemeyer's architecture. However, his response to the landscape is identical to that of both architects. Of the Niemeyer house, it has been said, 'Niemeyer let nature be his interior decorator'.[18] The same might also be said of Seidler's design (Fig. 5.42), as well as Neutra's, which both completely dissolve any visual barrier between the interior spaces and the landscape beyond. Also just as both the Neutra and Niemeyer houses fit with their respective natural settings – one an arid desert, the other a tropical forest – without pretending to be a part of them or concealing their sophistication, so does the Berman House respond to and compliment the bushland valley without submerging into it.

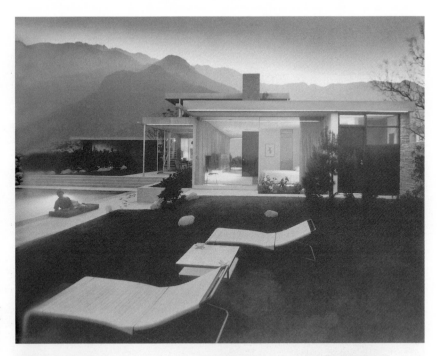

▶ **5.40** Richard Neutra, Kaufmann House, Palm Springs, California, 1947. General view. Photo: Julius Shulmann.

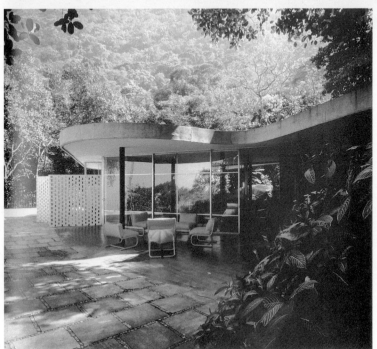

▶ **5.41** Oscar Niemeyer, House at Canoas, Rio de Janeiro, 1953. *Source: The House Book, 2001.*

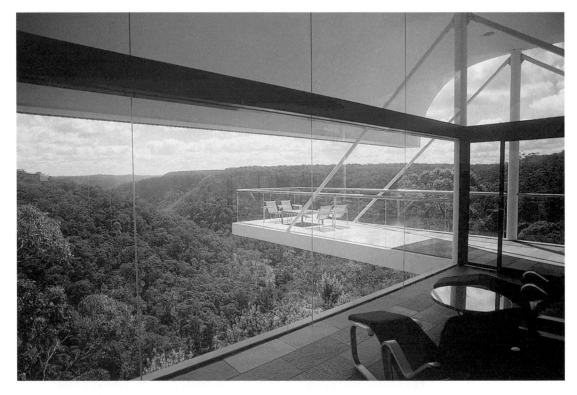

▲ **5.42**   Berman House, interior. Photo: Eric Sierins.

Each acts as a foil to the other, so much so that, were the house to be suddenly taken away, one cannot help but feel the valley itself would lose something in the act – just as if you took a fine bridge away from the river valley it enhances.

LOCAL OPPOSITION

It comes as a rude shock, therefore, to learn that this house, like many others designed by Seidler before it, initially met with objection by the local planning authorities, not for where it is situated – that was never a problem – but for the Modernist character of the design. That battle, like almost all the other similar contests Seidler has fought with the authorities throughout his career, was eventually won, and it is possible to exaggerate the actual effect of such official opposition over the long run.[19] Seidler's architecture has reaped many state and national, as well as international awards, and whilst he still considers himself something of an outsider, the enormous impact his work has had in Australia, especially in Sydney, is beyond question.

However, the opposition is not always confined to ill-informed officials and associated philistines. Ever since the Sydney School of architects found their collective architectural voices in the late 1950s, the Wrightian approach to the landscape – essentially submissive, rustic and neo-vernacular in character – has dominated local architects' imaginations as the embodiment of the Great Australian Dream.[20] This is hardly surprising. Wright's own utopian vision, Broadacre City, presents a rationalized model of dispersed living which differs only from the more mundane suburban reality in the average size of its plots (much larger – land was cheap back then), and in the uniformity of the architectural language (exclusively Wrightian, predictably).

The Sydney School and its later offshoots spawned much good architecture, providing a positive alternative, just as Seidler has done in his own way, to lamentable norms of design. However, welcome as these improvements are in the design of individual dwellings, they have generally not been accompanied by a parallel critique of the settlement patterns within which all these architects are working.

It must be added that in this matter architects are not alone in Australia. To a newcomer to the country, at least, it often seems as though a large part of the population, if not most of it, is in deep denial of its own urbanized and complex culture, preferring instead the comforting myths and popular images of a simpler life in the 'outback', embodied by the male bush worker.[21] The updated 'farmhouse' style of dwelling favoured by many designers panders to this rural, masculine self-image, as well as to both local and foreign concepts of a singular Australian identity.[22]

PRESSING PROBLEMS

However, what was once a desirable and affordable way of life for the majority during the long boom, is now literally costing the Earth – sustained in Australia, as in North America, only by heavily subsidized fuel prices for the thirsty automobiles which make the whole system run. While any raising of the standards of house design must be welcomed, it is difficult to see how improving the design of individual dwellings, no matter how many, will make any significant difference to the more pressing problems of the pressures on land, infrastructure and energy consumption which the Great Australian Dream has thrown up.[23]

Much else has also changed in Australia since 1970, aside from the rise in the (real) cost of fuel. The office towers Seidler designed in Sydney and elsewhere (Fig. 5.43) during the past three decades are themselves the outcome of a major shift in the structure of the Australian economy, like that in other developed countries, away from manufacturing towards services.[24] While the population has grown at a slower rate than of that in the long boom, it has also undergone radical changes in its composition, partly due to new immigration policies, and partly to social changes. As much as a quarter of Sydney's population is now of Asian origin – mostly from Asia Pacific – whilst the number of single parents and persons living alone has also risen sharply, in line with similar changes in Europe and North America.[25]

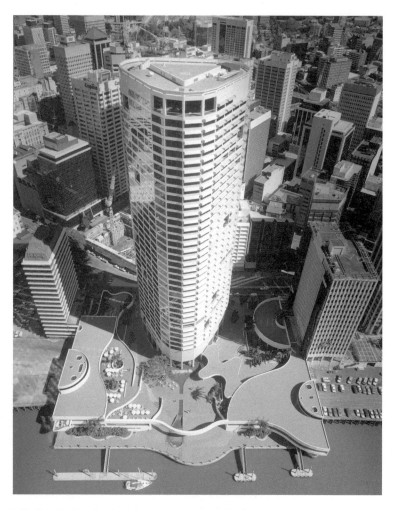

▲ **5.43** *Riverside Development, Stage 1, Brisbane, 1986. Photo: Eric Sierins.*

The change in the population mix also reflects a fundamental change in Australia's historical orientation, away from Europe and the mother country, towards its regional neighbours around the Pacific Rim, bringing with it new trading partners and political relationships.[26] All of these developments have had a marked impact on Australia's cities, creating new businesses and other opportunities, raising densities and generating new patterns of urban life, as well as demands for a greater variety of dwelling forms.

It is in this context that Seidler's Neue Donau Housing Estate (Fig. 5.44) in Vienna, together with his apartments in Sydney and experiments in low-rise,

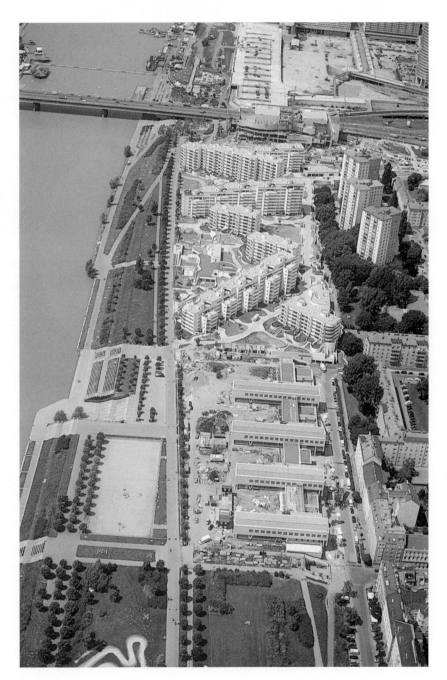

▲ **5.44** Neue Donau Housing Estate (upper half), Vienna, 2001. Photo: Eric Sierins.

medium-density projects, acquire a special significance. Inspired by the Victorian terraced houses of Sydney, the Yarralumya Group (Fig. 5.45), one of a series of related group projects dating back to the 1950s, combines the pleasures of owning your own plot with a stronger sense of place and community than suburban patterns can offer. Whilst the Vienna project was designed for a very different place and culture, it also embodies principles of social responsibility which Seidler believes are sorely lacking in Australia, where low-cost housing in the major cities is becoming increasingly scarce.[27]

NO DIVISION

Seidler himself continues to cater to the Great Australian Dream, helping his clients as best he can to realize that dream. However, his work on individual dwellings has been counterbalanced throughout most of his career by other equally important social commitments, not only to raising the standards of commercial architecture – at which he has few rivals anywhere – but, as the above

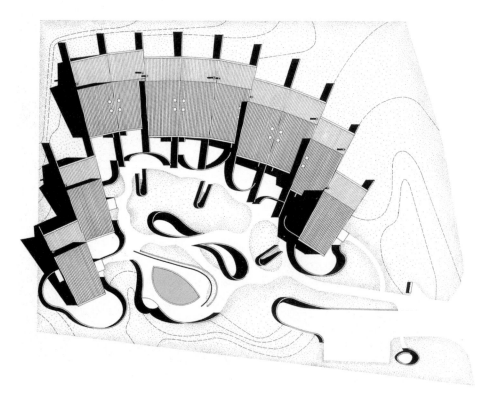

▲ **5.45** Group Houses, Yarralumya, ACT, 1984. *Source:* Harry Seidler Associates.

projects demonstrate, also to a search for higher quality living at high densities, and to improving the general quality of life in the city (Fig. 5.46).

For Seidler, there is no division between his single house designs and his other work. Each informs and sustains the other in a continuously fertile and critical exchange of ideas. As a result of that process, Seidler's later houses express an urbane quality which, while it may not conform to the rugged, rural image

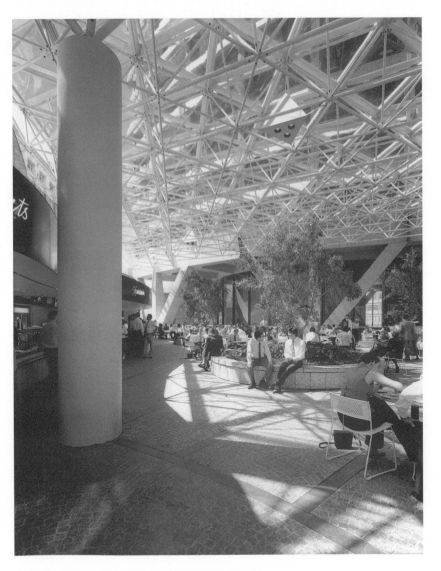

▲ **5.46** Grovesnor Place, Sydney, 1988. Photo: Max Dupain.

preferred by others, possibly better reflects the more complex realities of Australia's highly urbanized and rapidly changing culture.

Far from being the last of anything, Seidler is also best appreciated as one of those few designers who, by opening Modernism up to fresh influences and interpretations, both historical and contemporary, gave it new life during the period when it was most under attack. That larger battle – certainly more important than the minor local struggles Seidler has endured, though not entirely disconnected from them – is also now more or less won.[28] As one of the handful of architects of his own generation able to match a creative imagination with technical competence and flair, he will also surely come to be recognized, if he is not already, as one of the very first designers in the twentieth century able to fully realize the Modernist dream of the integration of art and technology – the ultimate integration of opposites.

6 MEDITERRANEAN MIX AND MATCH

HISTORIC CROSSROADS

Standing at the historic crossroads of the Mediterranean, between Sicily and North Africa, the island of Malta and its two smaller neighbours, Gozo and Comino (Fig. 6.1), have been inhabited since about 5 000 BC, the traces of which include some of the world's earliest known human constructions in stone.[1] They have been successively occupied thereafter by most of the region's dominant peoples: Phoenicians, Romans, Arabs, Normans, French, British – all took their turn at ruling the tiny but important group of islands.[2]

Few of these, however, left many permanent traces on the ground. Aside from the unique megalithic temples on Malta and Gozo – compact but immensely powerful curved structures predating Stonehenge (Fig. 6.2) – and some scattered Roman remains, what one sees today of the islands' major settlements and buildings is chiefly the two and a half-century legacy of the Knights of St John of Jerusalem.[3] Founded during the first Crusade to the 'Holy Land', the international religious and military order was driven out of its previous stronghold on the island of Rhodes by the Ottoman rulers of the Islamic Empire, resettling in Malta in 1530. The rocky and hilly land they found was not much to their liking, but it had two invaluable assets: the workable limestone of which the islands are composed provided abundant building material for fortifications; and an incomparable natural harbour on the eastern seaboard of Malta provided an ideal base from which the Knights could send forth their galleys to harass enemy shipping.

Following the 'Great Siege' of 1565, when the Ottomans failed to unseat the Knights from their new stronghold, a massive building programme of fortified settlements was begun in anticipation of further assaults.[4] The attacks never came, and with its new-found security and strategic importance as the home of the Knights, now amply supported by a grateful Europe, Malta enjoyed a period of unprecedented growth and prosperity.

Most of the important structures of this period still remain, from the fortified Renaissance city of Valletta (Fig. 6.3), the gridded capital of Malta laid across the resistant topography like San Francisco, to the many baroque churches built to

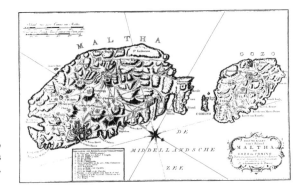

▶ **6.1** Islands of Malta. Map printed in Amsterdam by Is Tirion, 1761. *Source*: Q. Hughes, 1969.

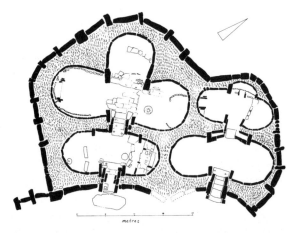

▶ **6.2** Temple complex of Ggantija, Gozo, Malta, *c.*3 600–3 000 BC. Plan. *Source*: A. Bonanno, 1997.

meet the needs of the rapid population growth which security and prosperity bred. All are built from the same cream coloured material of the islands, blending with the stone vernacular buildings and terraced walls of the open fields so as to blur the distinction between architecture and nature. Like some window into evolution, the islands offer the eye a graduated hierarchy from disorder to order: from the rock-strewn fields, to random rubble terrace walls, to the simple farm buildings of cut stone, to the step upon step of cubic dwellings piled up in the villages and towns, and finally, to the ornate shapes of the baroque churches which, happily, still dominate the skyline in most places, terminating the hierarchy and throwing it into reverse (Fig. 6.4). From entropy to negentropy, chaos to complexity, and vice versa, the whole monochrome progression thrown into stark relief by an intense sunlight, it is an impressive spectacle.

DRASTIC CHANGES

The British occupation that followed on from that of the Knights lasted nearly two centuries. However, save perhaps for the Nazi bombs the British presence

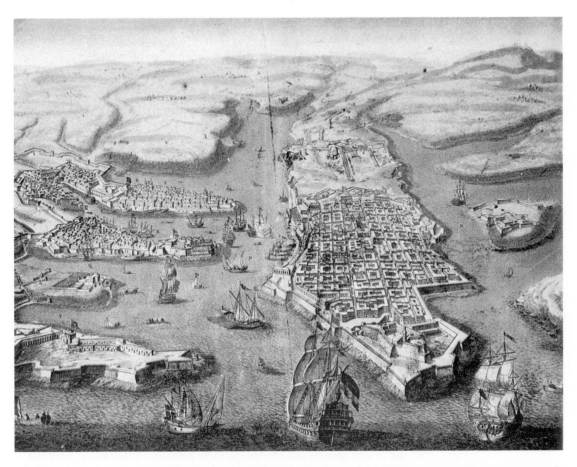

▲ **6.3** New City of Valletta, Malta, 1565–95. Engraving. Built soon after Great Siege, the baroque city was laid out by Italian planner Francesco Laparelli da Cortona. Grand Harbour is shown left of city. *Source*: The National Trust of Malta, 1976.

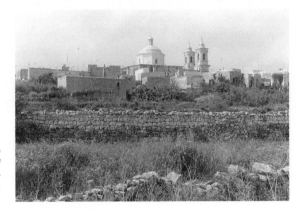

▶ **6.4** Malta's villages are typically situated on crests of hills or ridges and are dominated by Baroque churches. Photo: Author.

invited during World War II and a number of stone barracks built here and there, colonial rule had relatively little visible effect on this remarkable man-made landscape. Only later, with the coming of Independence in 1964 and the subsequent need to encourage tourism as an essential part of the new economy, did Malta begin its next transformation. From around 20 000 in 1960, the number of seasonal visitors to the island quickly rose to 730 000 in 1980, rising slowly thereafter to hold steady around the current figure of just over 1 million – more than double the permanent population.

While it has helped to bring prosperity to the island, the growth has not been without severe cost. Most of the new building has taken place in and around the densely populated historic towns and tourist centres on the lower levels of the eastern seaboard, swelling already crowded areas. Changes in domestic politics and the slow liberalization of the economy from the late 1980s onwards have had their own impact, creating new wealth but at the same time placing additional strains on the fragile environment (none of Malta's problems are unique, but the small size of the island greatly aggravates any failures – take any one common problem, whether it is waste disposal, overcrowding or traffic and multiply it by ten, and you get a good idea of the situation). Poor public transportation and a long neglected road system, plus a huge increase in private car ownership – now one car for every two persons – have combined to produce the highest density of automobile traffic per kilometre of road in the world. Though minute by comparison, Malta now suffers the same extreme environmental problems as the megacities of the developing world, with traffic threatening to bring parts of the island to a standstill during peak periods and polluting the once clear Mediterranean air.

All this drastic growth and change has sadly produced little new architecture of merit, and none yet to compare with the magnificent historical record.[5] Banal commercialism spliced with Postmodern kitsch predominates for most hotels and other building types, while the poor quality of new domestic architecture is only moderated by the almost uniform use of local stone, which helps blend it with the older settlements. The only distinguished design in the International Style, the former Hilton Hotel at St Julians Bay, was demolished years ago to make way for a much larger mixed development. Since Independence, only Richard England's Manikata Church[6] (Fig. 6.5), the Danish Village Hotel at Mellieha Bay, by Hans Munkhansen, and Ray Demicoli's own house at San Gwann hold up to close scrutiny, and rank among the best regional works of their time.

As in most parts of the developing world, the lessons of vernacular architecture regarding climate control have also been generally ignored. The result is that owners of new homes as well as businesses are increasingly reliant upon air-conditioning to maintain tolerable comfort levels in the hot summer months,

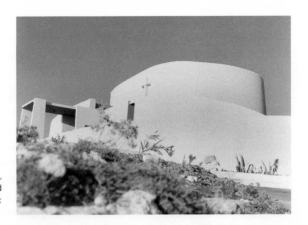

▶ 6.5 Church of St Joseph, Manikata, Malta. Richard England, 1962–74. Photo: Richard England.

when temperatures can reach over 40°C. The lack of any concerted government policy on energy conservation – compared with other Mediterranean countries solar energy is practically ignored in Malta, and, despite its obvious applicability, receives no government support or subsidies – coupled with widespread professional ignorance of and indifference towards sustainable design, have pushed energy demands and costs on the resource-strapped island to new highs.

OPEN DESIGN PHILOSOPHY

It is therefore with some relief as well as enthusiasm that one is able to report on a Maltese architectural practice that is bucking this dismal trend, and making a name for itself as regional leaders in sustainable design, as well as in other areas.

Architecture Project, or AP as they are called, was started up in 1991 by its four young partners, Konrad Buhagiar, David Drago, David Felice and Alberto Miceli-Farrugia, all graduates of the University of Malta save for Farrugia, who studied at Cambridge. Beginning, as most young practices do, with a few private commissions for individual houses, the practice quickly grew to embrace an unusually wide range of projects. They include the rehabilitation of historic buildings, shops and offices, apartment complexes and a terminal for cruise ships, plus a number of entries for foreign competitions along the way.

As the practice has grown and diversified, a novel, open design philosophy has evolved, which, while staying more or less within the broad traditions of Modernism, allows the partners to experiment freely with quite different approaches. Invariably, each project is treated on its own merits, involving a fresh examination of the programme going well beyond normal procedures. The very nature of the building type being looked at may be called into question, opening up new approaches and solutions. Rather than forcing new assistants to 'fit in', as most design partnerships do, creative responsibility is also readily given to newcomers whenever it is warranted. Unusually for a single practice, therefore, it is difficult to predict from one project to another what the next design might actually look like: '… the agenda of the office accommodates a new direction every time a new member joins the team'.[7]

At first glance, the wide range of projects shown here may therefore appear to have little in common. A number of relatively consistent themes are nevertheless apparent. An honest expression of materials and structure, together with a strong respect for how buildings work identify AP as Modernists, though not without qualification. Keenly aware of the fickle effects of time upon architecture, they reject any simplistic equations between form and use of the orthodox variety: 'given today's mixed imperatives, where rehabilitation and regeneration, epitomized by power stations being turned into art galleries, are now commonplace, the kind of deterministic thinking that turned such Modernist slogans as "form follows function" into dogma, is obsolete'.[8] Accordingly, much of AP's work, particularly in their rehabilitation projects, exhibits a self-conscious tension between form and use, in which neither quite gets the upper hand, nor gets forgotten.

A sensitive response to place and climate, rooted in a deep appreciation of the special character of Malta's own history and ecology, is also apparent in almost all AP's work, mediating their modernity without repressing it – historicism or facadism or any other Postmodern indulgencies are strictly *out*. Energy conservation is likewise a major priority, and has led to the use of innovative techniques of passive energy design. A clear articulation between public, private and semi-private spaces also typifies the residential projects. However, beyond these consistencies, the material fabric, spatial geometry and formal character of a project may vary wildly, according to the specific place and programme and who is involved.

INJECTING NEW LIFE

The inventive and free-wheeling spirit of AP's approach is clearly seen in their conservation and rehabilitation projects. With Malta's endless supply of historic buildings, many in poor condition, such projects constitute a vital part of the practice and are often used as a test-bed for injecting new life and ideas into the urban fabric.

Their first project of this kind, the Kenuna Tower (Fig. 6.6) in Nadur, Gozo, entailed the conversion of a 150-year-old structure built by the British forces as a semaphore station, into a modern telecommunications tower for Maltacom, a company providing cellular radio and maritime links. A simple stone tower, the original structure had no distinguishing features other than its spectacular placement on the edge of an escarpment. The town is one of the highest on the hilly island, and the tower has clear views all across Gozo and Comino and the seas in between towards Malta.

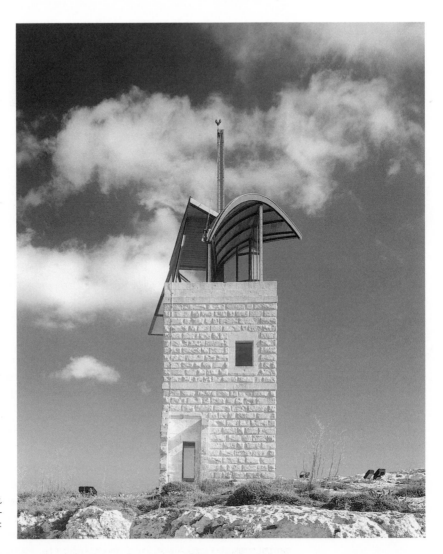

▶ **6.6** Kenuna Tower, Nadur, Gozo Island, Malta. Architecture Project, 1996–9. Photo: David Pisani.

AP have exploited the tower's full potential as a landmark, inserting a lightweight steel structure that pokes out of the top of the tower in a busy flurry of curved and pointed roof canopies and angled steel and glass walls, catching the eye from far away. Superficially, the irregular, alien forms of the new structure recall Coop Himmelblau's 1986 rooftop remodelling of an apartment block in Vienna. However, the functional and structural rationale of AP's design clearly separates them from the abstract preoccupations of those architects. Designed with London-based engineers Adams Kara Taylor, floors, roof and telecommunications equipment are all carried independently of the existing stone walls by a single

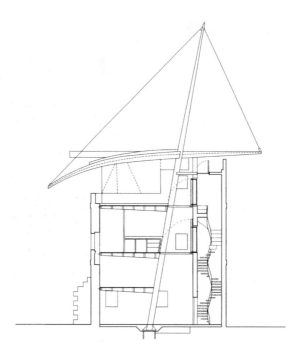

▶ **6.7** Kenuna Tower. Section.
Source: Architecture Project.

inclined steel column or mast, so that, should the need arise, the entire new structure and all its equipment could be easily removed or replaced (Fig. 6.7).

Their second major rehabilitation project involved the updating and adaptation of a block of eighteenth-century houses adjoining the Manoel Theatre[9] (Fig. 6.8), Valletta's principal cultural centre and a jewel of theatre design from the same period. Annexed by the theatre company over the years, the stone buildings provide various support activities and spaces, the most important of which includes an open, collonaded courtyard, part of the former Casa Bonici, the largest palazzo of the group. Situated on a prominent street corner and accessible from both outside and inside, the courtyard forms the heart of the scheme and serves as a circulation area, an extension to the theatre bar in the evenings, and a public café/restaurant and popular meeting place during the daytime.

Originally intended, as all such courtyards are, to provide both a shaded private outdoor space and open air lungs for the surrounding rooms of the palazzo, AP have designed an automated, retractable steel-framed roof which enhances the space's climate control functions and makes it usable in all weathers and seasons (Fig. 6.9a–c). Temperatures drop considerably overnight during the summer months and such courtyards are designed as cold air tanks, capturing the heavier night air, which slowly heats up and rises during the day, drawing fresh air through the surrounding rooms and drying out the porous limestone as it does so.

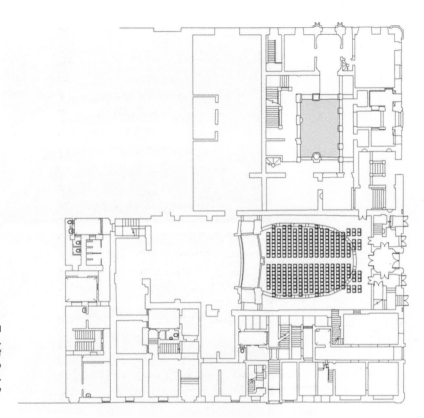

▶ **6.8** Mobile Roof, Manoel Theatre Complex, Valletta, Malta. Plan showing position of covered atrium adjacent to theatre. Architecture Project, 1995–7. *Source*: Architecture Project.

Comprised of parallel curved sections running on tracks concealed just below the parapet, each section has its own syncronized motor so that they can all be adjusted together to changing conditions: raised vertically and pulled back during the mild spring and autumn months; closed completely during the winter; or partly raised and covered in canvas to provide shade and ventilation during the summer. Metacrylic rather than glass is used for the transparent panels to reduce weight and the curved shape provides extra stiffness and helps to throw off rainwater. Designed with local engineers and made by a local steel fabricator, the motorized roof tested Maltese technical know-how.

HYBRID SYSTEM OF CLIMATE CONTROL

The adjustable roof of the Manoel Theatre courtyard was the first of a number of experiments with moving building parts which AP have designed, usually for environmental control but also for other purposes, which extend the adaptability of a building and its use. Automated vents located in the roof ridge also play a key role in the hybrid system of passive climate control devised for AP's most important rehabilitation project to date, the Malta Stock Exchange.[10] Housed in

(a)

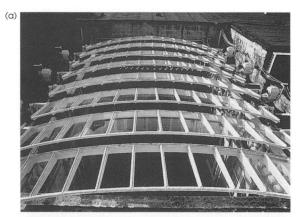

(b)

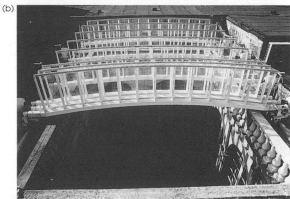

(c)

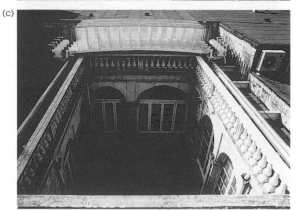

▶ **6.9** Mobile Roof, Manoel Theatre Complex. Roof with partly open fins (a), roof folded back (b), roof in fully retracted position (c). Photos: David Pisani.

the nineteenth-century British Garrison Chapel situated just inside Valletta's city walls (Fig. 6.10), the offices for the exchange are designed, like the Kenuna Tower, as a completely self-supporting steel-framed structure, with no outward or internal effect on the original shell. Comprising parallel steel frames four

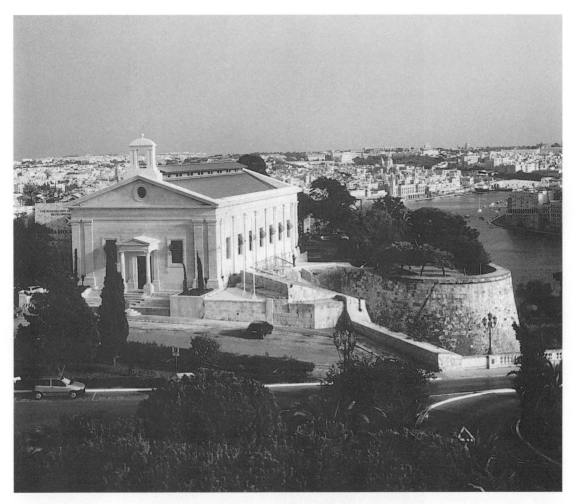

▲ **6.10**   Malta Stock Exchange, Valletta, Malta. View of British Garrison Chapel and Valletta fortifications with Grand Harbour beyond. Architecture Project, 1994–2001. Photo: David Pisani.

storeys high – three above ground and one below – running lengthways each side of the church, linked by pierced floors at ground and first level, the structure forms a five-storey high atrium from the conference centre at the lowest level to the apex of the timber roof, which was carefully restored. Cellular offices are grouped in the parallel blocks while open plan offices are provided in between and on the top floor, underneath the open roof structure (Fig. 6.11).

AP's collaborating environmental engineer in London, Brian Ford, had had previous experience of working in Malta with Peake Short on the 1994 Farson's Brewery extension,[11] which was also designed to be self-cooling. Since then Ford had designed a more advanced system of passive downdraught evaporative cooling (PDEC) for the Torrent Pharmaceutical Laboratory[12] in India, and done further

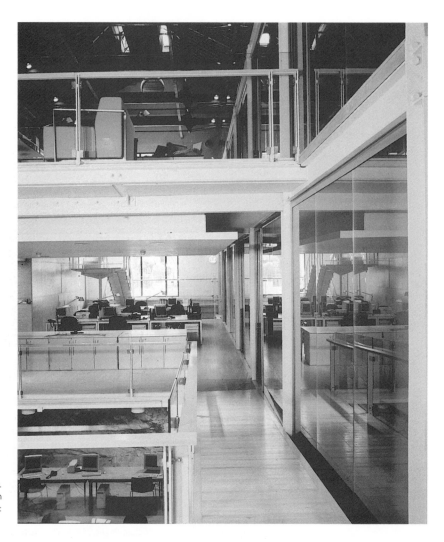

▶ **6.11** Malta Stock Exchange. Interior view of atrium with cellular offices to right. Photo: David Pisani.

research on the system in southern Italy. Using sprays of fine water particles to cool and increase the weight of warm air drawn in through towers or roofs, the system utilizes natural physics to move air through a building without mechanical assistance or noise.

Adapting the same system for the open spaces of the Stock Exchange, Ford combined it with a back-up system of chilled-water cooling coils also placed in the ridge, which performs in a similar way (Fig. 6.12). Conventional air-conditioning units are used for the cellular offices and the lower meeting and conference rooms. The performance of the hybrid passive system under changing conditions was accurately simulated in London using computational fluid dynamics

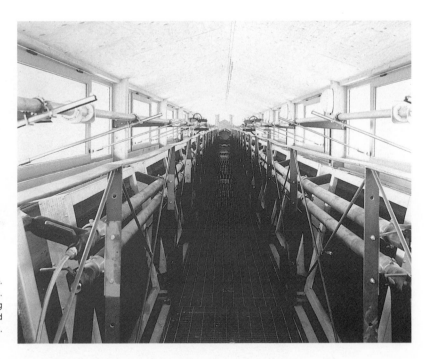

▶ **6.12** Malta Stock Exchange. Evaporative cooling system. View under ridge showing chilled water cooling coils and hydraulically operated vents. Photo: David Pisani.

(CFD) (Fig. 6.13a–c). Results so far indicate extensive savings on energy costs for an equivalent conventional system.

The extension to the branch of Marks and Spencer in Valletta also involved inserting a self-supporting steel structure into a stone shell, formerly an eighteenth-century house on the far side of Strait Street, a narrow way running along the back of the main store. Like the Stock Exchange, an atrium opens up the interior from ground floor to roof level, bringing natural light pouring down from the glazed upper walls and clerestory in the curved roof, which is further enhanced by wide glass strips in the floor edges around the open space. However, the treatment of the exposed, white-painted steel frame is far more lighthearted than in the former building and splits into angled 'branches' at each level, creating the effect of a series of steel 'trees' surrounding the atrium (Fig. 6.14).

More original still, the retractable steel and wooden bridge (Fig. 6.15) which links the two parts of the store across Strait Street at first-floor level is an extraordinary contraption that combines elements of the Maltese vernacular, and both ancient and modern technologies and materials. The entrance of the main store faces onto St Georges Square, a large open pedestrianized space situated on the principal thoroughfare through Valletta. It is assumed that most shoppers will continue using this entrance, which lies at a higher level than Strait Street, so a bridge connecting the two stores at an upper level was the obvious solution.

(a)

(b)

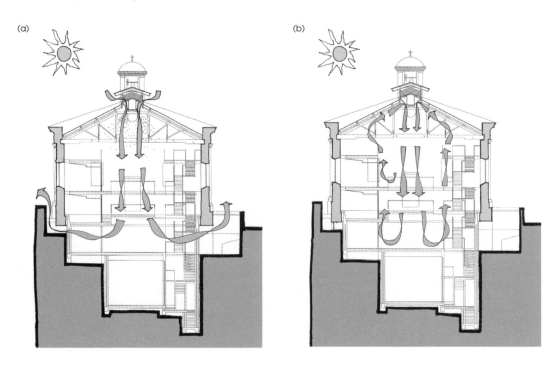

(c)

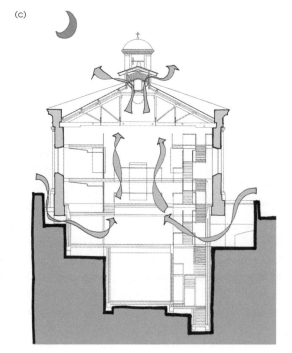

▲ **6.13a–c** Malta Stock Exchange. Hybrid evaporative cooling system: on dry summer days misting nozzles under open ridge induce downdraft driving air through building (a); when humidity exceeds 65 per cent vents close and cooling coils induce similar effect (b); air drawn through building by stack effect during night pre-cools building (c). *Source*: Brian Ford.

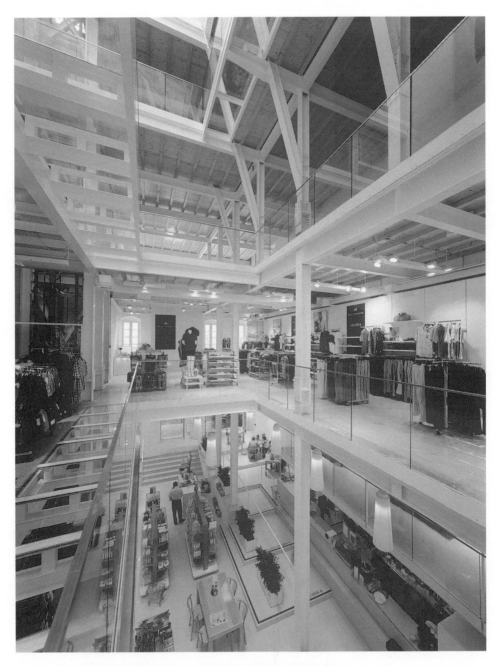

▲ **6.14** Marks and Spencer Extension, Valletta, Malta. Interior view of atrium. Architecture Project, 1996–2003. Photo: David Pisani.

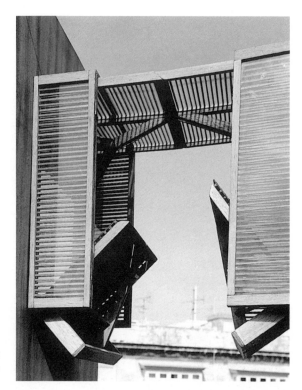

▶ **6.15** Marks and Spencer Extension. Folding footbridge. Model. Photo: David Pisani.

However, a permanent bridge would obstruct the view down the tall and narrow space of the long street – a defining characteristic of the city – so the bridge was designed to fold neatly in two halves back into projecting wooden boxes anchored by steel frames into the walls. When folded, the containers, which have hardwood frames and slats like the fully extended enclosed bridge, strongly resemble the traditional 'hanging balconies' (Fig. 6.16) which can be seen all over Valletta, and blend inconspicuously with the restored stone facades and wooden balconies of the original buildings. Not the least attraction of the eccentric design, the manually operated system of wires, pulleys and weights which enables the heavy bridge to be easily raised and tucked away, looks like something straight off Leonardo da Vinci's sketchpad (Fig. 6.17a and b). The ingenious system is cheaper, safer and more reliable than a comparable motor-driven system, which is what the architects first thought of.

VERNACULAR INFLUENCES

The bridge-balcony is only one of many references to the Maltese vernacular in AP's work. While the architects generally relish in sharp contrasts between modern and traditional materials and technologies, particularly in their rehabilitation projects,

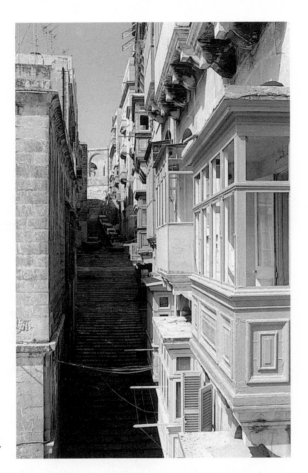

▶ **6.16** Hanging balcony, Valletta. Photo: Author.

their early house designs mostly exhibit a more conservative approach, in which vernacular construction techniques and other influences play a significant part.

Timber of any kind has always been a scarce commodity on the rocky Maltese islands and building timber was imported for beam supports and balconies. In addition, stone arches were widely used for supporting floors and roofs as well as openings for all forms of domestic architecture, from humble farmhouses to the grandest palazzos. The floors and roofs themselves were also traditionally made from stone slabs, so supporting arches were spaced closely together to reduce the span and carry the weight. The visual effect of the parallel arches on the internal spaces is very dramatic, and lends even the simplest vernacular dwelling a special dignity and character (Fig. 6.18).

Using similar construction methods, AP have designed several houses with a plan typology based on a repetitive system of parallel stone arches and vaults,

(a)

(b)

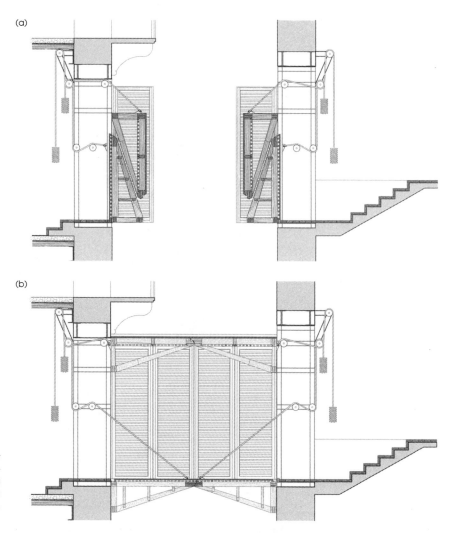

▶ **6.17** Marks and Spencer Extension. Retractable footbridge. Section showing bridge in open position (a); section in closed position (b). *Source*: Architecture Project.

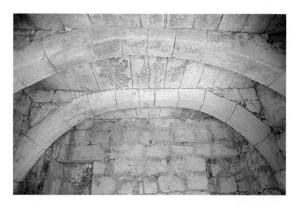

▶ **6.18** Vernacular stone house, Malta. Interior, showing vaulted roof construction. Photo: Author.

(a)

(b)

(c)

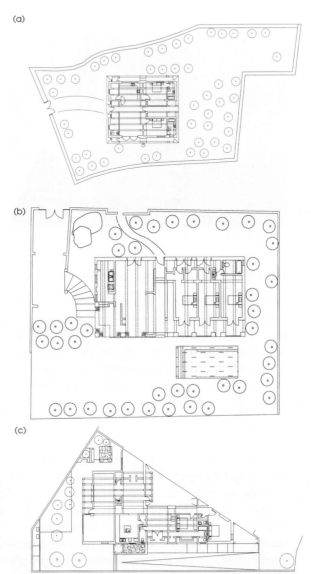

▶ **6.19** Comparative house plans: House for Grannie Nellie, San Pawl Tat-Targa, 1993–5 (a), villa on a Slope, Santa Marija Estate, Mellieha, 1993–6 (b), Victor Mangion's House, Kappara, 1997–2001 (c). *Source*: Architecture Project.

amounting to a distinctive architectural series in itself.[13] The House for Grannie Nellie at San Pawl Tat-Targa is typical of the series (Fig. 6.19a–c). For this relatively small house, all rooms have been grouped into two parallel spaces of equal width roofed by closely spaced stone arches in the traditional manner. However, whereas in vernacular architecture the segments on both sides of the apex would be infilled with the same stone to support a flat roof or floor above, the arches in this and AP's other houses in the series support parallel stone vaults (Fig. 6.20). While clearly reminiscent of vernacular building, the resulting interior

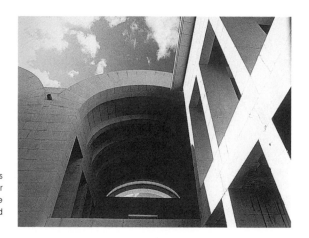

▶ **6.20** Victor Mangion's House. View of house under construction showing stone vaulting system. Photo: David Pisani.

volumes have an even stronger directional character and dignity, over and above that expected in what is otherwise a very simple dwelling.

AP's second major deviation from the traditional type is in their use of deep, hollow service walls to support the vaults and separate the main volumes. Also built from the same stone, these service spines vary in width, according to what they enclose: wardrobes and storage spaces, or bathrooms and stairways. The arrangement is clearly influenced by Louis Kahn's concept of 'served' and 'service' spaces, as well as by Christopher Alexander's and Serge Chemayeff's linear housing projects.[14] The parallel vaults also suggest miniature versions of Kahn's Kimbell Art Museum at Fort Worth, together with its Roman archetypes.

The Mews (Fig. 6.21), Kappara, a cluster of four houses linked by a central courtyard and a raised podium with parking underneath, was also partly influenced by local dwelling forms, though the aesthetic and construction techniques are quite different. Vernacular architecture mostly consists of isolated farmhouses or two-storey terraced dwellings with courtyards, tightly grouped together in the villages and towns, in typical Mediterranean fashion. However, since Independence and the increased mobility that has accompanied economic growth, the preferred dwelling form for the growing middle classes, like practically everywhere else, is the detached suburban villa with its own private garden and garage.

Located in an upmarket suburb a short distance inland from the east coast, the houses fit unobtrusively into their surroundings and look at first sight like an assembly of well-designed but otherwise conventional examples of the villa type (Fig. 6.22). The rendered concrete construction and early Modernist aesthetic, with its all-white, abstract cubic masses and sharp-edged horizontal and vertical planes, also place the houses firmly back with those classic designs by Gerrit Reitveld and other greats, which redefined the suburban villa as a Modernist icon. The knowing

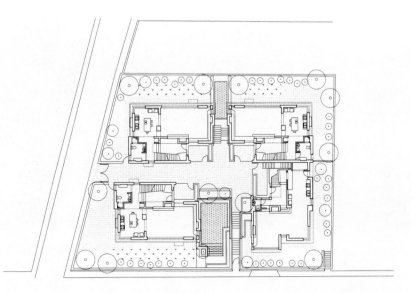

▶ **6.21** The Mews, Kappara, Malta. Ground floor plan. Architecture project, 1994–8. *Source*: Architecture Project.

Modernist nostalgia is complicated by the awareness – which a glance around the surrounding built-up hills readily confirms – that the cubic massing nods just as much towards the local vernacular as it does towards Modernist history (there is a play with history here also; as is well known, the Mediterranean vernacular had a strong influence on early Modernism). The stone-clad, inclined walls of the reinforced concrete parking podium also strongly suggest the solidly reassuring strength of the fortifications which are just as much a part of Malta's identity.

However, all is not quite what it seems. As well as taking up the gentle slope of the hill upon which the houses are situated, the podium provides the main visual clue to the social organization of the cluster, which is actually far from conventional. The length of street frontage on the site is sufficient for only two detached houses of average size and the plot would normally have been developed for two such houses with large rear gardens, similar to all the other villas in the area. Instead, with the developer's support, AP placed two more houses of the same size at the rear of the site, solving the problem of vehicular access and garaging with the parking podium, which also provides separate direct access for the occupants into each house from below.

The arrangement not only doubles the normal housing density – a useful as well as profitable measure in a small country with precious little open land left to build on. It also creates a rich spatial and social environment comprising private (the houses themselves plus their own corner gardens), semi-private (the central courtyard plus parking podium), and public (the street) domains, with a village-like ambiance. Exploiting natural airflows, AP also designed the houses and podium to behave in concord so that the cooler air which collects in the lower

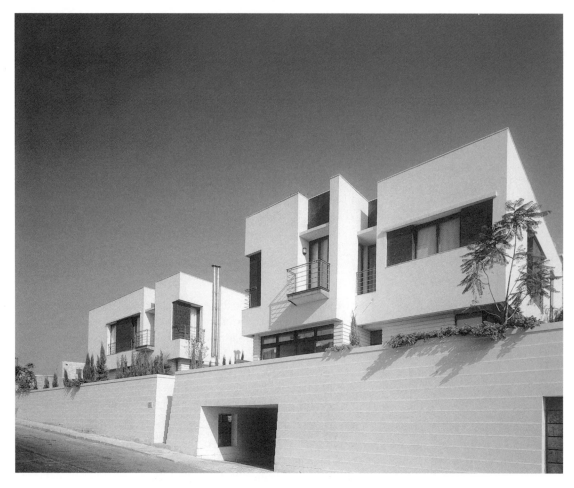

▲ **6.22** The Mews. View from street showing front two houses with semi-underground parking beneath. Photo: David Pisani.

level is drawn up by 'stack effect' through a series of vents and vertical spaces in each building, cooling and ventilating the interiors (Fig. 6.23).

NEW GEOMETRIES

If AP's domestic architecture represents the more conservative end of their practice, the most adventurous exercises are spread over a much wider range of projects, making it all the more difficult to pin the firm down to any single approach.

The design for a small retail outlet in the new Bay Street commercial centre in St Georges Bay for ALLCOM (Fig. 6.24), a retail subsidiary of Maltacom, was the first in a quite separate series of experiments in architectural form and geometry,

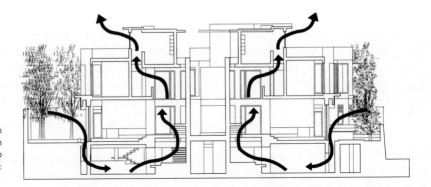

▶ **6.23** The Mews. Section showing natural airflow through parking podium and up through houses. *Source*: Architecture Project.

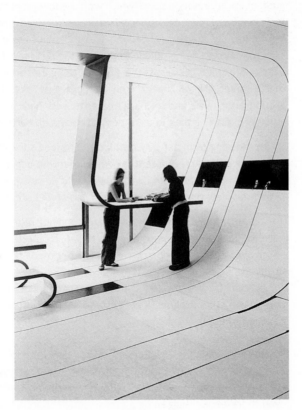

▶ **6.24** ALLCOM Showroom, St Georges Bay, Malta. Interior. Architecture Project, 1999–2000. Photo: David Pisani.

which defines AP in their most radical mode. Treating the floor, rear wall and ceiling of the shop like a single continuous surface – what AP call a 'giant billboard' – the designers have 'split off' strips of the same surface to form tables, seats and display shelves for mobile phones, creating the illusion of an all-embracing, smooth-surfaced cocoon. A changing lighting scheme and projected digital images onto the same surfaces enliven the whole experience.

However, AP's most extreme experiments with new geometries to date have been for two unbuilt projects, both of which were entries for international competitions. Notably, both designs were also produced with the assistance of Adams Kara Taylor and Brian Ford, AP's former collaborators on the Kenuna Tower and Stock Exchange, respectively. While there are common denominators, each project was nevertheless approached in a quite different way.

The first competition, for a new library for the University of Rostock, Germany, called for a strong visual and spatial connection between the new building and the student centre on the opposite side of the campus square. The need for ease of access to information and the various sections of the library also suggested the creation of an 'information spine' which would lead visitors through the building. Taking their cue from these two principal ideas, AP devised a novel method for generating the form of the library from the actual shape of the site itself. Cutting a piece of card to the exact same outline as the site, the designers first folded the card diagonally, then cut it twice across the diagonal, using the resulting strip to form the information spine (Fig. 6.25a–c). The effect is that, like the ALLCOM design, the ground-plane, walls and roof are treated as a continuous, though far more complex surface. Explaining their unusual design process, the architects claim:

> The resulting form not only contains the desired spine that links both ends of the building but also, because it is derived from the original flat shape of the site, is perfectly integrated with it. The library is, as a result, contained in a shell derived from an ideal geomorphic metamorphosis of the site itself.[15]

Translated into a curvaceous, undulating shell of reinforced concrete, the design makes a strong, even jolting impact (Figs. 6.26 and 6.27). However, the project, which was AP's most abstract design experiment to date, was not without its problems. Describing the design process for Rostock as primarily 'form-led rather than programme-led',[16] the partners concede they had difficulties with fitting all the complex functions into the shell, although they were all eventually resolved in the final scheme.

ETHEREAL STRUCTURE

AP's entry in the limited competition for a temporary Shelter for Five Twelfth Century Churches in Lalibela, Ethiopia, which received a special mention, looks even more exotic, suggesting a similar design approach was employed. However, according to AP, this was not the case. For all its striking appearance, the Lalibela scheme was mainly programme-led, and the billowing, irregular shapes of the cloud-like shelter derive directly from the unusual nature of the project and its site.

The competition brief called for protection of the sacred churches from the weather during restoration work, and shade and shelter for visiting pilgrims. The unique group of churches are all carved straight out of the rocky plateau

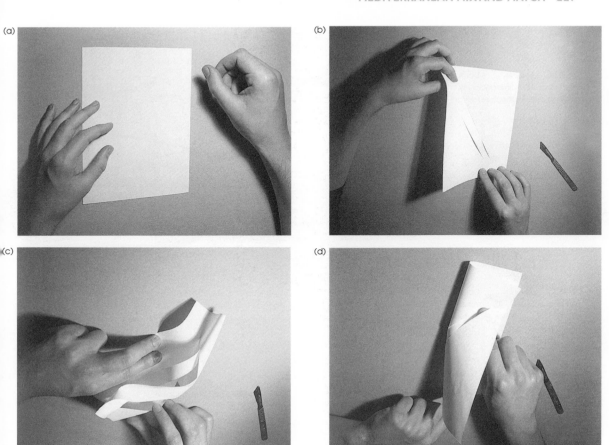

▲ **6.25** University Library Rostock, Germany, 2001. Sequence showing generation of curved building envelope: card cut to shape of site (a), folding across diagonal cuts (b), diagonal cuts manipulated to form ramped communication spine (c), completed envelope (d). Photos: David Pisani.

where they are, so that their roofs lie at the same level as the surrounding terrain, and are linked together below ground by a deep trench, also carved in the rock (Fig. 6.28). Rejecting any kind of solid structure which might intrude on the landscape or distract from the sunken churches, AP designed a semi-transparent membrane with a hollow double skin stretched over a demountable aluminium frame, hung from above by widely spaced, cantilevered struts (Fig. 6.29). Dramatically shaped like scyths and inclined backwards from their concrete pads, the aluminium supports are tied back into the ground to help counterbalance their load. This lightweight, ethereal structure floats over the church roofs, following the sloping ground while leaving the spaces beneath completely open: '…we thought it was essential that the intervention be perceived as a non-structure, an extension of the landscape itself or a secondary layer'.[17]

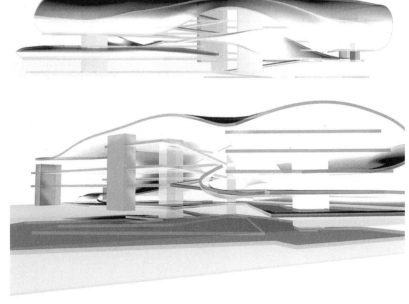

▶ **6.26** University Library Rostock. CAD 3D model. Exterior view. *Source*: Architecture Project.

▶ **6.27** University Library Rostock. CAD 3D model. Sectional view. *Source*: Architecture Project.

▲ **6.28** Temporary Shelters for Five Twelfth-Century Churches, Lalibela, Ethiopia. General view over site showing existing shelters over rock-carved churches. Photo: David Pisani.

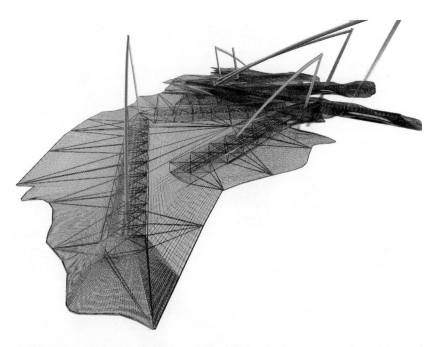

▲ **6.29** Temporary Shelters. Computer model of shelter showing primary and secondary roof structure with translucent hollow membrane. *Source*: Architecture Project.

Partly inspired by the large tents which are part of the local culture, local materials and technologies were nevertheless rejected early on since none could be used to create the large spans required. Instead, a waterproof, maintenance-free and transparent fabric made from glass fibre mesh was selected for the upper membrane, which allows 65 per cent of the natural light through while reducing glare and harmful UV rays. A perforated translucent tissue used for the lower membrane allows for the gentle passage of air through the hollow interior, cooling and ventilating the cushion-like structure and reducing upward wind forces.

The irregular outline of the structure, which looks as though it might have been randomly generated by computer in the fashionable manner, was, on the contrary, generated by a rational process of elimination and extension, whereby those parts of the site not requiring shelter were removed from the protected area, while those functions needing shelter in addition to the churches were covered. Thus, trees needing preservation, access points and areas for social and religious gatherings, views to and from the site as well as the collection of rainwater for reuse, all impacted on the final plan-form. Tests were also run to ensure that the final shape would encourage the flow of air beneath and through the structure. A lighting scheme designed by Franck Franjou in Paris, another regular collaborator, included

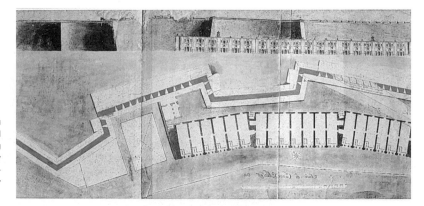

▶ **6.30** International Sea Passenger Terminal, Grand Harbour, Malta. Plan showing site with eighteenth-century waterline and baroque storehouses. *Source*: National Library of Malta.

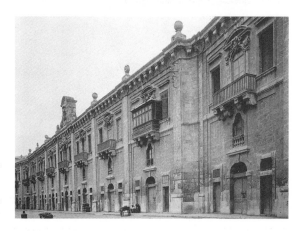

▶ **6.31** International Sea Passenger Terminal. Photo of baroque storehouses taken before WWII. *Source*: Heritage Malta/National Museum of Archeology.

strips of low-intensity, long-life cold cathode tubes placed between the two skins of the roof, so that the whole cloud-like formation would glow in the dark.

CONTINUOUS 'BUILD-SCAPE'

Whether built or unbuilt, in a short space of time AP have accumulated an impressive body of work, of which the above projects are only a selection. Other major projects now under development promise more, extending the range and scale of their architecture. The International Sea Passenger Terminal, Valletta, involves the building of a new terminal on the Grand Harbour to handle Malta's fast-growing cruise liner traffic around the Mediterranean, together with a new ferry terminal. The site at the foot of the city's bastions includes a crescent-shaped row of fine baroque storehouses (Figs. 6.30 and 6.31) along the waterfront, which are being restored and incorporated into the scheme. Together with the new buildings and towering bastions behind, they will provide

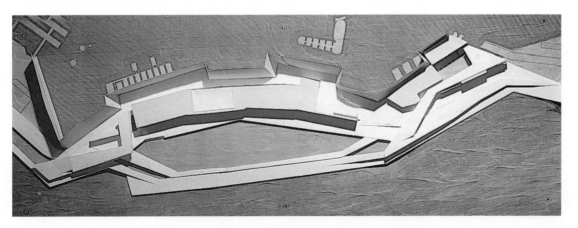

▲ **6.32** International Sea Passenger Terminal. Model. Architecture Project, 1999–. Photo: David Pisani.

an imposing backdrop to the activity along the waterfront and a suitably grand 'gateway' into the city. The original water line which was moved outward from the bastions in the nineteenth century will also be reopened, creating a small marina between it and the new causeway and restoring the close relationship of the baroque buildings to the harbour waters.

Conceived as a continuous 'build-scape', the whole site, including new buildings, pedestrian walkways, bridges and quays is treated as a single flowing plane, raised or ramped in some parts, lowered in others, or cut open to embrace the waters (Fig. 6.32). Like the former scheme in Ethiopia and some of AP's earlier projects, the Sea Passenger Terminal combines a sensitive approach towards the historical site and structures with a free-form geometry and spatial concept, exploiting the friction between the two.

THE DEATH OF STYLE?

However, it is not merely the range and diversity of AP's work that impresses most, but the refreshing open-mindedness and lack of dogma with which they approach every project (appropriately, the name AP chose for a recent exhibition of their work, was 'Open'). This produces what architects who are accustomed to identifying their own and others' work with a personal or preferred aesthetic, might find unsettling: an architecture of consistent high quality, but with no consistent formal or spatial vocabulary, or at least, not one that is recognizable throughout the work.

Now, while the architectural profession is replete with practices ready to produce any form or style at the drop of a hat, or rather a coin, AP's rigorous examination of each task from first principles generally exonerates them from accusations of that sort, though Rostok brought them unusually close to the 'form first' school. Neither does the less pejorative description, 'a style for the job' apply. AP do repeat certain construction techniques or typologies, most clearly in their use of the self-supporting frame in their rehabilitation projects, or vaulted plan forms in their houses, each of which comprises a consistent series which AP have reinterpreted time and again. However, the more irregular and curvaceous geometries and the idea of the lifted ground-plane appear in quite different sorts of projects, suggesting a semi-autonomous series of formal and spatial experiments in themselves, impacting on each project and programme in a different way.

Clearly, therefore, there are consistencies running through the work, but they are not of the easy, formal kind by which we instantly recognize so many star architects' designs. Rather, they manifest themselves, not in a single, unitary approach, but in a number of parallel series of different approaches and techniques, which sometimes converge and sometimes diverge in the work, as the situation varies. Paradoxically, if there is any one consistent theme which runs through all of these series, if not each and every building, it is sustainability, and the fact that sustainable design takes so many different forms in AP's mix and match approach makes nonsense of the idea that such architecture should have a consistent aesthetic or style.

If AP's work is anything to go by – and they are not alone in their approach – it may eventually be appreciated that an authentic organic architecture in our time is not necessarily one which imitates the forms or appearances of nature, but one which genuinely simulates evolution's organic processes of self-production and adaptation to different situations and places. While AP's architecture and methods and those of like-minded designers may not imply the death of style – it is probably too much embedded in architectural culture for that – they may hopefully herald the demise of its more restrictive and superficial manifestations. In particular, they suggest that architects committed to sustainable design need not necessarily enslave themselves to any one way of realizing that goal, but on the contrary, should be prepared to explore every possible means of achieving it, as diverse as the environments in which they live and work.

I

BIOTECH ARCHITECTURE: A MANIFESTO

WHAT IS BIOTECH ARCHITECTURE?

Biotech Architecture is *not* a style. It is a computer-centred *process* of architectural design, production and use.

Biotech architecture combines *global* technologies with *local* responses to site and social conditions.

Biotech architecture is *information* based, not *form* based. It does not prescribe what a building should look like, but rather how it should *behave*.

Biotech architecture uses *smart technologies* to achieve a dynamic, *interactive relationship* between a building, its users and its environment. In the near future, *smart materials* will be used to help achieve the same result.

Biotech architecture aims for customized design from the molecular level to the rooftop!

CAD + CAM = Craftsmanship. Biotech architecture takes the art and craft of building onto a new plane. It *resolves the alienation between humanity and machines*, which has plagued architectural ideology and practice since the industrial revolution, through *customized automation* and *human centred production systems*.

Biotech architecture presents *no artificial boundaries between architecture and nature*, or between human and organic growth and development. It embodies the same principals of *energy efficiency and dynamic balance* between different forms of life as those governing nature's own ecosystems.

Biotech architecture is synonymous with *sustainable design*. In Biotech architecture, the designer's remit covers the *entire foreseeable life cycle* of the building, from the production to the recycling of materials.

Customized architectural form and space – no matter how aesthetically pleasing they might be - *without* a related customized response to the local climate, is like a tree without roots. In Biotech architecture, energy conservation is as central to the architect's work as gravity is to the engineer's.

Biotech architecture is *self-organizing*. It is not a fixed or final product, but is more like a *biological organism*, continuously learning about itself and its surroundings, adapting to changing conditions and improving its own performance.

Biotech architecture is integral to the *electronic ecologies* of the future, upon which the very survival of the human race depends.

Self-organization does *not* mean 'out of control'. It means *no centralized* control! *Evolutionary planning*, which is based on self-organizing systems, comprises *multiple forms and levels of control and feedback*, providing mutual checks and balances dispersed throughout the affected population, both human and non-human. Like Biotech architecture, evolutionary planning is *holistic in conception* and *responsive in application*.

Biotech architectural design is a *total design approach* with continuous feedback from the production process to the design process and vise versa.

Biotech architectural design is *multi-disciplinary and network-based*. It entails coordinating a number of *simultaneous dialogues* with different people in different locations using complementary skills, covering all aspects of design, production and use, including *clients and future users* as far as possible.

Biotech architecture implies *integrated design*. It involves designing building, sub-systems and components all together in a *collaborative process* to achieve the *highest possible performance for the whole*.

The heart of the Biotech design process is the *virtual prototype*, which is both a design and communications medium. Used together with *rapid prototyping and virtual reality technologies*, Biotech architecture actively encourages full and open participation in design.

Biotech architecture embraces both the 'two cultures'. In Biotech architecture, art, science and technology are all enlisted toward achieving the same ultimate goal: *sustainable life upon Earth!*

Biotech architecture is *not dictated by architectural fashion* or limited to any cultural or professional niche, elitist or otherwise. It embraces *all forms of building and construction*, grand and humble, large or small, and *all forms of use*. Biotech architecture aims to *raise the general standard of environmental design for the benefit of all*.

Diversity is to Biotech architecture as *bio-diversity* is to nature. Innovation in design requires the *parallel development* of alternative approaches and *cross fertilization of ideas*, no less than evolution requires the multiplication and cross fertilization of biological species.

Biotech architecture demands *radical changes* in education and practice!

THE BIOTECH ARCHITECTURE WORKSHOP

The Biotech Architecture Workshop was created in 1996 in response to the *isolation, complacency and lack of vision*, which governs architectural education almost everywhere today.

The Biotech Architecture Workshop takes over where Modernism and Postmodernism left off! It accepts the original Modernist programme of *integrating architecture and industry*, but *rejects* the ideology of standardization and rigid mass-production technologies which went with it. It *accepts* the Postmodern critique of orthodox Modernists' aesthetic restrictions, but rejects the superficial focus on form for its own sake which Postmodernists encourage, both in education and in practice.

The Biotech Architecture Workshop values and respects *individual, social and cultural identities*. It teaches students in the use of *responsive technologies and flexible manufacturing systems*, which can be used to customize buildings for place, purpose and climate.

The endless possibilities offered by advanced tools of architectural production present entirely *new problems and decisions to make* for both teachers and students. The fact that something can be done – whether it is the production of a new form or the use of a specific technology or programme – does not necessarily mean that it should be done. The Biotech Architecture Workshop is concerned with educating students in *making the most appropriate and responsible choices for the task at hand*.

The Biotech Architecture Workshop rejects architectural elitism and the closed forms of communication and representation, which have moulded architectural education in the past century. It supports *accessible design processes and forms of representation*. Workshop projects are developed as multi-media presentations on Web sites and CDs, which are available to anyone who may be interested, architect or not.

The Biotech Architecture Workshop has no room for professional or academic divisions. It networks architecture students together with other students and professionals as well as practicing designers in multi-disciplinary *virtual workplaces, which simulate real-life working relationships*.

The Biotech Architecture Workshop promotes *mutually productive relationships between education, research, practice and industry*. The Internet offers new possibilities for *flexible, on-line collaboration* between students, practitioners and industry workers on real projects in real time, which have only just begun to be explored.

The Biotech Architecture Workshop restores the *essential connections between theory and practice* in architectural education, which have been widely neglected in the past, whether from ignorance of new production methods and technologies or ideological persuasion.

The Biotech Architecture Workshop eschews *ego-centred and exclusive approaches and projects*. Rather, it promotes approaches and projects which help to *raise the quality of the great mass of building types and structures, whether public, private or commercial, which comprise the built environment.*

II

BIRTH OF A CYBERNETIC FACTORY

As with the Hong Kong Bank, some of the greatest challenges and most advanced technologies in the construction of the Swiss Re and GLA involved the production of the cladding systems. Like Cupples, the fabricators for the bank's cladding, Schmidlin (Fig. AII.1), the Swiss-based company who made the cladding for both the London buildings, also had to upgrade their methods and technology to match Foster's own methods and requirements. A well-established leader in the field, Schmidlin already had a solid reputation for custom-made cladding systems, and were used to working closely with their architect clients. As a progressive company, they also used CNC machines in their production lines. However, like most manufacturers in the construction industry, prior to the Foster commissions, their operation was still based on the production of detailed drawings for every component in the traditional manner. In the same way, the CNC machines were manually programmed for each job, a laborious process requiring someone to translate the information from a drawing into appropriate data for the machine.

Also like Cupples, Schmidlin invested in new machinery at their Basel factory to cope with the Foster projects, including additional CNC machines. However, by far the greater investment went into software development. Uwe Bremen, Schmidlin's Head of Technology, soon recognized that the geometrical complexity of the cladding systems and huge number of variations ruled out conventional drawings, whether drawn by human hand or by computer. A single cladding element, i.e. a glazed frame in the GLA building, for example, is composed of over 200 components, including screws, etc., which all have to be

---

In his seminal paper, 'Towards the cybernetic factory', 1962, the British cybernetician Stafford Beer[1] described how computer-based production lines of the future would resemble responsive organisms, swiftly adapting to the needs of changing markets and individual customers. Following developments in other industries, flexible manufacturing systems are also now appearing in advanced sectors of the construction industry. The following unedited passage is abstracted from C. Abel, 'From hard to soft machines', 2004.[2]

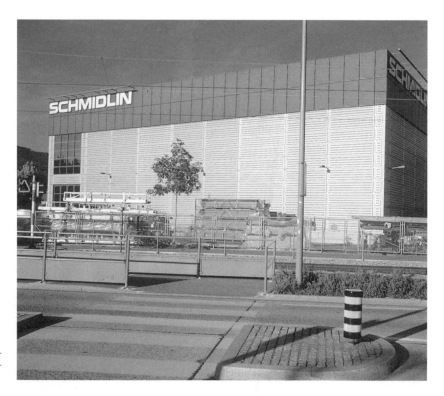

▶ **AII.1** Schmidlin AG Headquarters, Aesch/Basel, Switzerland. Photo: Author.

accounted for (Fig. AII.2). Half of these components, such as corner plates or glazing panels – only the profile is constant – also vary in some way from one element to the next. Often, the variations are too small to be noticed by eye, making it impossible to keep track of them with conventional methods. Multiply all those variations by 650 times for the whole cladding system – every single panel on the GLA is different by some degree – and you have potential chaos.

The transparency of both cladding and structure in each building – a defining characteristic of most of Foster's work – with all their highly visible connections, further complicated matters, since nothing could be hidden or fudged; everything had to be designed and made to the same high standards (Fig. AII.3). The helical structure and the cladding pattern of the Swiss Re also presented special problems of their own, since both offsets and diagonal crossing points as well as other details arising from the peculiar geometry had to be carefully worked out: the steel cladding of the helical frame, for example, also has a diagonal kink in it to accommodate the twisting of the structure around the circular plan (Fig. AII.4). The consultative process between Schmidlin's designers and Foster's project architects on the Swiss Re cladding alone lasted a whole year.

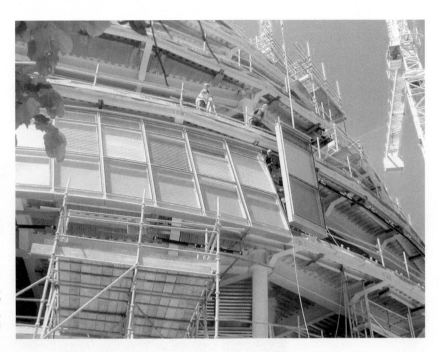

▶ **AII.2** GLA Headquarters, London. Installation of cladding. Norman Foster, 1998–2002. Photo: Nigel Young/Foster and Partners.

Although the Swiss Re was designed first, differences in the scale and programming of the two projects meant that the cladding contract for the GLA preceded that for the former building. The sequence was fortuitous, since it gave Schmidlin the opportunity to develop and refine their approach on the smaller contract before tackling the larger and more complex Swiss Re project. As it turned out, there were significant changes between the way each contract was handled, reflecting major differences in the production technologies employed. Taking the architects' initial surface coordinates as supplied in the Geometry Method Statement as their starting points, Schmidlin's cladding designers were able to translate their own designs for the GLA cladding into more detailed numerical data on the same spreadsheets (Figs. AII.5a–d). The same data were in turn fed directly from the spreadsheets into the programmes for the CNC machines without the need for any intermediary drawings.

While the use of the spreadsheets had the great advantage of eliminating the need for detailed drawings, the only way to check the accuracy of the final product for the GLA was to preassemble each element on an adjustable rig at the factory before delivery to the site – an effective but costly and time-consuming process in itself. Special dies also had to be made for testing the accuracy of some components, which could not otherwise be measured. While such methods were acceptable for the smaller GLA contract, the same approach would have resulted in unacceptable delays on the Swiss Re job.

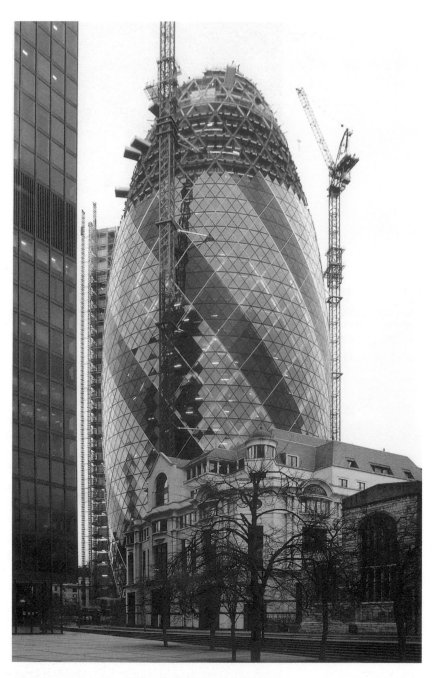

▲ **AII.3** Swiss Re, London, England. Installation of cladding. Foster and Partners, 1997–2004. Photo: Norman Childs.

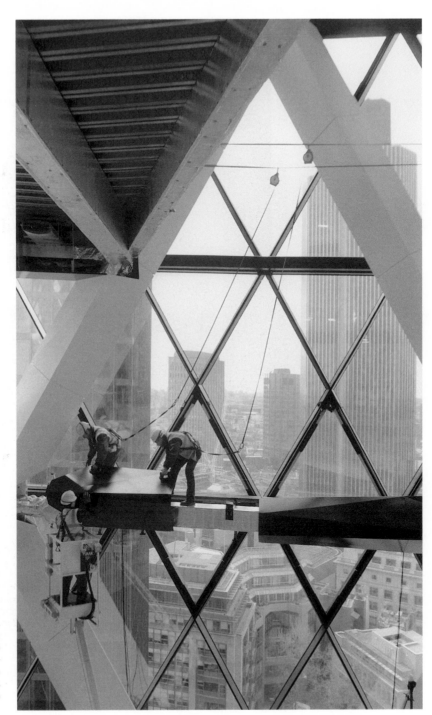

▶ **AII.4** Swiss Re, London, England. Diagonal kink in metal cladding of structure necessitated by twisting geometry is clearly visible from interior. Foster and Partners, 1997–2004. Photo: Norman Childs.

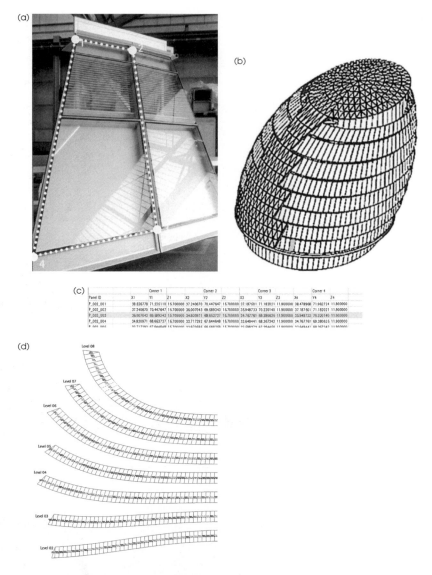

(a)

(b)

(c)

Panel ID	Corner 1			Corner 2			Corner 3			Corner 4		
	X1	Y1	Z1	X2	Y2	Z2	X3	Y3	Z3	X4	Y4	Z4
P_002_001	38.626278	71.226110	15.700000	37.240670	70.447647	15.700000	37.187601	71.182021	11.900000	38.478968	71.962724	11.900000
P_002_002	37.240670	70.447647	15.700000	36.007043	69.589343	15.700000	35.948233	70.220140	11.900000	37.187601	71.182021	11.900000
P_002_003	36.007043	69.589343	15.700000	34.830971	68.653737	15.700000	34.767761	69.380625	11.900000	35.948233	70.220140	11.900000
P_002_004	34.830971	68.653737	15.700000	33.711292	67.644648	15.700000	33.649441	68.367342	11.900000	34.767761	69.380625	11.900000
P_002_005	33.711292	67.644648	15.700000	33.670436	66.608366	15.700000	33.698273	67.364456	11.900000	33.649441	68.367342	11.900000

(d)

▲ **AII.5**   GLA Headquarters, London, England. Variations in size and geometry of cladding were precisely documented on spreadsheets: XYZ coordinates marked on corners of preassembled cladding units (a), 3D diagram of cladding (b), part of spreedsheet showing XYZ coordinates for four corners of each unit shown in photo (c), diagram showing variations of cladding units on main levels as laid out flat (d). Norman Foster, 1998–2002. *Source*: Foster and Partners.

Schmidlin's solution, as anticipated in the SMG template, was to create their own detailed 3D computer model of the cladding system, bridging spreadsheets and production line. Adapting existing software systems to the firm's needs, Schmidlin's computer staff built up a complete 3D model of the Swiss Re

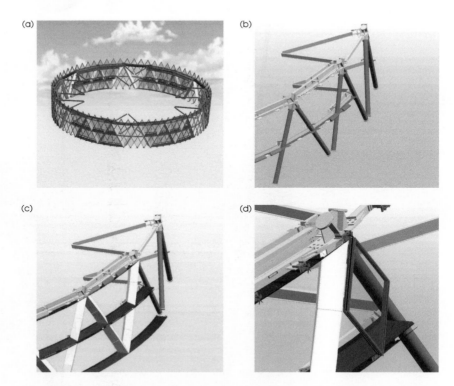

▲ **AII.6**   Swiss Re, London, England. Cladding systems for Swiss Re were designed and manufactured with customized 3D software: complete two-storey section of Swiss Re includes all cladding components including triangular floor edges around stepped skycourts (a), detail showing structure before cladding (b), detail showing partly clad structure (c), detail showing glazed unit in place (d). Norman Foster, 1997–2004. *Source*: Schmidlin AG.

cladding in two-storey sections, including every nut and bolt, enabling both architects and cladding designers to examine every facet of the system for accuracy or potential clashes, or any other problems in complete confidence, prior to actual production (Fig. AII.6). Like the spreadsheets, the 3D model also incorporated parametric features, enabling both Foster's and Schmidlin's people to make changes right up till the last moment, automatically updating the project data as needed.

Finally – and crucially for speeding up production – with the help of additional computer expertise, Schmidlin wrote their own special software linking the 3D model directly to the CNC machines on the production line, so doing away with conventional programming. From numerical spreadsheets, to 3D modelling, to the CNC machines on the factory floor, the entire process of production for the Swiss Re cladding was computer controlled in one form or another, each step being directly linked to the next (Fig. AII.7).

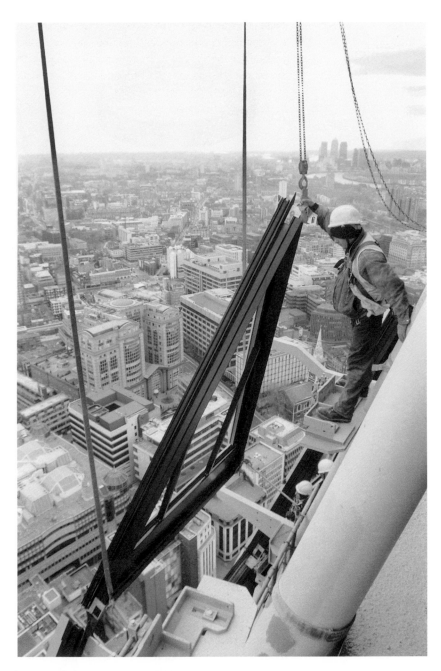

▲ **AII.7** Swiss Re, London, England. Glazed cladding unit being hoisted into place. Norman Foster, 1997–2004. Photo: Norman Childs.

The implications of Foster's and Schmidlin's joint achievements for the future of architectural production, and for the way we regard mechanized production in general, can hardly be overestimated. No longer the province of abstract theory or futurist speculation, the operational characteristics of Beer's cybernetic factory are clearly discernable in the computer-based design studios and production lines at Schmidlin.

NOTES AND BIBLIOGRAPHY

INTRODUCTION

1 Abel, C. (2003a). 'New Federal German Parliament, Reichstag, Berlin'. In Jenkins, D., ed. (2003) *Norman Foster: Works 4*, Prestel, Munich, p. 258.

2 Abel, C. and Seidler, H. (2003). *Harry Seidler: Houses and Interiors, 1 & 2*. Images Publishing, Melbourne.

3 Abel, C. (2000). *Architecture and Identity: Responses to Cultural and Technological Change* (2nd edition). Architectural Press, Oxford.

4 Venturi, R. (1966). *Complexity and Contradiction in Architecture*. The Museum of Modern Art, New York, p. 20.

5 Abel, C. (1979). 'The language analogy in architectural theory and criticism: some remarks in the light of Wittgenstein's linguistic relativism'. *Architectural Association Quarterly*, December, 1979, pp. 39–47. The same essay is republished under the title, 'Architectural language games', in Chapter 7, Abel, C. (2000, 2nd edition), Chapter 7.

6 Projections from authoritative sources of the consequences of global warming on the planetary environment over the coming decades paint a grim picture of potentially catastrophic effects. In their Special Report, the German Advisory Council on Global Change warns that a mere 1.4°C of further warming is tolerable, requiring cutbacks in carbon dioxide emissions globally by 45–60 per cent by 2050 and by industrialized countries by 20 per cent by 2020 relative to 1990 – targets far in excess of present commitments. Any further increases in temperature would drastically affect the already melting ice caps, eventually raising sea levels world-wide by as much as 30 feet, swamping many capital cities, including London, New York, Sydney and Tokyo. Even more disastrous is the possibility of a 'runaway greenhouse', where a self-reinforcing cycle of warming effects would eventually make life on earth untenable. German Advisory Council on Global Change (2003). 'Climate protection strategies for the 21st century: Kyoto and beyond', Press release, 25 November, http://www.wbgu.de. Also Lean, G. (2003). 'Melting ice will swamp capitals', *The Independent on Sunday*, 7 December, Home Section, p. 4. Also Monbiot, G. (2003). 'With eyes wide shut', *Guardian Weekly*, August 21–27, p. 13.

7   Abel, C. (2003b). 'Electronic ecologies', in Jenkins, D., ed. (2003) pp. 12–29.
8   Abel, C. (1997a). 'Networking the studio: architectural education and the virtual practice', *Environments by Design*, Vol. 2, No. 1, Winter 1997/98, pp. 71–85. The same paper is republished under the title, 'The Biotech Architecture Workshop', in Abel, C. (2000, 2nd edition), Chapter 6.
9   Abel, C. (1986a). 'Ditching the dinosaur sanctuary: seventeen years on', in *CAD and Robotics in Architecture and Construction*, Kogan Page, London, pp. 123–32. The same paper is republished under the title, 'Return to craft manufacture', *AJ Supplement*, 20 April, 1988, pp. 53–7. Also in Abel, C. (2000, 2nd edition), Chapter 4.

CHAPTER 1   ARCHITECTURE IN THE PACIFIC CENTURY

1   For earlier analyses of the region's economic strength and potential, see Organization for Economic Co-operation and Development (1992). *Long-term Prospects for the World Economy*. OECD, Paris. Also Coyle, W.T., Hayes, D. and Yamauchi, H., eds (1992). *Agriculture and Trade in the Pacific*. Belhaven Press, London. Also R. Hodder (1992). *The West Pacific Rim*. Belhaven Press, London.
2   Galtung, J. (1981). Untitled presentation to the Seminar on Appropriate Technology Culture and Lifestyle in Development, Science University of Malaysia (USM), Penang, 3–7 November.
3   Macintyre, M. (1985). *The New Pacific*. Collins/BBC, London. From address by Z. Suzuki, 'The Coming of the Pacific Age', at the East West Center, Hawaii, 16 June, 1982, as quoted in the introduction, p. 11.
4   Macintyre, M. (1985).
5   Thompson, W.I. (1985). *Pacific Shift*. Sierra Club Books, San Francisco.
6   Abel, C. (1986b). 'A building for the Pacific Century', *The Architectural Review*, Vol. CLXXXIX, No. 1070, April, pp. 54–61. For a later interpretation of related themes, see Buchanan, P. (1991). 'Pacific Rim and planetary culture', *The Architectural Review*, Vol. CLXXXIX, No. 1134, August, pp. 27–32.
7   For one of the more balanced overviews, see Atkinson, M. (1997). 'Asian tiger, tiger, burning not so bright', *The Observer*, 31 August, Business Section, p. 3.
8   Kattoulas, V. (1997). 'Asia: Not stalling, just shifting gears', *International Herald Tribune*, 10–11 May, p.13.
9   The Economist (1997). 'Asia's population advantage', *The Economist*, 13 September, p. 90.
10 Harris, S. and Klintworth, G., eds (1995). *China as a Great Power*. St Martin's Press, New York.
11 The term 'slash and burn' derives from the relatively small-scale practice of forest clearance by indigenous farmers in the region, who rotate between plots allowing the forest to heal itself in between. The far greater damage

done by commercial logging companies is, however, permanent, even without uncontrolled fires: once they are cut down and the remaining stumps are burnt, the slow growing hardwood trees are usually replaced with more profitable plantations of oil palm, or quick growing softwoods for paper and pulp, destroying the forest ecosystem forever. 'Smoky Southeast Asia', *International Herald Tribune*, 29 September, 1997, p. 8.

12 Higgens, A. (1997). 'Smog makes Asian tigers burn less bright', *The Guardian*, 26 September, World News, p. 9. Also, eds (1997). 'Health fears shrouded in haze', *The Guardian*, 27 September, World News, p. 3. Also eds (1997). 'Asia's heart of Darkness', *The Guardian*, 28 September. Reuters (1997). 'AUN sees long fallout from Asia fires', *International Herald Tribune*, 1 October, p. 2. Also Hiebert, M., Jaysankaran, S. and McBeth. J. (1997). 'Fire in the sky', *Far Eastern Economic Review*, 9 October, pp. 74–8.

13 Mawdsley, N. (1997). 'Indonesia aflame', *New Scientist*, No. 2105, 25 October, p. 51.

14 While Indonesia has laws with which to punish offenders, they have so far not been enforced. Gittings, J. (1997). 'Forest fire smog chokes SE Asia', *Guardian Weekly*, 28 September, p. 4.

15 In 1996 the UK – a favourite target for such charges – imported over 200 000 cubic meters of tropical timbers from Indonesia alone. Vidal, J. (1997). 'Poison fog blanket threatens world climate', *The Guardian*, 27 September, p. 3.

16 For this reason the new constitution recently voted for in Thailand, which was forced upon that country's leadership by the current economic crisis, is of special significance. Displacing the previous preferential system with more democratic and accountable procedures, the new reforms hold out promise of similar measures to come elsewhere in the region. Woollacott, M. (1997). 'Crisis that may force a change in those famous Asian values', *The Guardian*, Comment and Analysis, 30 August, p. 9. Also Bowring, P. (1997). 'Political Ripples in Southeast Asia', *International Herald Tribune*, 1 October, p. 8.

17 For a historical overview of the 'race for the clouds' and descriptions of these and other related skyscraper projects see Abel, C. (2003c). *Sky High: Vertical Architecture*. Royal Academy of Arts, London, 2003.

18 Gross national products (GNPs), even impressive ones like Southeast Asia's, are macro-economic measures and often obscure other more contentious factors, such as the distribution of wealth and problems of exclusion, not to mention the quality of the environment. For a wider view of development in the region, see Rigg, J. (1997). *Southeast Asia*. Routledge, London.

19 For a discussion of related patterns of innovation, see Chapter 2, this book.

20 Originally published in Abel, C. (1997b). *Architecture and Identity: Towards a Global Ecoculture*. Architectural Press, Oxford, p. 208.

21   For a critical analysis of the interrelations between urban and rural development and associated work and economic patterns, see Rigg, J. (1997).

22   For an example of CAP's approach, see Idris, S.M.M. (1990). *For a Sane,
Green Future*. Consumers' Association of Penang, Penang.

23   Domestic architecture, both traditional and modern, provides clear evidence of an archetypal Pacific House. Abel, C. (1994). 'Pacific House', *The
Architectural Review*, Vol. CXCVI, No. 1171, September, pp. 50–53.

24   See Chapter 16 in Abel, C. (2000, 2nd edition).

25   Jacques, M. (1997). 'Malaysia takes a leap into future', *Guardian Weekly*,
6 April, p. 23. Also Fuller, T. (1997). 'Malaysia's wired Super Corridor',
International Herald Tribune, 15–16 November, pp. 1 and 6.

26   A key plank in the Malaysian government's declared aim to turn itself into
a developed country by the year 2020, the Supercorridor appears so far to
have escaped any cutbacks. See Fuller, T. (1997). Also Hamid, A.S.A., ed.
(1993). *Malaysia's Vision 2020*. Pelanduk Publications, Petaling Jaya.

27   Similar predispositions towards clear-cut spatial patterns were observed
amongst Western architects by the urban theorist Melvin Webber in a
seminal essay on urban dispersal. Webber, M.M. (1964). 'The urban
place and the nonplace urban realm'. In *Explorations into Urban Structure*
(Webber, M.M., et al., eds), pp. 79–153. University of Pennsylvania,
Pennsylvania.

28   Tay, K.S. (1989). *Mega-Cities in the Tropics*. Singapore: Institute of Southeast
Asian Studies. KL LinearCity SDN BHD (1996). *KL LinearCity*. KL LinearCity
SDN BHD, Kuala Lumpur. Architectural Record eds (1997). 'A new record
for Kuala Lumpur? The world's longest complex', *Architectural Record*,
February, p. 30.

29   For an early critique of the megastructure idea and an argument for urban
dispersal, see Chapter 2 in Abel, C. (1997).

30   For a further discussion, see Chapter 18 in Abel, C. (2000, 2nd edition). See
also Abel, C. (2003c).

31   Radford, T. (1997). 'Around the corner: the 80mpg clean air engine', *The
Guardian*, 23 October, p. 3.

32   See note 30.

33   According to Tay Keng Soon, the difference in temperature in the tropics
can be as much as 5C higher for dense urban areas than for open countryside. Tay, K.S. (1989). Given this effect, it is unlikely that the inclusion of
vertical landscaping into the sorts of ultra-high density projects Tay advo-
cates would reduce this difference by any significant measure.

34   Abel, C. (1994). 'Verdant vertical living', *The Architectural Review*, Vol. CXCVI,
No. 1171, September, pp. 32–5.

35   For a detailed account of the architect's approach, see Yeang, K. (1996).
The Skyscraper Bioclimatically Considered. Academy Editions, London. Also
Yeang, K. (2002).

36 For a brief historical overview of the new tower type and its predecessors see Chapter 15 in Abel, C. (2000, 2nd edition). See also Abel, C. (2003c).

37 Many former colonial attitudes and practices have survived all too well in the way developed nations and multi-national corporations conduct their business with developing nations, and are at least partly to blame for the deteriorating environment. Raghavan, C. (1990). *Recolonization*. Third World Network, Penang. By contrast, both traditional and colonial architecture provides continuing inspiration for contemporary regionalists. See Chapters 12–18 in Abel, C. (2000, 2nd edition).

38 Kirby, J., O'Keefe, P. and Timberlake, L., eds (1995). *The Earthscan Reader in Sustainable Development*. Earthscan, London.

39 A report by the US Energy Department suggests that even without green taxes and other measures, research and development costs of new technologies to reduce carbon monoxide to 1990 levels by 2010 would be offset by energy savings alone. Hamilton, M.M. (1997). 'Technology can cut pollution', *Guardian Weekly*, 5 October, p.16. Other reports suggest that improving environmental practice is good for business as well as for the environment. Trapp, R. (1997). 'Don't let profits go up in smoke', *The Independent*, Section Two, p. 18.

40 Ekins, P. (1992). *A New World Order*. Routledge, London.

CHAPTER 2 CYBERSPACE IN MIND

1 Gibson's first and most frequently quoted novel, in which the term 'cyberspace' was originally coined, is Gibson, W. (1984). *Neomancer*. Ace Books, New York. For an example of Gibson's influence, see Benedikt, M., ed. (1994). *Cyberspace: First Steps*. MIT Press, Cambridge, MA. Related studies in cyberculture include Negroponte, N. (1995). *Being Digital: The Road Map for Survival on the Information Superhighway*. Hodder and Stoughton, London. Also Sardar, Z. and Ravetz, J.R., eds (1996). *Cyberfutures: Culture and Politics on the Information Superhighway*. Pluto Press, London. Also Dery, M. (1996). *Escape Velocity: Cyberculture at the End of the Century*. Hodder and Stoughton, London. Also Brown, D. (1997). *Cybertrends: Chaos, Power and Accountability in the Information Age*. Viking, London.

2 See Chapter 8 in Abel, C. (2000, 2nd edition).

3 Mitchell, W. (1995). *City of Bits: Space, Place and the Infobahn*. MIT Press, Cambridge, MA. Also Mitchell, W. (1999). *E-topia*. MIT Press, Cambridge, MA.

4 Mitchell, W. (1995), p. 8.

5 Mitchell, W. (1995), p. 131.

6 Time editors (1995). 'Welcome to cyberspace', *Time*. Special Issue, Spring.

7 Fleming, J., Honour, H. and Pevsner, N. (1999). *Penguin Dictionary of Architecture and Landscape Architecture* (5th edition). Penguin, London, p. 175.

8 Inoue, M. (1985). *Space in Japanese Architecture*. Weatherhill, New York and Tokyo.

9   Inoue, M. (1985), p. 144.

10 Kelly, K. (1994). *Out of Control: The New Biology of Machines*. Fourth Estate, London.

11 As Rene Descartes himself originally conceived of the difference between body and mind, all bodily movements were the outcome of mechanistic processes channelled through the nervous system, which he also conceived rather quaintly as a sort of a cross between an hydraulic system and a system of wires and pulleys. However, more complex forms of human behaviour, such as thought, speech and free will, were attributed to an independent soul. The former could be explained perfectly well according to the laws of causation, just like any machine. However, the latter could not, and was a matter for religious discussion only. See Copleston, F. (1963). *A History of Philosophy, Volume 4*. Image Books, New York.

12 Mitchell, W. (1995), pp. 14–15.

13 Heim, M. (1994). 'The erotic ontology of cyberspace.' In Benedikt, M., ed. (1994), pp. 59–80.

14 Heim, M. (1994), pp. 63–4.

15 Heim, M. (1994), p. 73.

16 Heim, M. (1994), p. 75.

17 Stone, A.R. (1994). 'Will the real body please stand up: boundary stories about virtual cultures.' In Benedikt, M., ed. (1994), pp. 81–118.

18 Tomas, D. (1989). 'The technophillic body: on technicity in William Gibson's cyborg culture'. *New Formations*, 8, Spring.

19 Stone, A.R. (1994), p. 107.

20 Stone, A.R. (1994), p. 112.

21 Kerr, P. (1995). *Gridiron*. Chatto & Windus, London.

22 Regarding the earlier comments on the popularity of baroque models for visualizing cyberspace, directors of sci-fi movies also invariably depict cyberspace as a dead straight and endless tunnel of space rushing towards us, lined with brightly coloured, electronic graffiti inspired by Kubrick's 'psychedelic' journey into a parallel universe in *2001*.

23 Kerr, P. (1995), p. 339.

24 Kerr, P. (1995), p. 367.

25 Ryle, G. (1949). *The Concept of Mind*. Barnes & Noble, New York.

26 Ryle, G. (1949), pp. 15–16.

27 Ryle, G. (1949), p. 25.

28 Ryle has often been dismissed as a behaviourist of the same school as James Watson and B.F. Skinner. See Watson, J.B. (1930). *Behaviourism*. W.W. Norton, New York, 1930, and Skinner, B.F. (1974). *About Behaviourism*. Alfred A. Knopf, New York. However, by externally observable behaviour Ryle included speech and the most complex as well as simpler forms of human expression. Nor does he ever suggest, as Watson,

Skinner and others did, that all behaviour could be reduced to mechanistic strings of stimuli and responses. Quite the contrary, he explicity describes intelligent behaviour in terms of individuals exerting control over their world: 'To be intelligent is not merely to satisfy criteria, but to apply them; to regulate one's actions and not merely to be well-regulated.' Ryle, G. (1949), p. 28.

29 Koestler, A. (1967). *The Ghost in the Machine*. Pan Books, London, 1967.
30 See, Von Bertallanfy, L. (1968). *General System Theory: Foundations, Development, Applications*. George Braziller, New York. Also, Koestler, A. and Smythies, J.R., eds (1969). *Beyond Reductionism: New Perspectives in the Life Sciences*. Hutchinson, London.
31 Koestler, A. (1967), p. 237.
32 Koestler, A. (1967), p. 238.
33 Koestler, A. (1967), pp. 243–4.
34 Koestler, A. (1967), p. 244.
35 Koestler, A. (1967), p. 244.
36 Koestler, A. (1967), p. 244.
37 See, for example, Lewin, R. (1993). *Complexity: Life on the Edge of Chaos*. Phoenix, London. Also Coveney, P. and Highfield, R. (1995). *Frontiers of Complexity: The Search for Order in a Chaotic World*. Faber and Faber, London.
38 Polanyi, M. (1967). *The Tacit Dimension*. Anchor Books, New York. Also Polanyi, M. (1958). *Personal Knowledge: Towards a Post-Critical Philosophy*. The University of Chicago Press, Chicago. Also Langford, T.A. and Poteat, W.H., eds (1968). *Intellect and Hope: Essays in the Thought of Michael Polanyi*. Duke University Press, Durham. Also Polanyi, M. and Prosch, H. (1975). *Meaning*. The University of Chicago Press, Chicago.
39 Polanyi, M. (1967), p. x.
40 For examples in architectural design see Chapter 9 in Abel, C. (1997).
41 Polanyi, M. and Prosch, H. (1975), p. 33.
42 Polanyi, M. (1967), p. 16.
43 Polanyi, M. (1967), pp. 15–16.
44 Polanyi, M. and Prosch, H. (1975), p. 36.
45 Norberg-Schulz, C. (1980). *Genius Loci*. Rizzoli, New York.
46 Polanyi, M. (1967), p. 16.
47 The spatial character of tacit knowing is clearly expressed in the following passage from a paper by Marjorie Grene: 'I attend from a proximal pole, which is an aspect of my being, to a distal pole, which, by attending to it, I place at a distance from myself. *All knowing, we could say, in other words, is orientation* (my emphasis). The organism's placing of itself in its environment, the dinoflagellate in the plankton, the salmon in its stream, or the fox in its lair, prefigures the process by which we both shape and are shaped by

our world, reaching out from what we have assimilated to what we seek.' Grene, M. (1968). 'Tacit knowing and the pre-reflective cogito.' In Langford, T.A. and Poteat, W.H. eds (1968), p. 35.

48   Polanyi, M. and Prosch, H. (1975), p. 36.
49   Novak, M. (1995). 'Liquid architectures in cyberspace.' In Benedikt, M. ed. (1995), pp. 225–54.
50   Novak, M. (1995), p. 241.
51   See also Chapter 1.
52   Castells, M. (1996). *The Rise of the Network Society*. Blackwell, Oxford.
53   Castells, M. (1996), p. 390.

CHAPTER 3   TECHNOLOGY AND PROCESS

1   Influential critiques of orthodox Modernism include, Venturi, R. (1966). *Complexity and Contradiction in Architecture*. The Museum of Modern Art, New York. Also Jencks, C. (1977). *The Language of Post-Modern Architecture*. Academy Editions, London. Also Watkin, D. (1977). *Morality and Architecture*. Clarendon Press, London.
2   Turbayne, C.M. (1971). *The Myth of Metaphor* (revised edition). The University of South Carolina Press.
3   Turbayne, C.M. (1971), ibid. Also Koestler, A. (1964). *The Act of Creation*. Macmillan, London. Also see Chapter 8, in Abel, C. (1997a). *Architecture and Identity: Towards a Global Ecoculture*. Architectural Press, Oxford.
4   Coplestone, F.S.J. (1963). *A History of Philosophy: Vol. 4*. Image Books. See also Chapter 2 this book.
5   The mechanistic view was prevalent amongst behavioural psychologists in the last century. See for example, Skinner, B.F. (1974). See also Chapter 2 this book.
6   The deterministic view underlying early Modernists' perception of history is analysed in Watkin, D. (1977).
7   Batchelor, R. (1994). *Henry Ford: Mass Production, Modernism and Design* (2nd edition). Manchester University Press, Manchester, p. 40.
8   Le Corbusier. (1927). *Towards a New Architecture*. Architectural Press, London.
9   Le Corbusier. (1927), p. 126.
10   Herbert, G. (1984). *The Dream of the Factory-made House*. MIT Press, Cambridge.
11   Heskett, J. (1980). *Industrial Design*. Oxford University Press, Oxford.
12   Drexler, R. (1973). *Charles Eames*. The Museum of Modern Art, New York.
13   Pawley, M. (1992). *Design Heroes: Buckminster Fuller*. Grafton.
14   Spaeth, D. (1985). *Mies Van Der Rohe*. The Architectural Press, London.
15   See Chapter 1, in Abel, C. (2000, 2nd edition). Also Russell, B. (1981). *Building Systems, Industrialization and Architecture*. John Wiley and Sons, Chichester.

16 See Chapter 1, in Abel, C. (2000, 2nd edition).

17 Prouve, J. (1966). 'Address delivered at the Symposium of the Union Internationale des Architects, held in Delft, The Netherlands, on 6–13 September 1964.' In *Int. Council for Building Research, Studies and Documentation-CIB*, eds (1966), p. 65.

18 For a comprehensive study, see Sulzer, P. (2000). *Jean Prouve Complete Works, Vols 1–4*. Birkhauser, Basel.

19 Abel, C. (1966). 'Ulm HfG, Department of Building.' *Arena*, Vol. 82, No. 905, pp. 88–90.

20 The work of these prominent architects has been widely published. Definitive monographs include Moore, R., ed. (2003). *Structure, Space and Skin: The Work of Nicholas Grimshaw & Partners*. Phaidon, London. Also, Buchanan, P. (1993–). *Renzo Piano Building Workshop: Complete Works, Vols 1–4*. Phaidon, London. Also, Jenkins, D. (2003–). *Norman Foster, Works 1–6*. Prestel, Munich.

21 Abel, C. (1989). 'From hard to soft machines.' In *Norman Foster: Buildings and Projects, Vol. 3* (I. Lambot, ed.) pp. 10–19, Watermark, Hong Kong. Also Abel, C. (1991). *Renault Centre: Norman Foster*. Architecture Design and Technology Press, London.

22 Abel, C. (1991).

23 See Chapter 1, in Abel, C. (2000, 2nd edition).

24 Einstein, A. (1961). *Relativity: The Special and General Theory*. Crown Publishers, London.

25 Capra, F. (1983). *The Turning Point*. Flamingo, p. 65. See also Capra, F. (1976). *The Tao of Physics*. Fontana.

26 The concept of a paradigm shift is due to Kuhn, T.S. (1970). *The Structure of Scientific Revolutions*. See also Chapter 11, in Abel, C. (1997a).

27 Abel, C. (1982). 'The case for anarchy in design research.' In *Changing Design* (Evans, B., Powell, J.A. and Talbot, R.J., eds) pp. 295–302, John Wiley & Sons, Chichester.

28 Capra, F. (1983), p. 66.

29 The science of cybernetics is generally credited to Norbert Wiener. For an early introduction, see Wiener, N. (1950). *The Human Use of Human Beings*. Sphere Books. Also Ashby, R. (1956). *An Introduction to Cyberbetics*. University Paperbacks, London. Also Beer, S. (1959). *Cybernetics and Management*. The English Universities Press, London. Also Pask, G. (1961). *An Approach to Cybernetics*. Hutchinson, London. Also Crosson, F.J. and Sayre, K.M., eds (1967). *Philosophy and Cybernetics*. Simon and Schuster, New York. Many of the basic concepts of cybernetics have since been absorbed into the more general field of complexity theory. See Chapter 2, note 37 in this book.

30 Abel, C. (1986b).

31 See Chapter 17, in Abel, C. (2000, 2nd edition). Also Abel, C. (2003b). Also Slessor, C. (1997). *Eco-Tech: Sustainable Architecture and High Technology*. Thames and Hudson, London. Also Behling, S. and Behling, S. (1996). *Sol Power: The Evolution of Solar Architecture*. Prestel, Munich. Also Travi, V. (2001). *Advanced Technologies: Building in the Computer Age*. Birkhauser, Basel.

32 Campbell, N.S. and Stankovic, S., eds (2001). *Wind Energy for the Built Environment: Project WEB*. BDSP Partnership with Imperial College, Mecal Applied Mechanics and the University of Stuttgart.

33 See Appendix I in this book.

34 Aukstakalnis, S. and Blatner, D. (1992). *Silicon Mirage: The Art and Science of Virtual Reality*. Peachpit Press, Berkeley CA. Also Zampi, G. and Conway, L.M. (1995). *Virtual Architecture*. B.T. Batsford. Also Schmitt, G. (1999). *Information Architecture: Basis and Future of CAAD*. Birkhauser, Basel.

35 Dickens, P.M. (1994). 'Rapid prototyping – the ultimate in automation.' *Journal of Assembly Automation*, Vol. 14, No. 2, pp. 10–13. Also Callicott, N. (2001). *Computer-Aided Manufacture in Architecture: The Pursuit of Novelty*. Architectural Press, Oxford.

36 GA eds (1998). *Guggenheim Bilbao Museao: Frank O. Gehry. GA Document No. 54*. See also Chapter 4 in this book.

37 See Chapter 5, in Abel, C. (2000, 2nd edition). Also Mitchell, W. (1995). *City of Bits*. MIT Press, Cambridge.

38 Abel, C. (2003).

39 The concept is defined in Abel, C. (1997a). See also Appendix I in this book.

40 Abel, C. (1997b).

41 See Appendix I in this book.

CHAPTER 4 FOSTER AND GEHRY: ONE TECHNOLOGY; TWO CULTURES

1 The work of both architects has been widely published. Comprehensive studies of Foster's architecture include Lambot, I. ed. (1989–). *Norman Foster: Buildings and Projects, Vols 1–4*. Watermark, Hong Kong. Also Jenkins, D. (2000). *On Foster. ...Foster On*. Prestel, Munich. Also Jenkins, D. (2002–). *Norman Foster; Works 1–6*. Prestel, Munich. Comprehensive studies of Gehry include Arnell, P. and Bickford, T. (1985). *Frank Gehry; Buildings and Projects*. Rizzoli, New York. Also *Frank O. Gehry: El Croquis 74–75*, 1995. Also Jencks, C. (1995). *Frank O. Gehry: Individual Imagination and Cultural Conservatism*. Academy Editions, London. Also Friedman, M., ed. (1999). *Gehry Talks: Architecture + Process*. Rizzoli, New York. Also Lindsey, B. (2001). *Digital Gehry*. Birkauser, Basel.

2 Quoted in Burns, C. (1990). 'The Gehry phenomenon'. In *Thinking the Present: Recent American Architecture* (Hays, K.M. and Burns, C., eds), pp. 82–3. Princeton Architectural Press, Princeton.

3   The close relationship between Gehry's early architecture and commercial advertising, with specific reference to the Chiat/Day Building, is clearly enunciated by Elizabeth Hornbeck: 'Unlike Apple's other outdoor advertisements, which can be seen around town, this ad is not located on a billboard. Instead, *Gehry's building itself becomes the billboard* (my emphasis), the carrier for this commercial message, inserting it in a public space which is otherwise relatively free of outdoor advertising.' Hornbeck, E. (1999). 'Architecture and advertising'. *Journal of Architectural Education*, September, p. 53.

4   See also Chapter 3 in this book.

5   Abel, C. (1989). The same essay is republished in Jenkins, D., ed. (2000), pp. 220–43. It is also republished in an extended form, including the passage presented in Appendix II in this book, in Jenkins, D., ed. (2004). *Norman Foster, Works 2*. Prestel, Munich. See also Chapter 3 in this book.

6   For a detailed study, see Abel, C. (1991).

7   For a detailed study, see Abel, C. (1986b). The same essay is republished in Jenkins, D., ed. (2000), pp. 132–49.

8   Suzuki, H. (1992). 'The fourth wave.' In *Century Tower: Foster Associates Build in Japan* (Davies, C. and Lambot, I.), pp. 10–17, Ernst & Sohn, Berlin.

9   For a detailed study, see Abel, C. (2004). 'Carre d'Art, Nimes, France, 1984–1993.' In Jenkins, D., ed. (2004).

10   According to Bruce Lindsey, despite increasing use of CAD/CAM techniques in the office Gehry still values the tactile qualities of physical models over any computer representation: 'Gehry does not like the way that objects look in the computer and feels that it takes the "juice" out of an idea.' Lindsey, B. (2001), p. 62.

11   Similar problems were encountered in the Lewis House project, which was also given the Catia treatment in the latter stages. Gehry argues that the main problem now is with the insurance companies, since his approach places increased liability on the architect. Friedman, M., ed. (1999).

12   Glymph was also joined in the early stages of the reorganization by Rick Smith, a consultant from IBM, and Randy Jefferson, who took a managerial role. They were also later joined by Dennis Shelden. Lindsey, B. (2001).

13   See Chapter 3 in this book.

14   According to Jean-Marc Galea (in interview with the author) at the Dassault Systemes HQ in Paris, the Catia system had also been used for a number of conventional building projects such as factories, prior to Gehry's use of it, as well as for other industries.

15   Friedman, M., ed. (1999).

16   For a detailed study, see Lindsey, B. (2001).

17   Gehry continued to rely on conventional techniques of model-making for projects well into his use of the Catia process. Stereolithography and other

rapid-prototyping techniques were only applied in more recent years and are still restricted on grounds of cost. Lindsey, B. (2001). Norman Foster also regularly uses similar automated modeling techniques in his own office.

18   Gehry, F. (1999). 'Commentaries by Frank Gehry.' In Friedman, M., ed. (1999), p. 176.

19   Gehry visited Aalto's office in 1972 and personally acknowledges his influence. Upon later meeting Aalto's widow, he declared: 'He is my hero.' Gehry, F. (1999), p. 43.

20   Aalto's habitual use of different planning geometries within the same design is analysed in Porphyrios, D. (1979). 'Heterotopia: a study in the ordering sensibility of the work of Alvar Aalto.' In *Alvar Aalto: Architectural Monographs 4*, pp. 8–19. Academy Editions, London.

21   Gehry often describes his work in similar terms: 'I guess the work has become a kind of sculpture as architecture.' Gehry, F. (1999), p. 49.

22   Friedman, M. ed. (1999), p. 18.

23   Abel, C. (1989). Also the extended version in Jenkins, D., ed. (2004).

24   Zaera, A. (1995). Information technology at Frank O. Gehry & Associates. *El Croquis*, 74–75, p. 152.

25   In conversation with the author.

26   According to Lindsey, 'The Lewis residence (1986–1995) changed the office.' Lindsey, B. (2001), p. 56.

27   For a detailed study, see *The ARAG Tower*. ARAG, Düsseldorf.

28   *El Croquis, 74–75* (1995).

29   Friedman, M., ed. (1999).

30   A brief mention of Gehry's approach to energy efficiency is made elsewhere: 'While Gehry eschews the term "green" as a designation, he does use intelligent siting, and massing, as well as computer simulations to make his buildings as environmentally conscious as possible.' Lindsey, B. (2001), p. 76. However, as with other accounts, no evidence is presented to suggest that energy efficiency plays any major part in shaping Gehry's architecture in the formative stages of the design process, except in those examples discussed in this chapter where Gehry reverts to more conventional forms.

31   See, for example, Abel, C. (2003b).

32   Abel, C. (2003).

33   For a detailed study, see Davies, C. and Lambot, I (1997). *Commerzbank Frankfurt: Prototype for an Ecological High-Rise*. Watermark/Birkhauser, Hong Kong/Basel.

34   Abel, C. (2003b).

35   As with all Foster's projects since the Commerzbank, extensive computer simulations were conducted by the London-based environmental engineers, BDSP, to test the energy efficiency of the design. Abel, C. (2003).

36   For a detailed account of the SMG's work, see Whitehead, H. (2004). 'Laws of form.' In *Architecture in the Digital Age* (Kolarevic, B., ed.), Spon Press, London.
37   Gehry, F. (1999).
38   The high cost of using the Catia system was a major factor in Whitehead's decision to use a different approach. Lindsey quotes a price of $70 000 per workstation for the Catia system in the early stages of use at Gehry's office, but suggests that costs have since reduced. Lindsey, B. (2001).
39   Despite the beneficial effects of using the Catia process, the economics of fabricating complex shapes remains a major factor in determining the degree of curvature in Gehry's designs: '....we know that if we use flat materials its relatively cheap; when we use single curved materials it's a little more expensive; and its most expensive when we warp materials. So we can rationalize all these shapes in the computer and make a judgement about the quantity of each shape to be used.' Gehry, F. (1999), p. 50. As a general rule, Gehry's design team keeps the most complex warped shapes, which can cost five times as much as single curves, down to just 5 per cent of the total number of curved shapes. Lindsey, B. (2001). Gehry also points to the work of Richard Serra, who also fabricates his large-scale metal sculptures from out of single curved materials based on ruled lines, as another influence. Gehry, F. (1999).
40   Whitehead, H. (2004). Also Appendix II in this book.
41   Gehry Technologies (GT) was launched on September 5, 2003. A joint venture with IBM and Dassault Systemes, GT was expressly created to provide expertise in the use of the Catia process and related services to industry members: 'Gehry Technologies aims to improve the way digital tools are developed and used by building professionals, and to foster changes in building industry practice through advances in digital technology'. Press release by Gehry Technologies, http://www.gehrytechnologies.com/GT-09-05-2003.html.
42   Abel, C. (2003b).
43   Abel, C. (2003b).
44   Abel, C. (1979). The same essay is also republished under the title, 'Architectural language games', Chapter 7 in Abel, C. (2000 2nd edition).

CHAPTER 5   HARRY SEIDLER AND THE GREAT AUSTRALIAN DREAM

1   For a comprehensive review of Seidler's early work, see Blake, P. (1973). *Architecture for the New World: The Work of Harry Seidler*. Horwitz, Australia, Sydney. For the later work see Drew, P. and Frampton, K. (1992). *Harry Seidler: Four Decades of Architecture*. Thames and Hudson, London. For the residential architecture, see Abel, C. and Seidler, H. (2003). *Harry Seidler: Houses and Interiors, 1 & 2*. Images Publishing, Melbourne.

2   Forster, C. (1999). *Australian Cities: Continuity and Change* (2nd edition). Oxford University Press, Melbourne.

3   Quoted in Indyk, I. (1984). 'Robin Boyd and the Australian suburb,' *UIA-International Architect*, Issue No. 4, p. 58.

4   Forster, C. (1999).

5   The story of Breuer's problems with the Cantilever House is told in Masello, D. (1993). *Architecture Without Rules: The Houses of Marcel Breuer and Herbert Beckhard*. W.W. Norton & Co., New York.

6   Abel, C. (2000, 2nd edition). Also Chapter 1 this book.

7   Numerous examples are presented in Taylor, J. (1990). *Australian Architecture Since 1960* (2nd edition). The Royal Australian Institute of Architects, Melbourne. The approach is best exemplified in the work of Glenn Murcutt. See Drew, P. (1985). *Leaves of Iron: Glen Murcutt; Pioneer of an Australian Architectural Form*. Angus & Robertson, Pymble.

8   Seidler, H. (1954). *Houses, Interiors and Projects*. Associated General Publications, Sydney, p. xx.

9   For an analysis of the conditions needed for efficient industrial production of buildings and the background to the industrialized building movement, see Chapter 1 in Abel, C. (2000; 2nd edition).

10 Seidler, H. (1954), p. xi.

11 Quoted in Drew, P. and Frampton, K. (1992), p. 120.

12 Underwood, D. (1994). *Oscar Niemeyer and Brazilian Free-form Modernism*. George Braziller, New York, p. 110.

13 The author is indebted to Konrad Buhagiar, Architecture Project, Malta, for his insights into baroque architecture, and for translating relevant passages concerning Borromini from Portoghesi, P. (1982). *L'Angelo della Storia: Teorie e Linguaggi dell'Architettura*. Biblioteca di Cultura Moderna Laterza, Rome.

14 Seidler, H. (1992). 'Planning and architecture at the end of our century.' In Abel, C. and Seidler, H. (1992), p. 383.

15 Frampton, K. (1992). 'Isostatic architecture, 1965–1991.' In Drew, P. and Frampton, K. (1992), p. 110. Frampton attributes the description to Philip Drew, who did not use those precise words but implied as much in his own essay on Seidler in the same book: 'The migration of an idea 1945–1976', pp. 14–31.

16 Wilk, C. (1981). *Marcel Breuer*. The Museum of Modern Art, New York, p. 108.

17 Scully, V. (1969). *The Earth, the Temple, and the Gods* (revised edition). Frederick A. Praeger, New York.

18 Underwood, D. (1994).

19 The problem, according to Seidler as well as other leading Australian architects, lies in the peculiarly rigid system of aesthetic control by local

authorities over new building applications (in addition to normal controls over height and setbacks, etc.). See Grennan, H. (2003). 'Mob rules', *Sydney Morning Herald*, May 29, domain section, pp. 6–8.

20 See note 7. For further examples see also Jahn, G. (1994). *Contemporary Australian Architecture*. Craftsman House, Roseville East.

21 Turner, G. (1997). 'Australian film and national identity in the 1990s.' In Stokes, G. ed. (1997). *The Politics of Identity in Australia*. Cambridge University Press, Melbourne. Turner suggests that while concepts of a singular national identity are slowly waning, Australian stereotypes survive even in such 'unconventional' movies as *Priscilla, Queen of the Desert*.

22 James Weirick, Professor of Architecture at the University of New South Wales, has suggested (in conversation) that the positive reception given abroad to Australian architecture of this kind is at least partly due to the fact that it reinforces prevailing – and patronizing – images of Australian culture, or the supposed lack of an urban culture; what might be called the 'Crocodile Dundee' syndrome.

23 Forster, C. (1999). Like a growing number of urbanists, the author concludes that, while strategies for sustainable growth vary, the most effective combine increased densities and concentrations of population in both old and new centres with increased investment in public transportation. See also Chapter 1 this book. Also Newman, P. and Kenworthy, J. (1999). *Sustainability and Cities: Overcoming Automobile Dependence*. Island Press, Washington. Also Abel, C. (2003c).

24 Eighty per cent of employment in Australia is now in the services sector – one of the highest percentages in the developed world – which by its nature requires concentrations of population in cities, further reducing the rural population. Rick Farley, 'The cities or the bush: is that the real problem?' In Irving, H., ed. (2001). *Unity and Diversity*. ABC Books, Sydney.

25 Forster, C. (1999).

26 Hudson, W. and Stokes, G. (1997). 'Australia and Asia: Place, Determinism and National Identities.' In Stokes, G., ed. (1997).

27 Forster, W. (2002). *Social Housing–Innovative Architecture*. Prestel, Munchen.

28 An indication of official winds of change was given by Bob Carr, Premier of New South Wales. Launching a new book on Seidler's work on 22 July 2002, at the RAIA Headquarters in Sydney, he remarked: 'Modernity becomes Australia.'

CHAPTER 6   MEDITERRANEAN MIX AND MATCH

1 Bonanno, A. (1997). *Malta: An Archaeological Paradise*. M.J. Publications, Valetta, Malta.

2 For a general history, see Blouet, B. (1981). *The Story of Malta*. Progress Press, Malta.

3   Hughes, Q. (1967). *The Building of Malta*. Alec Tiranti, London.

4   Hughes, Q. (1969). *Fortress*. Lund Humphries, London.

5   For an overview of Maltese architecture during this period see Hughes, Q. (1969). 'Malta past present and future.' *The Architectural Review*, July, pp. 2–81.

6   Abel, C. (1995). *Manikata Church: Richard England*. Academy Editions, London.

7   Abel, C. (2000). 'Open: the work of Architecture Project.' Introduction to the exhibition, Valletta, Malta, September 2000.

8   Buhagiar, K. (2002). Unpublished.

9   The editors (2001). 'Curtain call.' *The Architectural Review*, July, pp. 28–9.

10 The editors (2002). 'Evaporative cooling at Malta Stock Exchange.' *Ecotech*, 5 May (2001), pp. 14–17.

11 The Editors. 'The art of energy: Peake Short's Malta Brewery'. *Architecture Today*, No. 14, January 1991.

12 Chauhan, U. (1998). 'Rites of initiation.' *Indian Architect and Builder*, July, pp. 22–30.

13 The concept of a 'series' as used here is due to Kubler, G. (1962). *The Shape of Time*. Yale University Press. See also Chapter 11 in Abel, C. (2000, 2nd edition). *Architecture and Identity: Responses to Cultural and Technological Change (2nd edition)*. Architectural Press, Oxford.

14 Alexander, C. and Chemayeff, S. (1963). *Community and Privacy: Towards a New Architecture of Humanism*. Penguin Books, Harmondsworth.

15 From the competition entry.

16 In interview with the author.

17 In interview with the author.

APPENDIX II: BIRTH OF A CYBERNETIC FACTORY

1   Beer, S. (1962). 'Towards the cybernetic factory.' In *Principles of Self-Organization* (Von Forester, H. and Zopf, Jr. G.W., eds) pp. 25–89, Pergamon Press. For an analysis of the implications of Beer's concept and related technological innovations for architectural production see Abel, C. (1969). 'Ditching the dinosaur sanctuary.' *Architectural Design*, August, pp. 419–424. The same essay is republished as Chapter 1 in Abel, C. (2000, 2nd edition).

2   Jenkins, D. ed. (2004).

INDEX